Basic Knowledge Radiology

Martina Kahl-Scholz • Christel Vockelmann

Editors

Basic Knowledge Radiology

Nuclear Medicine and Radiotherapy With 215 Illustrations

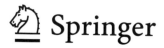 Springer

Editors
Martina Kahl-Scholz
Münster, Germany

Christel Vockelmann
Christophorus Clinics GmbH
Coesfeld, Germany

The translation was done with the help of artificial intelligence (machine translation by the service DeepL.com). A subsequent human revision was done primarily in terms of content.

ISBN 978-3-662-66350-9   ISBN 978-3-662-66351-6   (eBook)
https://doi.org/10.1007/978-3-662-66351-6

This Springer imprint is published by the registered company Springer-Verlag GmbH, DE, part of Springer Nature.
The registered company address is: Heidelberger Platz 3, 14197 Berlin, Germany

Dream your life nice and make those dreams a reality.
Marie Curie (1867–1934)

Preface

Modern medicine without imaging diagnostics and therapy is no longer imaginable in this day and age. Although every medical specialty deals "a little bit" with the imaging procedures of its own spectrum, the radiologists' and nuclear medicine specialists' claim is to have an overview of the diagnostics necessary for the problem and to keep an eye on the secondary findings, which may become the main findings for the patient.

At the same time, the fields of radiology, nuclear medicine, and radiotherapy remain in constant flux due to technical developments. Due to the diversity and the increasingly strong interventional field (especially in radiology), the areas are far from a "work in the dark closet."

In particular, the radiologist treats patients of any age and with almost any disease. So one is something like a specialized all-rounder. But there is also a need for specialization: pediatric radiology, neuroradiology, or interventional radiology require special knowledge and skills. Nuclear medicine specialists and radiologists work closely together to offer patients the best possible diagnostics in PETCT examinations. And the constant technical development also demands continuous training for colleagues who have been working in the profession for many years.

In the course of your studies, you have certainly had some contact with X-rays, nuclear medicine, or radiation therapy. But how does it all actually work? And why does the nuclear medicine doctor get upset about your blood pressure medication before the kidney scintigraphy? Why does the MTRA stop her when she walks into the MRI? And why doesn't the radiotherapist want to give radiation to the demented patient for whom surgery seems far too costly? We want to answer these and other questions and share our enthusiasm for our specialties with you.

With the basic knowledge of radiology and imaging procedures, we want to give you an overview of diagnostic and therapeutic options for the most common diseases. In doing so, a book alone cannot claim to be complete; it is not for nothing that the libraries of the radiology departments tend to be the most extensive ones in a hospital. But we want to lay a starting point for a very interesting field of medicine, from which you can at least go the first part of the way. This includes the correct use of the methods with knowledge of the advantages and disadvantages and the correct description of the findings. The evaluation of the same is also in the professional everyday life often a rereading in thick special tomes and the discussion of the possible diagnoses with colleagues of their own and the treating specialty.

Special thanks go to our author colleagues, without whom this book would not be equipped with so much expertise: Dr. Blum, Dr. Kremers, Dr. Wenker, Dr. Heilsberg, and Dr. Münstermann. We would also like to thank our colleagues Heinrich Rühe, Madlen Hagemann, and Dominika Kotas, as well as Dr. Matthias Göb, who actively supported us in compiling the images.

Further thanks go to the staff at Springer-Verlag, above all to Mrs. Rose-Marie Doyon in project management, for the opportunity to make this book a reality and for the corresponding support.

We welcome suggestions and comments from you to further develop the book and adapt it to the needs of our readers.

We hope that this book will be a valuable companion for you as a student in clinical traineeship or PJ and also as a resident in radiology, nuclear medicine, or radiotherapy in your everyday student and professional life.

Christel Vockelmann
Coesfeld, Germany

Martina Kahl-Scholz
Münster, Germany
January 2017

Contents

II   Disease Patterns

III   Testing

        Mirja Wenker, Martina Kahl-Scholz, and Christel Vockelmann

Editors and Contributors

About the Editors

Martina Kahl-Scholz
is a medical doctor and graduate pedagogue. She did her doctoral thesis in radiology and discovered her passion for this broad subject. Together with Dr. Vockelmann she has already published several books in this medical branch.

Christel Vockelmann
is chief physician of the radiology department of the Christophoruskliniken Coesfeld, Dülmen and Nottuln. She is also a member of the PJ examination board. In addition to being the editor of Fachwissen MTRA, Dr. Vockelmann can look back on co-authorship of several books.

Contributors

Ursula Blum   Practice for nuclear medicine, Mühlheim an der Ruhr

Guido Heilsberg   Clinic for Radiotherapy and Radio-Oncology, Klinikum Dortmund gGmbH, Dortmund

Martina Kahl-Scholz   Münster

Carla M. Kremers   Radiological Clinic, Christophorus-Kliniken GmbH, Dülmen

Esther Münstermann   Clinic for Radiotherapy and Radio-Oncology, Klinikum Dortmund gGmbH, Dortmund

Christel Vockelmann   Christophorus Clinics GmbH, Coesfeld, Germany

Mirja Wenker   Radiological Clinic, Christophorus-Kliniken GmbH, Coesfeld

Basics

Contents

Physical Basics

Martina Kahl-Scholz and Christel Vockelmann

Contents

© Springer-Verlag GmbH Germany, part of Springer Nature 2023
M. Kahl-Scholz, C. Vockelmann (eds.), *Basic Knowledge Radiology*,
https://doi.org/10.1007/978-3-662-66351-6_1

1

Ionizing radiation is used for the early detection and diagnosis of diseases by imaging techniques and for the treatment of malignant tumors. The physical principles, the origin of the different types of radiation and their interaction with matter will be examined in more detail in the following sections. Special attention will be paid to the radiation protection of the examiner.

1.1 Radioactivity and Its Interactions

In order to understand how we use different types of radiation in the diagnosis and therapy of diseases, but also what dangers emanate from the various types of radiation, we must first take a look at the physical and chemical fundamentals. This includes the characterization of atomic nuclei, which are made up of protons and neutrons. Protons and neutrons are called nucleons. The **mass number A** is the number of nucleons (that is, protons and neutrons) in the nucleus. The number of protons in the nucleus gives the **atomic number Z**. Atomic number Z and mass number A occur repeatedly in the following section, since both numbers change with the different types of decay.

❯ Atomic number Z corresponds to the number of protons in the nucleus. Mass number A corresponds to the number of protons and neutrons in the nucleus.

1.1.1 Radioactive Decay Modes

Radioactivity is produced by the emission of radiation through spontaneous nuclear transformations. In this process, radionuclides change from an unstable to a stable state while releasing energy. Depending on the type of decay, the energy is emitted in the form of particle or electromagnetic radiation. The unit of radioactivity is **Becquerel (Bq)**. Antoine-Henri Becquerel discovered uranium at the end of the 19th century.

❯ The type and energy of the emitted radiation is characteristic for each radionuclide.

■ Alpha Decay (α-Decay)

In heavy nuclides, α-radiation is produced by the emission of an α-particle consisting of two protons and two neutrons. This causes Z to decrease by two, A by four. In addition, two electrons leave the atomic bond. The α-particle is accelerated by the released energy. The amount of this kinetic energy is the same for each α-particle, so it is monoenergetic radiation. Due to the large mass of the α-particles, they are rapidly decelerated by matter, i.e. also by the body, and release their energy directly to the tissue. As a result, the affected cell is severely destroyed. Because of this pronounced effect, α-radiation is almost no longer used in medicine. α-radiation can already be shielded by a simple sheet of paper.

■ Beta-Minus Decay (β⁻-Decay)

β⁻ emitters are used in medicine for nuclear medical therapies. The treatment of benign and malignant thyroid diseases with iodine[131] (^{131}J) is particularly worth mentioning here. The range of the β⁻-radiation is higher than that of the α-radiation, but it is not sufficient for diagnostic applications, where an image of the radiation outside the body is to be captured. In atomic nuclei with a high neutron excess, a neutron is converted into a proton, an electron (β⁻-particle) and an antineutrino. Thus the additional proton increases Z by 1, A does not change. The β⁻ particle and the antineutrino leave the nucleus, and the kinetic energy released is distributed between them. So the β^--particle can have energy values between zero and maximum energy, we do not get monoenergetic radiation but a continuous energy spectrum. The antineutrino has an extremely small interaction with matter, but must be taken into account in the energy balance of the β^--decay.

■ Beta-Plus Decay (β^+-Decay)

The radiation produced by β^+ decay is used in medicine primarily in positron emission tomography (PET). The most commonly used emitter is [18] fluorine.

In atomic nuclei with an excess of protons, a proton transforms into a neutron, a positron (β^+-particle) and a neutrino, Z decreases by one, A remains constant. β^+-particle and neutrino leave the nucleus. As in β^--decay, the released kinetic energy is distributed with a continuous spectrum. The neutrino interacts negligibly with matter, but must be taken into account in the energy balance of the β decay.[+]

As an antiparticle, the positron has only a short lifetime and unites with a free electron of the environment within microseconds. Near the nucleus, the mass of both particles is converted into two photons, which fly apart at an angle of 180° and with an energy of 511 keV per quantum (annihilation radiation). The β^+ decay can therefore only occur if the energy difference between mother and daughter is 1022 keV.

■ Electron Capture

If the decay energy at proton excess is smaller than 1022 keV, electron capture occurs instead of β^+-decay. An electron from the near-nuclear shell migrates into the nucleus and combines with a proton. A neutron is produced and a neutrino leaves the nucleus, Z decreases by one. A does not change. The electron gap is filled by an electron from an outer, higher-energy shell, and when it bounces back, the energy released from the energy difference between the two shells is emitted as characteristic X-rays. Some nuclides used in nuclear medicine diagnostics are produced by EC e.g.[201] Thallium. If the atomic number of the nuclide is below 30, the energy is mainly transferred directly to electrons. These so-called Auger electrons leave the atomic bond.

■ Internal Conversion/γ-Radiation

After a nuclear transformation, a residual energy often remains in the daughter nucleus for a short time, the nuclides are excited or metastable. This residual energy is released via two competing processes.

On the one hand, the excitation energy of the nucleus is transferred directly to an electron of the shell. If the binding energy of the electron is exceeded, the electron leaves its place. The resulting gap is also filled with an electron of a higher, more energetic shell; again, depending on the atomic number, characteristic X-rays or the emission of Auger electrons are produced.

However, the energy released when the nucleus is excited can also be emitted as electromagnetic radiation in the form of gamma quanta of equal or different energy. A gamma emitter frequently used in nuclear medical diagnostics is[99m] Tc.

1.1.2 The Physical Half-Life

Another characteristic quantity of a radioactive substance is the so-called **physical half-life**. In this period of time, half of the originally existing atoms have decayed. Depending on the substance, the physical half-life ranges from fractions of seconds to billions of years.

1

1.1.3 Physical Interaction Processes of Electromagnetic Radiation with Matter

Interaction of Photon Radiation with Matter

The interaction of photons with matter, including the patient, attenuates the radiation intensity in proportion to the material thickness d and the attenuation coefficient μ. Mathematically, the relationship is expressed in **Lambert-Beer's law:** $I(d) = I(0) \exp(-\mu d)$. The attenuation coefficient μ depends on the material and its nuclear charge number Z and on the energy E of the photons. The attenuation of the radiation occurs by absorption (photoelectric effect and pair formation) and by scattering (**Compton effect**).

> ❯ Attenuation = Absorption + Scattering

▪ Photoelectric Effect

In the energy ranges of up to 100 keV used in radiology, the photoelectric effect is the basis for image formation. The X-rays emitted from the X-ray tube are attenuated by tissues such as bone and soft tissue with their different densities according to Lambert-Beer's law. The resulting radiation image has different shades of gray due to the different attenuation.

> ❯ The more energetic the photon radiation, the weaker the contrast, as the attenuation decreases with increasing beam energy.

In photoabsorption, the total energy of the photon radiation is transferred to an electron of the atomic shell of matter. The shell electron is either excited and thus raised to a shell of higher energy or ionized and knocked out of the atomic shell. Ionization occurs when the energy of the photon exceeds the binding energy of the electron to the nucleus. The difference between the binding energy and the energy required for ionization is transferred to the photoelectron released from the atomic shell as kinetic energy.

> ❯ The higher the residual energy, the more the photoelectrons are emitted in the direction of the primary beam.

In order to be able to delimit hollow organs and vessels in the native X-ray image, the patient is given a so-called positive contrast medium with a high atomic number (J: $Z = 53$; Ba $Z = 56$...), which absorbs the X-rays more strongly than the surrounding tissue. In nuclear medicine, the scintigraphic image is produced by the unscattered photons emerging from the body.

When electrons excited by the photoelectric effect jump back to their original orbit and release the energy again, this is called **classical scattering.** The emitted photon radiation has the same energy and therefore also the same frequency as the original radiation. If the frequency is in the range of visible light, we can see these light quanta as luminescence. Luminescence is the basis of the imaging plate technique, with which the resulting radiation image is stored as an X-ray image that we can use. Barium halides, for example, are excited in the imaging plate, which is in the X-ray cassette, by means of a photoelectric effect. A laser in the readout unit causes the previously held electrons to fall back to their original state and the imaging plate lights up, producing the X-ray image.

▪ Compton Scattering

The Compton effect describes a scattering of the photon, which gives only a part of its energy to the shell electron of the outer shell. The photon itself is scattered with the residual energy in a changed direction. Secondary electrons of lower energy are scattered in the lateral direction, the higher the residual energy, the more the secondary electrons are scattered in the forward direction. These scattered photons degrade image quality in diagnostic imaging and therapy. These scattered photons are captured by scattering beam grids (▶ Chap. 2) made of lead lamellae; in nuclear medicine, the corresponding counterpart is the placement of a corresponding energy window to capture low-energy scattered photons.

■ Pair Formation

The pair formation effect occurs at high photon energies from 1022 keV. Near the nucleus, the photon forms a pair of an electron (negatively charged) and a positron (positively charged). The atomic nucleus remains unchanged. The formed pair annihilates with an electron of the absorber in two annihilation quanta of 511 keV each. This effect of energy dissipation plays an essential role in radiation therapy when ultra-hard photons are used.

1.1.4 Interaction of Particle Radiation with Matter

The energy output of electrically negative particles to matter can be achieved by ionization, generation of deceleration radiation and excitation. The energy output of the electrons is proportional to the density of the matter, in contrast to photon radiation, the range of the electrons is finite. The occurring interactions of the particle beams with the matter depends on mass and charge of the particle, which is determined by its rest mass and velocity.

❯ As a rule of thumb, the range of electrons in centimeters in tissue-equivalent matter (water) corresponds to half the energy in MeV.

Electrons are used in the radiotherapy of superficial tumors. The depth of treatment and thus the protection of the underlying tissue is achieved by the appropriate choice of electron energy.

Neutrons and protons are used to treat deeper tumors. These procedures are technically very complex and therefore only available at specialized centers. Neutrons and protons emit their energy at a certain resonance energy of the tissue. As long as this resonance energy is exceeded, they penetrate deeper into the tissue with little energy release. When the initial energy has decreased to the level of the resonance energy, the energy delivery to the tissue increases and the tissue in the target area is destroyed.

❯ – The higher the number of atoms present, the more interaction processes occur. The attenuation depends on the density and thickness of the matter irradiated.
 – The probability of photoabsorption occurring depends on the atomic number of the matter being irradiated and thus also on the number of electrons available.
 – High-energy radiation penetrates matter without significant photoabsorption.

1.2 X-Rays

In contrast to radio waves, for example, X-rays are very short-wave and therefore have a high frequency. X-rays are generated in an evacuated glass bulb, the X-ray tube, which contains a cathode and an anode. Two different types of voltage are applied to the tube: a heating voltage for the cathode and a high voltage between the cathode and the anode. Due to the thermoelectric effect, the heating voltage initially causes an electron cloud to "evaporate" at the cathode. This is accelerated to the anode by the high voltage applied (20,000–200,000 volts). When the electrons hit the anode, there is an abrupt deceleration of the electrons, and the kinetic energy of the electrons is converted into X-rays, electromagnetic waves and heat. In addition, direct interactions of the electrons with the anode material occur.

1

❯ The higher the atomic number of the anode material and the higher the high voltage with which the electrons are accelerated towards the anode, the higher the yield of X-rays.

The energy of the accelerated electrons before impacting the anode is given by:
1. the number of electrons accelerated to the anode, i.e. evaporated from the cathode, and
2. from the tube voltage, which accelerates the electrons towards the anode.

The unit of this energy is the electron volt (eV).

❯ One eV is defined as the energy absorbed by an electron when it is accelerated during the free passage of a voltage of 1 V (without resistance in vacuum).

Two types of X-ray radiation are produced: **X-ray deceleration radiation** and **characteristic X-ray radiation.**

The deceleration of the electrons at the nucleus produces **X-ray deceleration radiation.** Some electrons release radiation as soon as they hit the anode, others penetrate deeper into the electron material, whereby they have already lost part of their energy and only generate **X-rays** afterwards. This process explains why the X-rays produced have different wavelengths. The amount of X-rays produced depends on how much the electron is decelerated. The immediately produced X-ray deceleration radiation has a smaller wavelength than the radiation produced by the initially decelerated electrons.

X-rays of different wavelengths produce a gapless, continuous X-ray deceleration spectrum that is independent of the anode material. Short-wave radiation can penetrate matter better than long-wave radiation. In practice, it is possible to produce shorter-wave X-ray radiation, which can penetrate matter better, by applying a higher pick-up voltage (**high voltage**) to the generator.

Characteristic X-ray radiation is produced in addition to X-ray deceleration radiation and is a so-called **line spectrum**, which is exclusively dependent on the anode material. The characteristic line spectrum is, so to speak, the **fingerprint of the anode material.**

This line spectrum is produced by the knocking out (**ionization**) or **excitation** (lifting to a higher energy level) of electrons from the two inner shells of the atoms of the anode material. The empty spaces on the inner electron shells are filled up again from the outside, the released energy is released in the form of characteristic X-rays, which are clearly defined according to their wavelength.

❯ In an X-ray tube, only 1–2% of the X-rays are produced; the rest of the energy of the accelerated electrons is converted into heat.

Gamma rays have the same properties as X-rays. The two types differ only in the place of their origin and energy.

❯ While X-rays are produced in the atomic shell, gamma rays are produced by radioactive decays in the atomic nucleus.

X-ray quanta have an energy of 100 eV to 200 keV. For gamma quanta, this range extends from about 1 keV to several MeV.

❯ X-rays, together with α-, β- and γ-rays, belong to the group of ionizing rays. This means that all these types of radiation interact with matter.

1.3   Dose Terms

When dealing with ionizing radiation, one encounters a myriad of dose terms where one can quickly lose track. Let us try to bring some order into the many terms and to understand when we need which terms.

1.3.1 Kerma = Kinetic Energy Released in Matter

Photon and neutron beams, i.e. indirectly ionizing beams, release charged particles, so-called **secondary particles.** Kerma is therefore dependent on the irradiated medium. The sum of the energy transferred during the first impact corresponds to the kerma. Kerma is expressed in **Gray (Gy).** In medical dosimetry, the kerma corresponds approximately to the absorbed dose.

1.3.2 Ion Dose

The ion dose describes the electric charge of the ions of the same sign, which are produced by ionizing radiation in a certain mass. The unit of ion dose is **coulomb per kilogram.** In the past, the ion dose was expressed in X-rays.

❯ Rod dosimeters or ionization chambers measure the ion dose.

❯ Ion dose rate describes the absorbed ion dose per time unit

1.3.3 Absorbed Dose

The absorbed dose is the basic quantity in dosimetry. It describes the absorbed radiation energy in relation to the irradiated mass.

Dose = absorbed energy / mass

Unit of absorbed dose is also **Gray (Gy).** In older books you may come across the term **rad (rd),** which was used until 1985. A conversion is made as follows:

One rd $= 0.001\,\mathrm{Gy} = 0.001\,\mathrm{J^* kg^{-1}}$

The absorbed dose cannot be measured in the body. Therefore, the ion dose is measured in an air-filled ionization chamber, from which the absorbed dose for specific materials or the human body can be calculated.

1.3.4 Equivalent Dose

The dose equivalent describes the absorbed dose multiplied by a weighting factor. This takes into account the relative biological effectiveness (RBE) of the absorbed type of radiation. Since the weighting factor has no dimension, the unit of dose equivalent is the same as that of absorbed dose, i.e. joules per kilogram. However, to avoid confusion with the absorbed dose, the equivalent dose is expressed in **sieverts (Sv).**

❯ Equivalent dose rate describes the equivalent dose absorbed per unit of time.

Let us return to the **relative biological effectiveness.** The different types of radiation show different biological effects. The RBE is defined as the ratio of the absorbed dose of a reference radiation, which causes a certain biological effect, to the dose of another radiation, which leads to the same biological effect on the same object.

The RBE thus correlates to the energy transfer of the radiation to the irradiated object. The measure for this is the **linear energy transfer (LET).** This is an indirect measure of the number of ionizations per path length. Radiation of heavy, charged particles exhibits a higher linear energy transfer, i.e. it generates a large number of ionizations and triggers more biological effects on the irradiated object. In addition to the type of radiation, the linear energy transfer also depends, of course, on the irradiated object.

❯ The RBE increases only up to a maximum at about 100–200 keV/μm, and then drops sharply. The reason for this is the so-called overkill. More energy is transferred to the cell than is necessary for inactivation.

After these theoretical basics, we come to values that are important in daily practice. These are partly displayed directly on the devices and are also subject to documentation according to the X-ray ordinance.

1.3.5 Incident Dose

This describes the dose in Gy, that is measured "free air" without stray bodies. By **scattering bodies** are meant phantoms or also patients, which would lead to a scattering of the radiation. The incident dose depends on the focal distance, energy (in X-rays kV and filter) and the dose rate. The field size has only little influence.

1.3.6 Surface Dose

Now the patient or a phantom comes into play. In addition to the incident dose, the backscatter from the irradiated object, e.g. the patient, is added to the surface dose.

On the inlet side, the backscattering can be up to 50%. The backscattering is strongly dependent on the field size.

In radiotherapy, the surface dose at the exit side is also important, as this must be taken into account in the case of opposing fields. More on this later.

1.3.7 Deep Dose

The depth dose describes the dose at a certain body depth, measured from the irradiation surface. The relative depth dose indicates the ratio of a depth dose to the dose maximum in percent. The depth dose is particularly important in radiation therapy, since here a specific dose at a specific location in the body, e.g. a lung tumor, is targeted for therapeutic success. At the same time, surrounding healthy tissue should of course not be damaged.

The dose distribution at depth is caused by three effects:

1. the weakening in the tissues,
2. the dose decrease due to the distance increasing with depth,
3. added scattered radiation.

Scattered radiation also plays a role in the depth dose. Therefore, there is also a dependence on the field size here.

1.3.8 Dose Area Product

As the name suggests, the dose area product (DFP) is the product of dose and area. This is the dose value that is calculated, for example, during a normal X-ray examination of the lungs and must be documented in accordance with the X-ray Ordinance.

It gets a bit more complicated, because the dose is sometimes given in cGy, sometimes in µGy and also the unit for the area can be given e. g. in m^2 or $cm.^2$

The conversion is implemented as follows:

$$1 cGy\, cm^2 = 10\, mGy\, cm^2 = 0.1 dGy\, cm^2$$
$$= 1 Gy\, m^2 = 10^{-6}\, Gy\, m^2$$

Occasionally, the term area dose product with the abbreviation FDP is also used as a synonym.

1.3.9 Dose Length Product

The dose length product (DLP) is the equivalent of the dose area product for computed tomography. The product is formed from the dose in a slice, the weighted CTDI (Computed Tomography Dose Index), and the number of slices. The CTDI is necessary because, in contrast to projection radiography, the patient is exposed to X-rays from all sides. The CTDI is determined with the aid of water phantoms that simulate the conditions of the human body as accurately as possible.

The dose terms DFP and DLP used so far do not ultimately say anything about how dangerous or harmless the radiation used is for the patient. In order to be able to make a statement about this, one must know which organ regions have been exposed to the radiation.

1.3.10 Organ Dose

Organ dose stands for the absorbed dose to an organ or body part in Gy, multiplied by a radiation weighting factor. This depends on the type of radiation used. Actually, you already know this from relative biological effectiveness. In contrast to the experimentally scientifically determined relative biological effectiveness, the radiation weighting factor is determined by legal standard. It is not yet assessed how radiation-sensitive the corresponding organ is.

1.3.11 Effective Dose

The effective dose takes into account the sensitivity of the individual organs. The effective dose is determined by the sum of the organ dose multiplied by the tissue weighting factors. The tissue weighting factors are calculated and determined by the International Radiation Protection Commission (IRCP).

The following table shows some examples of tissue weighting factors (■ Table 1.1).

■ **Table 1.1** Examples of tissue weighting factors

Organs and Tissues	Tissue Weighting Factor
Gonads	0.08
Rred bone marrow	0.12
Chest	0.12
Skin	0.01
Brain	0.01

The sum of all tissue weighting factors is 1.

By calculating the effective dose, radiation exposures can be compared with each other.

Numerous computer programs are now available for estimating the effective dose.

1.3.12 Personal Dose, Local Dose and Body Dose

According to the Radiation Protection Ordinance and the X-ray Ordinance, it is generally required that body doses are determined for persons who are in controlled areas. For the whole-body dose, a homogeneous radiation exposure of the entire body is assumed. The mean value of the equivalent dose for the head, torso, upper arm and thigh is then calculated. For partial body doses, the mean value of the equivalent dose in an organ or body part is determined. These values are important in occupational radiation protection. Here, limit values are specified both for the whole-body dose and for partial-body doses.

However, the problem with partial body doses and also whole body doses is that these values cannot be measured directly. Therefore, simpler measurands (local dose and personal dose) are defined as a proxy, which allow an estimation of the effective dose if required.

■ Local Dose
Here, the equivalent dose for soft tissue is measured at a specific location.

■ Personal Dose
Measured at a representative site on the body surface, the personal dose represents the equivalent dose to soft tissue.

> The personal dose is determined on the basis of the X-ray badge. You should wear this ventrally on your torso. If you work in controlled areas, the badge belongs on your clothing under the lead apron.

1.4 Effect of Ionizing Radiation on the Organism

As the tragic and well-known events from Japan and Ukraine, among others, have shown, ionizing radiation is very dangerous for humans. Both accidents released radioactive iodine and cesium – both are beta emitters that are incorporated and thus trigger more interactions in the organism.

1.4.1 Radiation Effects

The effect of the different types of radiation depends on the frequency of the radiation and the associated interaction processes which the types of radiation enter into with matter. These are based on the elementary processes of excitation and ionization.

During excitation, an atom is moved to a higher energy state by supplied energy. In this process, a shell electron of an inner shell is lifted to a higher shell. Within a very short time, the excess energy is usually released again by emitting electromagnetic wave radiation. The excited atoms are very reactive and can enter into chemical reactions which are relevant for the effect of the radiation on the organism as a whole.

Ionization describes the absorption or release of an electron and the associated disturbance of the equilibrium of charges in an atom. This can occur either by impact ionization, i.e. direct ionization (a charged particle hits a shell electron and releases energy) or by absorption and thus indirect ionization (electromagnetic waves or neutrons hit an atom and their energy is absorbed, releasing an electron from the atomic bond).

When passing through matter, the electromagnetic radiation is weakened by absorption of the energy. This absorbed part of the radiation, whose energy has thus been transferred to the matter that has been radiated through, is relevant for the effect on the body.

The properties of the different types of radiation also play a major role when considering the effects of radiation on the human organism. One measure of the damaging effect is the Linear Energy Transfer (LET), which describes how many ionizations a radiation quantum can trigger on its way through tissue.

$$LET = lost\ of\ energy(keV)\ /\ flight\ distance(\mu m)$$

Particle radiation is one of the densely ionizing types of radiation that are hardly scattered but trigger numerous ionizations. X-rays (photon radiation), on the other hand, trigger comparatively fewer ionizations, but are more strongly scattered and thus also influence surrounding cells.

The Linear Energy Transfer corresponds to the physical consideration of the radiation effect. Relative biological effectiveness (RBE) describes the potential health hazard posed by different types of radiation. The RBE factors relate the biological effects obtained by using the same dose in Gray:
- X-rays: 1
- Gamma radiation: 1
- Beta radiation: 1
- Neutron radiation (depending on energy): 5–20
- Proton radiation: 5
- Alpha radiation: 20

The effect radiation can cause in the organism depends on several factors:
- Which tissue is irradiated?
- What dose was administered?
- What is the LET/ionization density of the radiation?

For this reason, the effects of radiation accidents such as those in Fukushima or Chernobyl are also not comparable with their use in medicine. Irrespective of this, such events and their effects serve to research the consequences of radiation.

All these results are used by professional societies for the assessment of necessary limit values for e.g. foodstuffs and the development of medical applications.

A distinction is made between two types of radiation effect:

Stochastic Radiation Effect

Stochastics involves probability calculations. For the effect of ionizing radiation, this means: Theoretically, every X-ray quantum can trigger a damaging event. The more X-ray quanta hit the organism, the higher the probability of a "hit".

This stochastic radiation effect is the basis for the top priority of radiation protection:

❯ "As Low As Reasonably Achievable" (ALARA principle)—only as little radiation as absolutely necessary may be used, as there is no threshold dose for a specific radiation damage.

For everyday medical practice, this means: Can I carry out the diagnosis without X-rays (i.e. sonography, magnetic resonance imaging)? Have I observed all the preliminary examinations? Do I need the X-ray examination at all, or am I only "interested" in it, but the treatment of the patient does not change?

When performing the examinations, the same applies: Which area do I need to examine? Can I narrow down my radiation field? Can I reduce the dose for the question?

Typical stochastic radiation damages are **gene and cell mutations** that lead to tumors and hereditary diseases only years after exposure.

Deterministic Radiation Effect

Deterministic radiation effects occur above a certain dose. We know, for example, after how much radiation the healthy skin reacts with a skin reaction (erythema), there is a **threshold dose**. This is defined for each tissue. From the point of view of radiation protection, deterministic damage must not occur. From the point of view of therapy, however, it is precisely this damage that is "desired", since research results can prove when the threshold dose of a tumor is also reached.

In radiotherapy, deterministic damage is specifically inflicted on malignant tumors. In order to successfully combat a tumor, a compromise must be found between the safe destruction of the tumor and the still tolerable side effect of the surrounding tissue.

As early as the 1930s, Hermann Holthusen, a radiologist from Hamburg, illustrated this in the diagram named after him. He described that one can never strive for 100% tumor control, as the side effect rate of 50% is then also too high. The therapy should be directed in such a way that one achieves 85–90% tumor control with 5–10% side effects to be expected.

1.4.2 Phases of the Radiation Effect

In connection with health damage caused by ionizing radiation, keywords such as "radiation-induced tumor" or "mutations in the offspring" are used. This suggests that after exposure to radiation, an effect cannot be observed immediately, but may occur many years or even generations later.

In order to explain this effect, one must first deal with the temporal sequence of the radiation effect.

The phases of the radiation effect can be divided into four phases.

Physical Phase

In this phase, the absorption of the radiation in the tissue takes place in fractions of a second (10^{-16} s). It is the starting point for all further processes, since only the absorbed energy triggers an effect in the organism. The absorption leads to ionizations, molecular excitations and heat.

1

Physical and Chemical Phase

This phase describes the chemical reactions and associated damage (direct and indirect) to the molecules. Direct damage is caused by loss of bonding electrons in the molecules, causing them to break apart. Indirect damage is caused by radicals, which are chemically very reactive substances. These reactions also take place in the body in times far below one second (10^{-6} s).

This phase is also called the radiochemical phase. The free radicals are formed by the radiolysis of the water. Since the human cell consists of about 80% water, radiation energy has plenty of points of attack here.

Biochemical Phase

In the biochemical phase, which is in the seconds to minutes range, there are damaging changes to organic molecules, which particularly affect cell DNA. As a result of radiolysis, radicals are formed, including H_2O_2 (hydrogen peroxide), which is a powerful cell toxin.

Which radicals are predominantly formed and how strong their effect is also depends on the Linear Energy Transfer (LET). The higher the LET, the:
- more H_2O_2 is formed,
- less the presence of the oxygen plays a role,
- the radical yield is lower,
- higher is the direct number of hits on the cell and thus a higher number of non-repairable cell damages.

The radicals primarily attack the DNA of the cells and cause various types of damage there. In basic experimental research, the following damage can be determined so far:
- Base modifications and base losses
- Changes in sugar molecules
- Single and double strand breaks
- DNA crosslinks
- Multiple DNA alterations (bulky lesions)

▪▪ Irradiation Damage

After irradiation with 1 Gy of X-rays, the following damage can be found in a cell:
- 1000–2000 base changes
- 500–1000 single strand breaks
- 800–1600 changes in sugar molecules
- 150 crosslinks
- 50 Double strand breaks and bulky lesions

Sophisticated safety systems exist in the cells to repair damage and thus prevent mutations.

Most of these repairs are completed in 6–8 h. Some, quick repairs take place in 10–20 min, others need the full repair time of a few days. About 95% of all damage can be repaired.

❯ As a rule of thumb, after 2 h most of the possible repair processes on normal tissues are completed, after 6–8 h. This temporal relationship is significant for the planning of a radiation therapy, if one wants to destroy tumor tissue and spare normal tissue.

All unrepaired damage can lead to cell death or mutations and thus to tumor disease.

Biological Phase

The last phase of the radiation effect is the biological phase, which cannot be limited in time, in which mutations, changes in metabolism or cell death can occur at the cellular level. Such changes often only become visible after decades through the development of malignant tumors or even in subsequent generations if damage has been inherited.

Serious radiation effects on the cell include various forms of cell death:
1. **Loss of function in cells that** are in the G0 phase and are no longer able to divide, e.g. nerve cells, muscle cells.
2. **Reproductive cell death**, the cells lose their ability to divide, e.g. hematopoietic stem cells.

3. **Interphase death** affects cells that are just between two mitoses. The cell dies in a few hours and does not reach the next mitosis.

In radiotherapy, the relationships between dose, cell damage, repair processes, temporal dependencies and cell survival curves are represented in various models (e.g. multitarget model, linear-quadratic model) in order to determine the ideal therapy for the individual patient.

Not all tumor cells behave in the same way. There are particularly radiation-sensitive tumors (e.g. leukemia) and those that require higher treatment doses (e.g. bone sarcomas). Since in comparatively radiation-resistant tumors the surrounding tissue is also exposed to radiation, the radiation sensitivity of a tumor can be increased, e.g. chemotherapy.

Practice Questions

1. Briefly describe what is meant by photoelectric effect, Compton effect and pair formation.
2. What is meant by incident dose, surface dose and depth dose?
3. What is the difference between deceleration X-ray and characteristic X-ray radiation?
4. What is the Relative Biological Effectiveness (RBE)?
5. What are stochastic and what are deterministic radiation damages?

Solutions ▶ Chap. 27

Conventional X-ray Diagnostics

Christel Vockelmann

Contents

© Springer-Verlag GmbH Germany, part of Springer Nature 2023
M. Kahl-Scholz, C. Vockelmann (eds.), *Basic Knowledge Radiology*,
https://doi.org/10.1007/978-3-662-66351-6_2

The chapter "Conventional X-ray diagnostics" deals with the origin of X-ray radiation, the structure of the X-ray tube and the possibility of regulating the type and amount of radiation. Furthermore, the formation of the digital X-ray image as well as the processing of the images are dealt with, and special devices of conventional X-ray diagnostics are described as examples. Furthermore, you will find an overview of the basic specifications of the guidelines of the German Medical Association for conventional X-ray diagnostics.

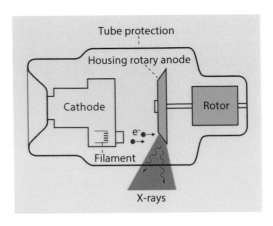

Fig. 2.1 Schematic structure of an X-ray source. (From Hartmann et al. 2014)

2.1 Design and Operation of an X-ray System

An X-ray system always consists of the following components:
- an **X-ray source** that generates the beams,
- an **X-ray generator**, which supplies the X-ray source with high voltage,
- an **X-ray application device** used for positioning the patient, and
- an **X-ray image converter** (X-ray film, detector,…).

2.1.1 The X-ray Source

Structure of the X-ray Tube

An X-ray source is a cathode source and consists of a negatively charged cathode and a positively charged anode. By heating the cathode, electrons can be released from the cathode. Due to the different charges between the cathode and the anode, these electrons are then accelerated towards the anode and finally hit the anode where, among other things, X-rays are produced (**Fig. 2.1**).

Since the electrons would be slowed down and deflected in normal air, the cathode and anode are located in an evacuated, i.e. airless, glass bulb. This glass bulb is located in an oil-filled radiation protection housing. The oil serves to protect against the high voltage and to dissipate heat to the outside. The protective housing also shields the parts of the X-ray radiation that do not exit through the radiation exit window. Below the radiation exit window is a legally required filter made of 1.5 mm thick aluminum. This filters out the radiation that is unable to penetrate the body due to its energy.

■ The Cathode

The cathode consists of one or two filaments which are heated by the so-called tube current. The heat causes the electrons to oscillate (thermal electron emission) and they can be released by the voltage triggered between the cathode and the anode. The filaments are mainly made of tungsten, since tungsten has the highest melting point of all metals (3680 K = 3406.85 °C) and the electrons can also be released relatively easily. The released electrons or the electron cloud is now accelerated towards the anode.

Since the electrons would travel undirected in the direction of the anode, they are focused by a Wehnelt cylinder. This cylinder is located in the immediate vicinity of the cathode. By applying a negative charge, the exit of the electrons can be regulated and the direction of flight focused.

■ **The Anode**

When the electrons hit the focal spot (also called focus) at the anode, various processes or even interactions occur. Only 1% of the energy is converted into X-rays, 99% of the energy is released into heat.

Because of the large amount of heat generated, the anode must be made of a particularly heat-resistant and thermally conductive material. Here, too, **tungsten** or a tungsten-rhenium mixture has proven to be ideal. In order to distribute the heat generated over a large volume, rotating anodes are used in X-ray diagnostics. The anode is shaped like a plate and is rotated by an electric motor (typical speed: approx. 3000 rpm). This heats not only a single point, but an entire circular path. Since the electrons always "destroy" tiny parts of the anode, this distribution also prolongs the life of the anode.

Nowadays, the entire plate is no longer made of tungsten, but consists of molybdenum and graphite to optimize heat distribution (composite anode). Only the focal spot track is still made of tungsten.

■ **Focal Spot/Focus**

Since X-rays are generated in the X-ray tube not only at one point but on a surface, the phenomenon of the penumbra occurs (■ Fig. 2.2). On the X-ray image, the image of details becomes blurrier due to this phenomenon.

In order to reduce the area as much as possible, two tricks are used:
1. By bevelling the edge of the plate, not only a more favorable change in the direction of the radiation is achieved, but also an optical reduction in the size of the focal spot, depending on the angle of the bevel.
2. The tubes usually have two different sized cathode filaments, the large and the small focus. The small focus allows a higher spatial resolution, but is not as powerful.

The Depth Stop with Light Sighting

The depth diaphragm is mounted below the X-ray protection housing.

In the upper area of the depth stop, there are additional filters that can be moved into the beam path either manually or electronically. These filters have the same task as the filter located directly at the beam exit win-

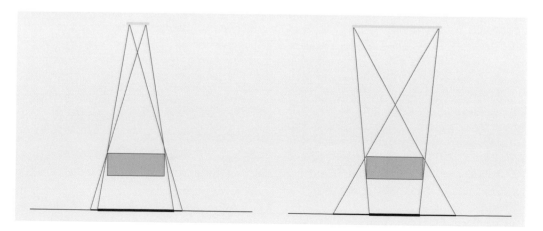

■ **Fig. 2.2** Penumbra as a function of focal size. (From Hartmann et al. 2014)

2

dow. The low-energy radiation components that do not contribute to imaging are filtered out. This is also referred to as "hardening" of the radiation.

The depth diaphragm contains adjustable lead blades that block the X-rays. A distinction is made between the near-focus and near-object apertures. While the **near-tube** diaphragms shield the radiation that has not originated directly at the focus (extrafocal radiation), the **near-object** diaphragms serve to adjust the field size, i.e. the area to be examined.

In order for this field to be visible, a transmissive mirror is placed in the beam path of the X-rays, which is illuminated by a light bulb. The deflected light field is visible below the depth stop and corresponds exactly to the radiation field of the X-ray tube. The depth diaphragm is also rotatably attached to the protective housing in order to optimally adapt the field to the exposure.

An area dose meter is attached to the exit window of the depth aperture.

2.1.2   The X-ray Generator

The main component of a generator is the transformer.

With a **single-phase generator,** "gaps" in the applied tube voltage occur again and again due to the blocking of the negative voltage. Now one can convert this negative part by means of a rectifier. But even then the effective voltage is still full of gaps (**two-phase generator**). If a three-phase supply is chosen (this consists of three alternating voltages which are applied to the coil in a time-shifted manner), these gaps become smaller, but there is no constant voltage in the X-ray tube (**three-phase or six-phase generator**).

Since these fluctuations in the tube voltage deteriorate the quality of the resulting X-rays to the detriment of the patient, these generators are no longer approved for use in human medicine.

Nowadays, only so-called converter or high-frequency generators are used. In principle, the tube voltage is generated according to the same principle. By means of electronic circuits, however, a much more uniform tube voltage is achieved and can also be adapted to the characteristic curves of the tube in order to ensure an optimum yield of radiation.

Tube Voltage

The voltage applied between the cathode and anode is used to control the speed of the electrons and thus the energy with which these electrons hit the anode. Due to the effects mentioned above, the radiation becomes more energetic (**beam quality**).

> Higher-energy radiation has a shorter wavelength than low-energy radiation. High-energy (or as it is called in radiology "harder") radiation can penetrate dense structures more easily than lower-energy ("soft") radiation.

These differences are used, for example, to make the ribs appear almost transparent on an X-ray of the thorax. This makes it easier to assess the lungs.

Since the radiation produced in the tube consists primarily of deceleration radiation, an increase in voltage does not only lead to an increase in energy. Due to the higher-energy electrons, more radiation is also produced at the lower energy spectrum. The voltage therefore has a disproportionate influence on the amount of radiation (◘ Fig. 2.3).

Tube Current

With the heating current applied to the cathode, the amount of radiation can be dosed.

> A high current releases more electrons, which can migrate to the anode: thus one increases the amount of radiation (radiation quantity).

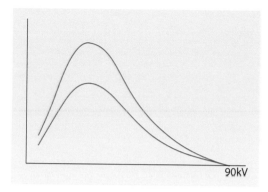

Fig. 2.3 Radiant energy as a function of current intensity. (From Hartmann et al. 2014)

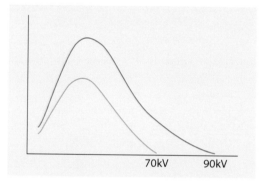

Fig. 2.4 Radiant energy as a function of voltage. (From Hartmann et al. 2014)

The amount of radiation is largely proportional to the current intensity (**■** Fig. 2.4).

The tube current at the generator is usually controlled by adjusting the current-time product, i.e. the amount of charge.

Dose

The dose is always a mixture of tube current and voltage. If, for example, the voltage is increased for a forearm exposure, the resulting radiation can travel more easily through the bones. Thus, less radiation is needed for the X-ray image than if a radiation is selected, a large part of which "gets stuck in the bone".

> The higher the voltage, i.e. the harder the radiation, the less detail can be seen of the bone structures.

It is therefore necessary to choose the optimal mix between radiation quality and quantity for each body region.

Exposure Point System

If you want to set the voltage (kV) or the amount of charge (mAs) for an X-ray exposure on the X-ray generator, the first thing you notice is that this setting can only be made in certain stages. These individual steps are called exposure points (BP). The values of these steps depend on the X-ray tube and can differ from one X-ray system to another.

Automatic Exposure Control

A more precise setting of the dose can be achieved with the automatic exposure control.

2.1.3 Mapping Laws

As is known from natural light, the known laws also apply to X-rays:

Ray Theorem

The X-ray image is always a central projection with the focus as the center (**■** Fig. 2.5). The X-rays represent an object (G) on a projection surface (B) (film, detector). Here, the beam coming directly from the focus and located in the center of the irradiated field is called the central beam. The beam that strikes the irradiated surface perpendicularly is called the perpendicular beam.

With such a type of projection, the law of mapping applies:

In X-ray imaging, the distance g is called the **focus-object distance** and the distance b

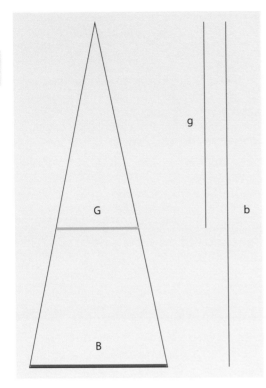

Fig. 2.5 Ray set/central projection. (From Hartmann et al. 2014)

is called the **focus-film distance** (FFA). The distance B-G is called **object-film distance** (OFA). The variable V indicates the magnification of the image.

> The greater the object-to-film distance, the larger the object is imaged, with all objects in an image plane being magnified equally.

In principle, one always wants a representation in the X-ray that is as accurate as possible in terms of size. Unfortunately, this cannot be achieved because the patient has a certain thickness. When setting the image, care is therefore taken to ensure that the region to be assessed is close to the film in order to achieve a sharp and accurate image. (Sternum in prone position, spine in supine position, …).

In some radiographs, these imaging laws are exploited. In mammography (▶ Chap. 3),

for example, a specific region is enlarged by enlarging the OFA.

When taking a thoracic image, one would like to image the heart as accurately as possible. However, since the heart is always at a certain distance from the film, the FFA is enlarged to reduce the magnification factor ($1.10 \text{ m}/1.10 \text{ m} - 0.20 = 1.22 \rightarrow 2.0 \text{ m}/2.0 \text{ m} - 0.20 = 1.11$).

Projection/Parallax

With a central projection it also happens that two objects lying on top of each other cannot be distinguished. This is particularly problematic when these objects appear in the same image size due to their size and position.

However, if the focus is now shifted in a plane, the object in the image plane also shifts (parallax shift, ◘ Fig. 2.6). In this way, objects can be "free projected" in an X-ray image, i.e. the objects that were previously displayed on top of each other are then displayed next to each other.

Distortion

Since an X-ray image is a projection, it is unfortunately the case that objects are only displayed in their full extent if they are perpendicular to the central beam. If the object is not perpendicular, it will be displayed foreshortened. If it is not in the central beam, the size representation also changes (◘ Fig. 2.7).

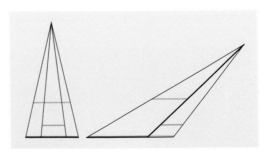

Fig. 2.6 Projection at parallax shift. (From Hartmann et al. 2014)

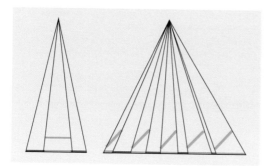

■ **Fig. 2.7** Projection under distortion. (From Hartmann et al. 2014)

Law of Distance Squared

One of the most important physical laws in radiology is the distance-squared law. It states that as the distance (r) increases, the dose/intensity (I) decreases squared.

This law is of particular importance in the field of radiation protection.

2.1.4 Quality of the X-ray Image and Quality Improvement Measures

The Good X-ray Image

What makes an X-ray image a good X-ray image? Regardless of the body region to be examined and the structures to be depicted, the image should have homogeneous, sufficient exposure and good contrast.

An image is homogeneously exposed when the average blackening corresponds to a medium grey tone, i.e. when bright and dark areas in the image can be recognized evenly. Only in this way can the complete grey spectrum be used for display. It is therefore important to select the tube current, the exposure time and the quality of the radiation (tube voltage, kV) optimally.

For the representation of structures you need a sufficiently high contrast between the details.

❯ The harder the radiation, the easier it is to penetrate dense structures, which can lead to these differences in density being displayed with similar brightness. The mnemonic "kV makes gray" describes exactly this fact: that at high kV values the image consists of relatively equal shades of gray.

Another quality feature of a good X-ray image is the sharp representation of the structures.

Motion Blur

Although X-ray diagnostics work with relatively short exposure times, motion blur can occur in the image. **Good patient care** can already improve the quality of the image by actively ensuring that the patient maintains a calm and constant posture/position during the exposure. Sometimes it is advantageous to perform an X-ray exposure lying down rather than sitting down, as the patient can be positioned more stably and unconscious movements can be avoided.

The well-known breathing command of radiology: "Breathe in, breathe no more!" serves to **minimize movement**. Thus, not only the optimal position of the lungs is ensured during lung inhalation, but of course also the movement of the lungs is reduced.

In some images, on the other hand, one takes advantage of the motion blur. When taking an image of the cervical spine from the front, the lower jaw would cover the vertebral bodies. By moving the lower jaw quickly ("jaw flap"), it is possible to partially prevent this overlapping by "blurring" the lower jaw on the image.

Scattered Beam Reduction

In an X-ray image, not only the direct radiation that passes through the body contributes to the imaging, but also the radiation scattered in the body. This scattered radiation causes the structures in the image to no longer be clearly displayed. In order to improve the image quality, this scattered radiation should therefore not hit the detector.

The amount of scattered radiation is directly dependent on the tube voltage, the patient thickness and the field size.

Image Noise in Digital X-ray Images

The advantage of a digital X-ray image is that almost every X-ray image results in a usable image due to the high sensitivity of the digital sensor technology. This technology is much less sensitive to deviation in the amount of radiation than the "old" X-ray film. While overexposure, i.e. too much radiation, does not harm the quality of the image, underexposure results in an image that shows much less detail. This phenomenon is also called **image noise.**

This noise is not always immediately visible on the preview monitors of the X-ray systems. For this purpose, the **dose indicator** exists in digital imaging technology, which,

however, was developed by each manufacturer itself and therefore cannot be transferred from one system to another.

2.1.5 Setting Up a Bucky Workstation

The conventional X-ray workstation is often called the Bucky workstation (◻ Fig. 2.8). Dr. Gustav Peter Bucky was, among other things, a radiologist and developed the principle of the "floating" table top and the scattered radiation grid.

Bucky Table

The table on which the patient lies during the examination is called a bucky table. The special feature of this table is that the table top can be moved in all directions.

Grid Wall Stand

The grid wall stand is primarily used for recording while standing or sitting. Here, the height-adjustable grid drawer is located behind a plate.

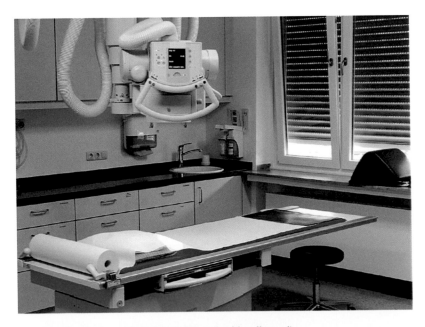

◻ **Fig. 2.8** Example of a Bucky workstation (table and grid wall stand)

Tripod

The X-ray tube or, more precisely, the X-ray protection housing with depth diaphragm is often located on a so-called ceiling pendant. The ceiling pendant consists of two vertical rail systems attached to the ceiling, to which a telescopic arm is attached.

2.1.6 Mobile X-ray Equipment

Mobile X-ray units are used in the intensive care unit or in the operating theatre. Generator and tube are mounted on a mobile unit. Through the use of converter generators, these units have become smaller and can be operated with a normal mains voltage or even battery.

2.1.7 Special Radiation Protection Measures

Direct Radiation Protection

- Shielding

When an X-ray is taken, the patient must of course be exposed to the X-rays. However, if possible, all parts of the body that are not being examined should be shielded from the radiation. Most aids for this purpose are made of lead or lead compounds ("lead rubber"). Depending on the organ being examined, the patient can be protected in various ways. In particular, the organs that are sensitive to radiation should be protected. First of all, these are the gonads, i.e. the ovaries in women and the testes in men. But also the small intestine and the hematopoietic tissue are particularly sensitive to radiation.

> Since many cells in children are still growing, children are generally more sensitive to radiation than adults and therefore require special protection.

When exposing the extremities, the patient should ideally always wear a lead apron or a lead gown. Infants can also be completely wrapped in so-called radiation protection wraps.

When exposing the chest area, a half apron (gonad protection apron) or a radiation protection skirt must always be worn to protect the lower half of the body from radiation.

For exposures of the pelvis or hip, you can no longer put on a half-gun, as this would cover the bone. There are special lead covers for these exposures, depending on gender.

In male patients, the guidelines of the German Medical Association prescribe (in the case of gonadal admission) that the testicles are protected by a testicular capsule) which completely encloses the testicles.

For women, a so-called ovarian protection should be used, which can be applied either indirectly or directly. The indirect protection is attached with a splint or a magnetic holding system below the depth diaphragm and placed by means of the light visor in such a way that the ovaries are covered in the lower pelvic region. The direct ovarian shield is placed on the patient's lower abdomen. For images while standing, this can be fixed by means of a belt.

During the X-ray exposure, all persons except the patient should leave the room. In addition, the doors of the examination room should also be closed in order to shield against possible stray radiation. If a person is required to hold the patient during the X-ray exposure, this person should always be protected with a radiation protection apron. In pediatric radiology, there are additional special radiation protection walls made of lead or lead glass for the person holding the patient during standing radiographs.

- Insertion

One of the most effective methods of minimizing X-ray radiation is to fade in the radiation field.

> The smaller the irradiated field, the less dose reaches the patient and the less scattered radiation is produced in the patient.

2

This means that the overlay not only protects the patient, but also provides a better quality X-ray image.

■ **Additional Filters/Compensating Filters**

Filters were mentioned at the beginning of this chapter. These also contribute to the radiation protection of the patient. The filters in the depth diaphragm harden the rays so that the radiation that does not contribute to image formation does not reach the patient in the first place.

■ **Radiation Quality**

The dose for the patient can also be minimized by changing the radiation quality. Whereas a few years ago, for example, the fingers were X-rayed with a voltage of 44 kV, the Medical Association now prescribes a voltage of at least 50 kV. This makes it easier for the rays to pass through the bones and the current intensity can be reduced. With the introduction of digital imaging techniques, the lower contrast resulting from the higher voltage can be increased by suitable image processing.

Indirect Radiation Protection

Before taking an X-ray, i.e. emitting radiation, it is important to check the preconditions for this.

❯ It should always be checked whether an X-ray of the same region has already been taken beforehand. In this way, any unnecessary duplicate examinations can be avoided.

Viewing the preliminary images is also very important because this is the only way to select the correct imaging technique. For patients with hip prostheses, it may be necessary to select a different cassette format for the hip images in order to be able to image the complete prosthesis.

Radiation protection also includes avoiding erroneous images. The applied radiation should always result in a meaningful, diagnostic image. Therefore, careful and concentrated work is important in radiology. Thanks to digital imaging, the number of false exposures has decreased, but these are also possible here, for example, due to incorrect setting technique or too low a dose.

According to the X-ray Ordinance, the **justifying indication**, i.e. the reason for this examination, must be carefully examined before each examination. Particularly in the case of children, it must be considered whether an X-ray image must be taken or whether other examination methods such as an ultrasound would be sufficient to answer the question.

2.2 Digital Image Processing

One of the greatest advantages of digital radiography is the **linear sensitivity** of the imaging plate and solid-state detector. This means that there are virtually no more false exposures, as good imaging can be achieved with the digital systems even with too little or too much radiation. However, there is a small limitation in the lower dose range. If too little image information (in the form of light pulses) is available, a noisy image is produced.

Digital images also offer the possibility of processing them after they have been taken. In the following chapter, you will learn about some of these options.

2.2.1 Matrix

A digital image consists of many individual **pixels**. These are arranged in rows and columns, this arrangement is then called a **pixel matrix** or **matrix** for short (◘ Fig. 2.9). Depending on the system, an X-ray image consists of between 1024 × 1024 and 4096 × 4096 pixels. One speaks of a 1024 pixel matrix or a 4096 pixel matrix.

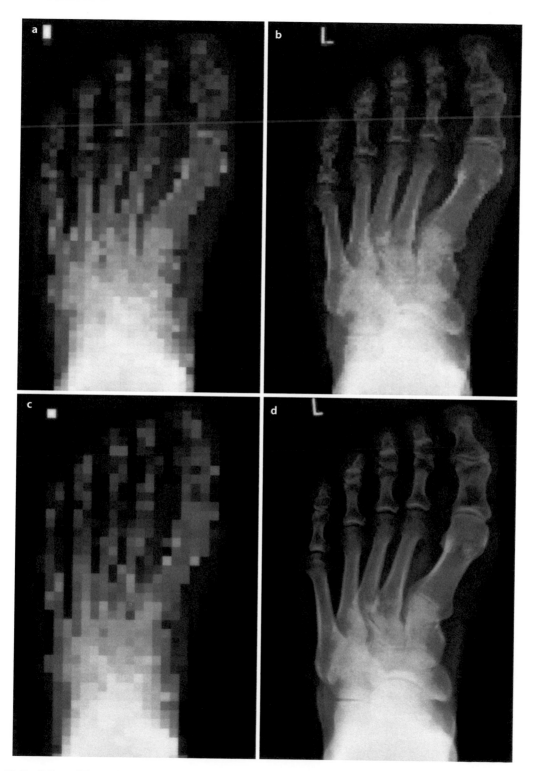

Fig. 2.9 **a–d** Examples of different image matrices. (From Hartmann et al. 2014)

2

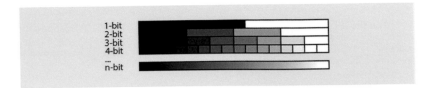

◘ **Fig. 2.10**   Examples of the different color depths. (From Hartmann et al. 2014)

❯ The larger this matrix is for the same image size, the more accurate the image representation.

2.2.2 Color Depth

A specific color is stored for each pixel. This color information depends on the so-called color depth of the image. If only the information 1 (white) or 0 (black) is stored for each pixel of an image, the color depth is said to be one **bit** (◘ Fig. 2.10). However, since the X-ray image does not only consist of black or white, but of different shades of gray, each pixel is described with a certain value, which describes the gray value between black and white.

With a color depth of 1 bit, only two color values, black and white, can be displayed ($2^1 = 2$ colors), with a color depth of 2 bits, four colors can be stored ($2^2 = 4$), and so on. The image that is created at the detector has a color depth of 14 bits, i.e. it contains 16,384 gray values.

2.2.3 Error Correction

As soon as you take a digital X-ray image, it is processed by the acquisition system itself in the first step. The so-called **raw image** is analyzed directly by the acquisition system. First, image errors are corrected, i.e. pixels that do not "fit" the environment due to detector errors or measurement errors are replaced by the average value of the surrounding pixels. Such mismatched pixels can be those that are permanently interpreted as black or white, but also pixels that do not respond to radiation as efficiently as those surrounding them. These errors can be detected during the calibration of the system. The result of this calculation is called a **"pre-processed image"**.

The next processing step is a so-called **histogram analysis**. Here, the brightness distribution of the complete image is analyzed. The software used is precisely adapted to the type of detector used and cannot simply be exchanged. The histogram analysis makes it possible to detect direct radiation and scattered radiation and to use this information to improve the contrast of the image accordingly.

Practice Questions
1. Name the main technical components of an X-ray system.
2. What is meant by "image noise"?
3. What is the law of mapping?
4. Which measures count as direct radiation protection?
5. What is a matrix?

Solutions ▶ Chap. 27

Mammography

Christel Vockelmann

Contents

© Springer-Verlag GmbH Germany, part of Springer Nature 2023
M. Kahl-Scholz, C. Vockelmann (eds.), *Basic Knowledge Radiology*,
https://doi.org/10.1007/978-3-662-66351-6_3

The chapter "Mammography" describes which technical means of a mammography device are used to achieve the special requirements of an X-ray mammography. The effects of compression and magnification in mammography are also discussed.

3.1 Design and Function of a Mammography Device

A cathode ray also works in mammography. However, since in mammography, on the one hand, the finest microcalcifications and, on the other hand, breast and fat tissue have to be distinguished from each other, particularly soft, low-energy radiation is required. For this purpose, mainly molybdenum anodes are used in order to make use of the part of the characteristic X-ray radiation (17.5 and 19.6 keV). Unlike conventional X-rays, the hard radiation is reduced by filters.

3.1.1 The Heel Effect

If we now look at the distribution of the resulting X-rays at the anode, we find that there is a certain distribution (Herzt's dipole) (■ Fig. 3.1).

Due to this special distribution and due to the slope of the anode and the resulting self-absorption, a characteristic intensity distribution occurs within the field. The radiation decreases in the direction of the cathode. This phenomenon is called the Heel effect. The mammography tube is therefore constructed in such a way that the cathode is located close to the thoracic wall, since the breast is thicker and denser here than close to the mammilla.

❯ The Heel effect refers to the anode-side dose drop.

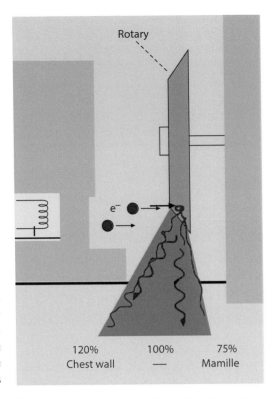

■ **Fig. 3.1** Schematic of the Heel effect. (From Hartmann et al. 2014)

3.1.2 Compression, Scattered Radiation Reduction

Thin objects cause less scattered radiation than thick objects. This dogma is exploited in mammography. The breast is clamped and compressed in the mammography device. This simultaneously minimizes the overlapping of the different structures as well as the motion blur. Another effect is that due to the compression, the breast has at least approximately the same thickness both near the thoracic wall and near the mammilla, thus achieving **homogeneous exposure of** the image (■ Fig. 3.2).

❯ Due to the compression of the breast, the tissue is distributed homogeneously both thoracic and mammillary and can thus be assessed more precisely.

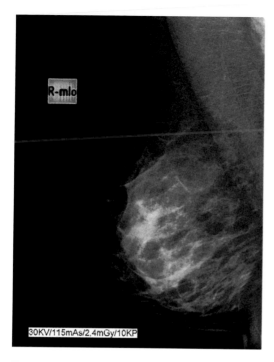

R-mlo

30KV/115mAs/2.4mGy/10KP

◻ **Fig. 3.2** Mammography image

A scattered radiation grid is also used in mammography. Unlike in conventional X-ray, however, a much more complex grid movement is necessary so that the grid is not imaged in the image due to the soft radiation.

3.1.3 Magnification Mammography

In magnification mammography, the distance between the breast and the image receiver is increased. Due to the imaging laws (► Chap. 2), this results in an enlargement of the structures, e.g. in order to better recognize the shape of microcalcifications, even if the geometric blurring becomes somewhat greater. In addition, the grid can be dispensed with in the enlarged image, since the scattered radiation is already too far attenuated and no longer reaches the image receiver.

3.1.4 Automatic Exposure Control

An automatic exposure system can also be used in mammography. Here, care must be taken to ensure that the measuring chamber is placed in projection onto the gland body. Depending on the size of the mamma or also in the case of breast implants, manual exposure is therefore also frequently selected in order to avoid incorrect positioning of the measuring chamber and thus incorrect exposure of the mammogram.

3.1.5 Image Receiver, Image Viewing

As in conventional X-ray, mammography devices are nowadays equipped with digital image receivers. The requirements for spatial and contrast resolution are significantly higher here. Pixel sizes between 0.05 and 0.1 mm are required for the correct delineation of fine connective tissue strands and microcalcifications.

In order to be able to use this matrix size for diagnostic purposes, appropriate monitors are required. While 2-megapixel monitors are sufficient for conventional images, 5-megapixel are required for mammography.

Practice Questions
1. What is meant by the Heel effect?
2. Why is it necessary to compress the breast during mammography?
3. What is magnification mammography?

Solutions ► Chap. 27

Transillumination

Martina Kahl-Scholz

Contents

© Springer-Verlag GmbH Germany, part of Springer Nature 2023
M. Kahl-Scholz, C. Vockelmann (eds.), *Basic Knowledge Radiology*,
https://doi.org/10.1007/978-3-662-66351-6_4

This chapter deals with the basic operation of fluoroscopy equipment and its application in medicine.

The fluoroscopy technique is used for:
— Reduction of bone fractures,
— Examinations of the gastrointestinal tract and other body cavities using contrast media,
— Examinations of vessels also with contrast media,
— Placement of probes or drains in the body.

Of particular importance is the consideration of real-time processes in the study of the swallowing act.

The X-ray contrast media used are adapted to their field of application (▶ Chap. 9).

> ❯ In fluoroscopy, the use of contrast agents allows structures to be depicted that are otherwise difficult to visualize due to the small differences in density compared to the surrounding tissue.

4.1   Image Intensifier (BV)

The image intensifier consists of an evacuated, i.e. airless, glass or metal bulb. The slightly curved entrance surface of the X-rays is coated with a luminescent material (caesium iodide). This layer produces a **luminescent image** when the radiation hits it. A photocathode is applied directly to this luminescent layer, which emits electrons corresponding to the luminescence image, the so-called **"electron image"**. These electrons are accelerated towards the anode by the applied voltage of approx. 25 kV–35 kV.

Further electrodes are attached to the outer wall inside the glass bulb. Their negative charge ensures that the free electrons are focused on a specific point (= **electron optics**).

Beyond the focal point, the electrons also strike the output screen, and the resulting luminance image is brighter, inverted, and reduced in size.

This change in brightness is caused by the acceleration of the electrons inside the image intensifier and by the higher electron density in relation to the area compared to the input screen.

> ❯ The resolution plays a big role. If the layer is too coarse, small details can easily get lost.

Depending on the circuit of the electron optics, the scale of the **electron** optical **reduction** can be changed by shifting the focal point. Thus, only a small area of the input screen can be displayed on the output screen to show details.

The image of the output screen is recorded by a camera and displayed on a monitor. This is done by means of a so-called **tandem optics**, i.e. two lens systems that forward the image of the output screen to the camera system.

The image of the fluoroscopy is displayed on a monitor in the examination room. Due to the **"Last-Image-Hold (LIH)"** function, the last image on the monitor is retained and can be digitally stored, thus replacing an additional X-ray image.

Since the image should be constant during fluoroscopy, regardless of the area being fluoroscoped, the electronics on the output screen also control the generator power of the X-ray tube, among other things.

> ❯ Because of the automatic dose control, never hold or place a lead glove or other opaque object (e.g., scissors, etc.) in the radiation path. This procedure increases the X-ray dose for the patient and the examiner, as the generator regulates the dose upwards until the object is transilluminated.

4.1.1 Structure of A Fluoroscopy Unit

A fluoroscopy system consists of an X-ray tube, a patient positioning table, an image receiver and (in the case of digital systems) an evaluation unit.

In the meantime, mainly under-table units are used, in which the tube is located below the table. For optimal adjustment, either the table can be moved or the X-ray unit can be moved above the patient. In addition, the entire system consisting of the target unit, tube and table can be tilted so that examinations can be performed with the patient standing (e.g. swallowing studies) or with the patient in the head or foot down position (e.g. phlebography—examination of the deep leg veins).

❯ In a fluoroscopy-only unit, the tube image receiver unit cannot rotate around the patient. To take a lateral image, the patient must rotate on the table.

Practice Questions
▶ Chapter 5

Angiography, Rotational Angiography/Angio-CT

Martina Kahl-Scholz and Christel Vockelmann

Contents

© Springer-Verlag GmbH Germany, part of Springer Nature 2023
M. Kahl-Scholz, C. Vockelmann (eds.), *Basic Knowledge Radiology*,
https://doi.org/10.1007/978-3-662-66351-6_5

This chapter deals with the basic operation of angiography equipment and its application in medicine.

A further development of the classic fluoroscopy **unit** is the **angiography unit** with the so-called **C-arm**. The image receiver and the X-ray tube are connected by a semicircular rail, which is anchored to the rest of the system by means of a holding module. This holding module can rotate and can also be moved so that the tube can move sideways along the patient (= images in all spatial directions are possible).

For viewing the fluoroscopic images, there are at least two monitors at the so-called traffic light. On one screen the fluoroscopic image can be seen, on the other previous images can be displayed, which the radiologist can use for orientation during the angiography.

The C-arm can either be floor-mounted or suspended from a ceiling pendant. Some systems have two C-arms, the so-called biplanar angiography systems. These C-arms can be positioned independently of each other. The advantage of these systems is that the radiologist can use two images from two spatial directions for orientation during an angiographic intervention. This enables him to better assess the course of the vessels.

5.1   DSA Technique

DSA, digital subtraction angiography, is an application that is primarily used for imaging vessels using contrast medium. This can be done either by injecting the contrast agent directly into the punctured vessel (e.g. in phlebography) or by inserting catheters into the vascular system and injecting the contrast agent "on site".

Subtraction requires at least two X-ray images: one image without contrast medium and one or more images with the contrast-filled vessel. The first image is called the **mask,** which is subtracted from the subsequent images. This subtraction eliminates the image portions of the mask from the subsequent image that have **not** moved in the time between images. Only the changed image parts are still visible (◘ Figs. 5.1 and 5.2).

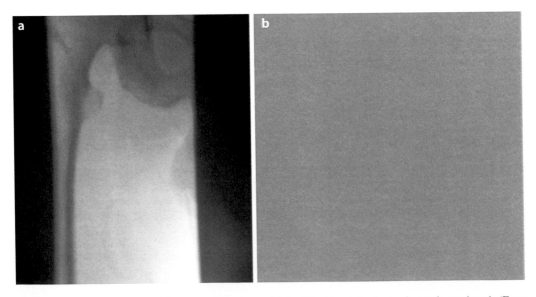

◘ **Fig. 5.1 a,b** Mask image without contrast agent with itself subtracted: A grey image is produced. (From Hartmann et al. 2014)

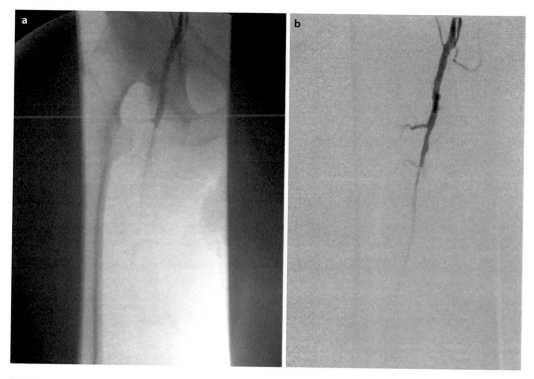

If contrast medium is already present on the mask image, this portion of the image is displayed white in the subtraction image.

❯ For a good subtraction, it is important that the mask image "fits" the subsequent images as exactly as possible, i.e. that the image area does not change, i.e. that the patient does not move.

If the patient has moved, the mask can still be shifted accordingly (= **pixel shift**, □ Fig. 5.3).

Since the contrast medium continues to flow normally in the vessel with the injection and is diluted by the blood, only a limited area of the vessels is always visible during the serial image. This can be sufficient for small examination areas for orientation, but larger ones cannot be assessed in their entire length in this way or used for the examination procedure.

For this purpose, the subtraction images are summed up or "appended" to each other. In this way, not only the main stem of the vessel, but also all the secondary branches are visible in the image.

Such a **summation image** can be placed semi-transparently on the fluoroscopic image for better orientation, so that the examiner can see the course of the vessels on the monitor even without further administration of contrast medium (so-called **roadmapping**).

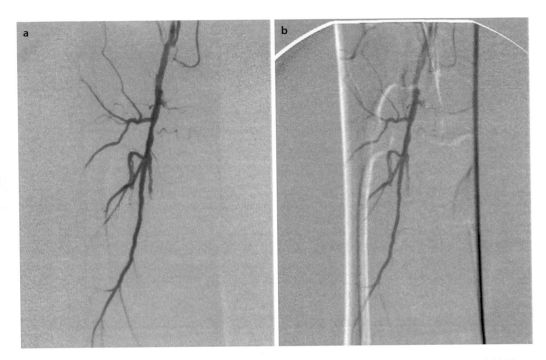

◘ Fig. 5.3 a,b   Subtracted image with and without motion correction (pixel shift). (From Hartmann et al. 2014)

5.2   Angiography-CT Rotational/ Angio-CT

In order to better visualize the position of the vessels, especially in the head region, modern angiography systems are able to produce a so-called rotational angiography. In this case, the C-arm moves around the patient by approx. 200° (manufacturer-dependent) during the series sequence. The result is a raw data set of 180–560 individual images. From this data set, CT-like slices can be calculated by means of back projection and a 3-dimensional vascular image can be calculated. These methods are used, for example, in neurointerventions to find the best working projection for the treatment of aneurysms. Another field of application is transarterial chemoembolization of the liver for the treatment of hepatocellular carcinoma

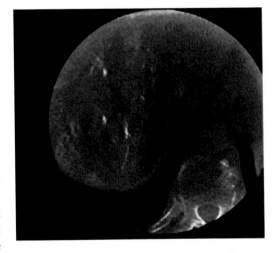

◘ Fig. 5.4   Example of a dynamic sectional view

(HCC). Here, the calculation of a sectional image can ensure the correct distribution of medication and the avoidance of incorrect embolization (◘ Fig. 5.4).

5.3 Seldinger Technique

In addition to the equipment technology, the examination technique plays a major role in angiography. The basis for this is the Seldinger technique. Sven-Ivar Seldinger was a Swedish radiologist who developed a technique for puncturing blood vessels in the 1950s. The central point here is the Seldinger wire over which each step of the procedure is performed (◻ Fig. 5.5). After puncturing the artery with a hollow needle or a needle with a removable inner stylet, a wire is advanced into the vessel. Often the wire is bent in a J-shape at the tip to avoid vascular injury. Catheters, locks, balloons or stents are then inserted via this wire. Depending on the task, there are various special wires, e.g. for recanalization of occlusions or particularly soft ones for probing aneurysms.

> The golden rule is always to hold the end of the wire in your hand so as not to lose the wire in the jar.

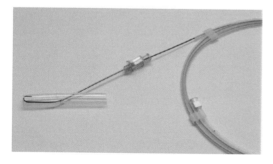

◻ **Fig. 5.5** Seldinger system

Therefore, changing catheters requires a wire that is at least 2.5 to three times as long as the catheters. This means that you often "fight" with 3 m long wires.

Locks, catheters and also many balloon and stent catheters are so-called **"over-the-wire"** catheters. With these, there is a lumen through which the wire runs from the beginning to the end of the catheter.

In the meantime, there is also the alternative of the **monorail system** or also **"rapid-exchange catheter"**, especially in neurointervention. With these catheters (especially balloons and stents), the wire is only guided through a second lumen of the catheter for the first 20–30 cm, after which it runs freely parallel to the catheter. In addition to the shorter wires, this also allows a faster catheter change, but the guidance of the catheter is somewhat worse, since the wire reinforcement is only given at the catheter tip.

Practice Questions

1. What are the main questions for which fluoroscopy is used?
2. What is meant by a "last image hold"?
3. What is the advantage of the C-arm?
4. What is the DSA suitable for?
5. What is a Rapid Exchange Catheter?

Solutions ▸ Chap. 27

Computed Tomography (CT)

Mirja Wenker

Contents

© Springer-Verlag GmbH Germany, part of Springer Nature 2023
M. Kahl-Scholz, C. Vockelmann (eds.), *Basic Knowledge Radiology*,
https://doi.org/10.1007/978-3-662-66351-6_6

Computed tomography (CT) produces sectional images using X-rays. Since computer tomographs are available in almost all hospitals and radiology practices and the examination time is very short, CT is the method of choice in emergency diagnostics. The patient is exposed to radiation and the attenuation is determined. This produces images of different structures that are free of superimposition and allow spatial delineation in all planes. Organs and pathologies can thus be precisely assigned and their extent determined.

6.1   History

The history of computed tomography began in the early 1970s with Sir Godfrey Hounsfield, who developed the first computed tomograph. For this he received the Nobel Prize in 1979. Hounsfield received financial support from the record company EMI, which among others had the Beatles under contract. For this reason the first scanner was also called EMI scanner, with which skull CT's could be accomplished. Since computers were not well developed at that time, the resolution was low (matrix 80×80) and the examination time very long (about 10 min/image). However, it was possible for the first time to diagnose large brain processes without operating on the patient. Larger tumors and hemorrhages could be delineated and ventricular width assessed. Today, in honor of Hounsfield, the units of attenuation are given in **Hounsfield Units (HU).**

6.2   Design and Operation of A Computer Tomograph

The CT scanner itself consists of the **table** and the **gantry.** The gantry is the heart of the tomograph. The X-ray tube, aperture

system, detector system, cooling system and mechanical elements are located under the cover. The entire gantry can be tilted horizontally up to ±30 °. In a CT, the tube-detector systems rotate around the patient with a weight of 2–3 t (in dual-source systems even 4–5 t). This creates immense centrifugal forces. The X-ray emitter of a CT is a rotating housing emitter. Here, the entire housing, i.e. anode and cathode, rotates around the patient.

X-rays are emitted continuously during the rotation. After penetrating the patient, the X-rays are detected on the opposite detector. Different tissue with different densities is located in the beam path. These density differences are registered or measured. This weakened radiation, which has penetrated the patient, is converted into electrical signals. Behind the detector system there is the DAS (= Data Acquisition System) to record the signals. These are passed on to the computer where the generation or reconstruction of the digital images takes place. Both - the power supply of the tube and the forwarding of the detector signals - are carried out via slip rings.

6.3   Investigation Techniques

6.3.1 CT Sequence

The first technique developed is sequential recording technique. It is also called "step and shoot". Transversal/axial exposures are performed slice by slice. A table movement is necessary between two exposures. The amount of data to be reconstructed is small and can be done immediately. The examiner can therefore view the images directly. However, the disadvantage is the long examination time. Since the data acquisition is not continuous, there is a risk of not capturing the smallest details between two slices. There is no possibility of three-dimensional representation.

Nowadays, sequential CT is mainly used for interventions and prospectively triggered cardio-CTs. Even cranial CTs are still acquired sequentially in some cases today in order to avoid exposing the lenses of the eye, which are very radiation-sensitive structures, to the direct beam with a tilted gantry. However, modern equipment techniques are increasingly replacing this technique with spiral scans.

6.3.2 CT Dynamic

Dynamic CT images are also mainly taken using a sequential technique. However, only a selected slice position is continuously recorded. This makes it possible, for example, to perform flow measurements and thus to depict and assess physiological processes. These measurements can only be made with the aid of contrast media. The blood flow is displayed by the contrast medium, so that the kinetics are recorded and measured. This makes it possible, among other things, to make statements about organ perfusion or the cardiac output rate. The dynamic CT examination plays an essential role for acute stroke patients. Lysis therapy can be effective up to 4.5 h after the onset of the first symptoms; therefore, a patient with suspected stroke must undergo imaging as soon as possible. Computed tomography can detect the area of the brain that is poorly perfused by measuring the perfusion of the brain and identify the artery that should supply this area.

Another dynamic imaging technique is **bolus triggering**. The contrast agent accumulation in the focused vessel lumen is continuously measured at a selected slice position. If a preset and predetermined density (HU) is reached, the device starts automatically and acquires images of the desired region.

6.3.3 CT Spiral/CT Singleslice (SS-CT)

New possibilities were opened up by the introduction of spiral CTs in the early 1990s. Data acquisition was no longer "only" sequential, but also spiral, also called helical or helical. The patient is acquired throughout the volume with continuous table advancement and continuous tube rotation, and there are no data gaps. A detector array acquires the data. The region to be examined can be covered very quickly by spiral acquisition. This shortens the examination times to such an extent that the examination can be performed within one breathing phase. The amount of contrast medium can also be reduced automatically. The volume coverage is now seamless and allows the possibilities of overlapping reconstruction, so-called multiplanar reformation (2D) and 3D imaging.

6.3.4 CT Multislice (MS-CT)

In 1998, the first multislice CT came onto the market. It was a so-called "4-slice", as four detector rows were available. With a tube rotation around the patient, four slices could be recorded directly. Thus a larger volume coverage took place. The volume acquisition was therefore faster, which shortened the examination times, which in turn led to a reduction in contrast medium. Another advantage of the multislices is the post-processing. By stringing together several detectors, an isotropic voxel geometry can now be achieved. Isotropic means that all edge lengths are of the same length. This is important for the 3D display, because it allows the step-free display of reconstructed images in all spatial planes without continuity interruptions.

❯ The smaller the voxels, the better the spatial resolution.

However, as the slice thickness decreases, the signal-to-noise ratio deteriorates and the radiation dose to the patient increases.

Detector Design

The introduction of the multi-line technique, in which several detector rings are placed opposite the X-ray source, allows the acquisition of several layers simultaneously. The detector lines do not have to have the same width. There are two types of detectors.

■ Adaptive Array Detector

In the "Adaptive Array Detector", the detector chambers become wider and wider towards the periphery. This leads to the possibility of interconnecting individual elements and lines. Thus, the option of different layer thicknesses exists.

■ Fixed Array Detector

With the "Fixed Array Detector" there are fixed sizes of detector elements per detector row. By selecting certain detector lines, the layer thickness can be determined.

6.3.5 CT Dual-Source (DS-CT)

In the DS-CT, there are two tubes in the gantry at a 90° angle with two associated, opposing detectors. The tubes work in parallel, but can be operated with different energies. The first tube has with 80 kV a lower voltage than the 2nd tube with 140 kV. Some manufacturers allow the use of different tube voltages with only one tube, this technique is called Dual-Energy.

Two images are created. The different tube current results in different attenuation values. Since the tube current is automatically adjusted, there is no increased radiation exposure. The acquisition time is very short due to two separate acquisition units. This is a distinct advantage for spatial resolution, especially for involuntarily moving organs such as the heart. However, the dual-source technique offers further possibilities and advantages:

— The two images with different energies can be added together to produce a "mixed image" equivalent to a 120 kV image.

— Iodine can be accurately detected and subtracted from both images, resulting in a "native" image, i.e. as if the examination had been performed without KM. Thus, separate native images are no longer necessary beforehand. It is used, for example, in liver and kidney diagnostics.

— As an alternative to the virtual removal of iodine information from the image, this information can also be color-coded, e.g. in the evaluation of myocardial ischemia, i.e. reduced blood flow to the heart muscle, or pulmonary perfusion, i.e. blood flow to the lungs.

— Besides iodine, other materials can also be differentiated and characterized by this so-called material decomposition, e.g. ureteral stones.

The use of different energies is also made possible in current device generations, depending on the manufacturer, by modulating the tube voltage or a special detector configuration ("double-layer detector").

6.4 Important Parameters in Spiral CT

6.4.1 Pitch Factor

The pitch describes the **relationship between table feed and detector width**. It is calculated with **p (pitch = table feed/number of simultaneously detected detector lines) x** slice **thickness.**

With a pitch = 1 the volume is recorded without gaps, with a pitch > 1 the data helix is pulled apart. Mathematically, one still obtains a complete data set with a lower image quality but also lower radiation exposure. With a pitch < 1 the volume is acquired overlapping. The pitch regulates the speed of the table feed and thus also the duration of the examination.

6.4.2 Collimation

Collimation describes how **thick or thin a slice** is selected along the z-axis, i.e. the longitudinal axis of the patient's body. Collimation is achieved by a system of apertures and detector elements. The **apertures** serve to focus the radiation and to reduce scattered radiation in front of the detector. The choice of collimation determines the activation of the detector rows and the detector elements. The detector **elements** have different sizes. The layer thickness is influenced by the choice of detectors and can subsequently be reduced to a maximum of the size of the smallest detector element.

6.4.3 Tube Voltage (kV)

The tube voltage is applied between the cathode and anode and determines the penetration capability of the radiation through the matter. Values between 70 and 140 kV can be selected in steps, depending on the manufacturer. Higher kV values mean a hardening of the X-ray radiation, which means that it penetrates tissue types with higher absorption better and causes less scattered radiation. For examinations of the parenchyma, 120 kV tube voltage is usually selected, for CT angiographies (CT-A), i.e. vascular imaging, or bony examinations and examinations of children, 80 kV is usually selected. An increase in tube voltage has a disproportionate effect on the radiation dose. A change of the tube voltage from 100 kV to 140 kV with otherwise unchanged parameters leads to a 4-fold higher dose.

6.4.4 Tube Current-Time Product (mAs)

The tube current has a linear relationship to the radiation dose; doubling the tube current also doubles the radiation dose.

> ❯ The thicker the object being transmitted, the more mAs are required to ensure adequate image quality.

Since bone absorbs or scatters the radiation more, a higher tube current must also be used in body regions with more skeletal parts, such as the shoulder girdle or the pelvic skeleton. This is usually done using automatic dose modulation in order to obtain a homogeneous image quality of the examination (▶ Sect. 6.9.1).

6.4.5 Scan Time (S)

It indicates the actual examination time and depends on the scan distance, the pitch and the rotation time.

> ❯ The longer the scan time, the slower the examination and therefore the higher the dose.

For examinations that involve increased motion artifacts (thoracic CT with respiratory movements, abdominal CT with intestinal peristalsis and pulsation artifacts through the aorta), it is advantageous to select the scan time as short as possible. This can also reduce image blurring caused by involuntary patient movements.

6.4.6 z-sharp Technology

Spring focus, also called flying focal spot or double-z-sampling, is a novel technology. The electron path is deflected by an electromagnetic field so that two focal spots are formed on the anode. The distance between the two focal spots is half of the thinnest collimation selected, so there is an offset, but also an acquisition overlapping by half. With a 64-slice CT, double the volume coverage can be achieved, i.e. 128 slices can be acquired. The overlapping acquisition technique results in a higher spatial resolution, because the image information is added to the same slice.

6.5 Parameters for Image Reconstruction

6.5.1 Layer Thickness

The slice thickness in which the images are to be reconstructed can be chosen by the examiner. It can be minimally equal to the thickness of the smallest detector element and is determined by the choice of collimation.

6.5.2 Increment

The degree of overlap in the reconstruction of the individual slices is determined by the selection of the increment. An increment of 20–30% should be selected for further 3D post-processing.

6.5.3 Convolution Kernel, Reconstruction Filter or Algorithm

This is a computational algorithm that is used to highlight certain structures during reconstruction. The edges of the bony structures and lung structures in the lung window are emphasized with a sharp convolution kernel so that they can be precisely delineated and assessed. The smallest details are shown with sharp separation. In soft tissue imaging, i.e. parenchymal organs, a soft kernel is

selected and the image is optically smoothed. The detail detectability of structures with small density differences is improved.

6.5.4 Windowing

The human eye has only a limited perception, even the best radiologist cannot distinguish significantly more than 60 gray values. Therefore, a narrowing down of the grey values is carried out with the help of windowing. The range of gray values depends on the region or organ to be examined, depending on where the focus lies. The focus is referred to here as "Center (C)". The spectrum of gray values used is called "Window Width (WW)". The Center is the "zero point" of the window. Thanks to this setting, one can refer to the density of the interested organs and delimit and judge them.

6.5.5 z-Interpolation

After or during a spiral acquisition, this measuring principle is carried out by software in the background and only enables the complete data acquisition. Due to a spiral, no complete 360° acquisition takes place. Data within a 360° rotation that lie outside an image plane are "copied" to an image plane, the z-axis, by z-interpolation. This is done by using a computational algorithm to calculate a second spiral that is 180° to the measured spiral. The scanned spiral and the calculated spiral together provide 360° coverage on a plane. Since the pixels have small distances to each other, this provides a good spatial resolution. In addition, the motion artifacts that occur due to the permanent table movement are eliminated. After the z-interpolation the next calculation is performed. The mean values of the image points are determined for image reconstruction/image calculation.

6.6   Image Formation

The patient is positioned isocentrically on the table, i.e. the object to be imaged is always in the center of the beam path during imaging and rotation. This is a very important point for dose control, spatial resolution and thus image quality. First, an overview image, a **topogram** or **scout**, is taken. With its help, the area to be examined is defined and delimited. The data acquisition is carried out with the preset parameters and the data is forwarded to the computer. After z-interpolation, the mean values of the image points are determined. This raw data forwarded to the computer, the attenuation values from all angles, is also called a **sinogram**. The result is a blurred image. The filtered back projection is necessary for a detailed recognizability.

6.6.1   Filtered Back Projection

The main role here is played by the selected convolution kernel. Depending on the convolution kernel, the edge emphasis is enhanced by means of mathematical algorithms. For this purpose, a negative filter is assigned to each voxel in the edge region. After subtraction of filter and measurement data, the edge region is signal-free. This results in edge accentuation and sharper imaging and delineation. The choice of a stronger edge emphasis increases the image noise.

6.6.2   Iterative Reconstruction

This computational process plays an important role in modern computed tomography. It is used for noise reduction, which means that all examinations are performed with a lower dose. Noise had previously greatly affected images with lower doses and degraded image quality. With iterative reconstruction, the noise is "calculated away" and the image impression remains the same. In the best case, a **dose reduction of**

50–60% is achieved, depending on the examination region and object.

The noise or better signal-to-noise ratio (SNR) is the quality criterion of CT images. It is measurable and should be between 12–15 HU. The measurement is made in the peripheral area of the CT image, outside the object, practically in the air.

> ❯ The less radiation is incident, the fewer X-ray quanta hit the detector elements. This increases the noise and the poorer the image quality.

So more radiation is needed, the tube current must be increased. It is important to know that there is an exponential relationship between the mAs and the noise. So to halve the noise, a fourfold of mAs must be used.

6.6.3   Hounsfield Scale

The density values of individual structures and objects in computer tomographic examinations are measured and an image is calculated from them. The different density values are displayed in different grey scales. These scaled values are called Hounsfieldunits (HU) after the inventor of the CT. The reference values for water and air were set at room temperature. For water the value is 0 HU, for air −1000 HU. Bone, although not a reference value, is still important and ranges from +1000 to +3000 HU.

The spectrum of the Hounsfield scale ranges from −1024 to 3071 HU. The human eye cannot differentiate this amount of grey levels. That is why the window technique was introduced.

6.6.4   Window Technology

The window technique is used to limit the number of gray values (❑ Fig. 6.1). The setting and narrowing down refers to the HU of the object of interest and is done by the

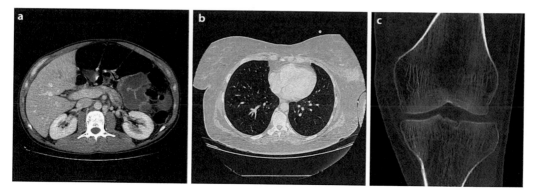

Fig. 6.1 **a** Soft tissue window. **b** Lung window. **c** Bone window

combination of Center (C) and Window Width (WW). The center, also called window location, sets the center of the window width (WW). It is approximately at the density value of the object of interest. The Window Width, also called Window Width or just Window, specifies the range of gray values that will be used to differentiate the structures. It determines the distribution of gray values from white to black.

6.7 Post-Processing

This refers to the post-processing of the acquired data in 2D or 3D representations. These are not used for primary diagnosis, but can be used for better visualization. The object can be viewed in all planes and at any angle. The calculation should be done using very thin, axial slices and there should be an overlap, i.e. the increment should be chosen at least 20% smaller than the slice thickness. This avoids a step-like representation (step artefacts) of the object.

6.7.1 2D Representation

■ Multiplanar Reconstruction (MPR)

This post-processing is a standard part of every examination. The axially acquired data are displayed coronally and sagittally (■ Fig. 6.2), so that the findings can be made in all planes. The curved MPR is a special form of MPR. Objects that are not straight can be displayed straight thanks to this method. This is used, for example, in vascular examinations in order to better visualize the course.

■ Maximum Intensity Projection (MIP)

In MIP, the structures with the highest density in each slice are determined and displayed in an enhanced form. This method is usually not used in the axial images, but is intended for coronal and sagittal images. The axial datasets are the ones relevant to the findings. The slice thickness is usually chosen thicker than in MPR, because the accumulation of the denser structures leads to higher intensity and representation of the same. Areas of application include thoracic CT in the lung window (■ Fig. 6.3) or all vascular examinations.

■ Minimum Intensity Projection (minIP)

In this case, the highest density is not determined and amplified (MIP), but the lowest. The rest of the principle is the same as for the MIP. The representation of the chochlea can be done, for example, with this projection.

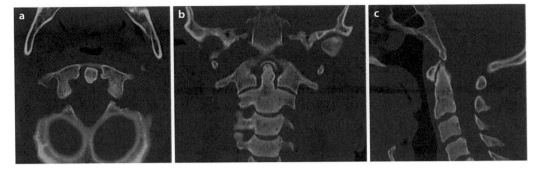

Fig. 6.2 **a** Axial layer plane. **b** Coronal MPR. **c** Sagittal MPR

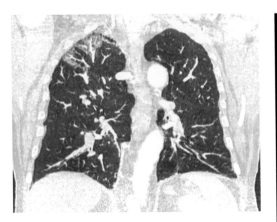

Fig. 6.3 MIP in the lung window

6.7.2 3D Representation

- Shaded Surface Display (SSD)

The 3D surface representation can be used for surgical planning. It restricts the representation of a bone surface (**Fig. 6.4**) to certain Hounsfield values above a threshold value. Under certain viewing angles and a hypothetical light source, which the computer uses for shading, the surfaces appear plastic.

- Volume Rendering (VR)

This is a color assignment and transparency of the individual CT values (**Fig. 6.5**).

Furthermore, it is possible to measure distances and angles as well as to carry out calcification of vessels or bone density measurements.

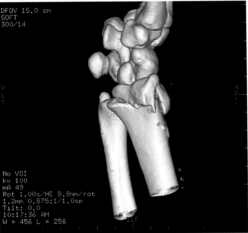

Fig. 6.4 SSD of the distal forearm bones and wrist joint

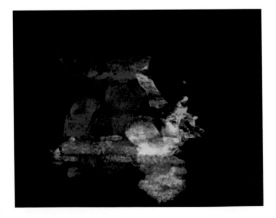

Fig. 6.5 VR of the vessels in the upper thoracic region

6.8 Artifacts

Artifacts are image disturbances that can reduce the assessability of the images or even prevent them altogether. Different types of artifacts are distinguished, which can occur both patient-based and physical-technical.

6.8.1 Movement Artefact

This image disturbance (◼ Fig. 6.6) is caused by movement of the patient, such as breathing. It can be either voluntary or involuntary. The patient may need to be sedated briefly for the examination.

6.8.2 Pulsation Artefact

These occur involuntarily, such as the heartbeat, vascular pulsations or the peristalsis of the intestines.

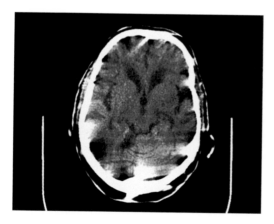

◼ **Fig. 6.6**   Cranial CT with motion artifacts

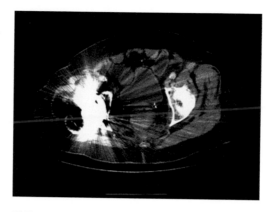

◼ **Fig. 6.7**   Metal artefacts due to implanted hip TEP

6.8.3 Metal Artifact

Metal in the examination field causes detail obliteration (◼ Fig. 6.7). Therefore, all removable metal parts should be removed from the examination region before the examination. If a metal part cannot be removed, e.g. in the case of hip TEP, a higher tube voltage can be selected directly in order to reduce the artefacts.

6.8.4 Partial Volume Effect/Partial Volume Effect

This effect occurs when two adjacent objects in a layer show massive density differences (◼ Fig. 6.8). In this case, the mean value of the measured attenuation values is converted into a gray value for the image display. This can be prevented by choosing thinner layers.

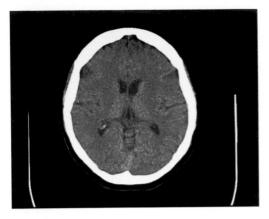

◻ **Fig. 6.8**   Incised sulcus right frontotemporal

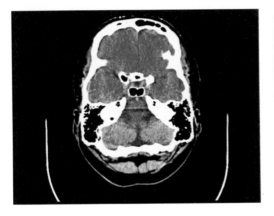

◻ **Fig. 6.9**   Hardening artefact in the area of the brain stem

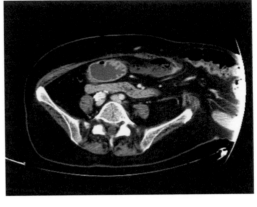

◻ **Fig. 6.10**   Exceeding the measurement field in a patient with a large abdominal wall hernia

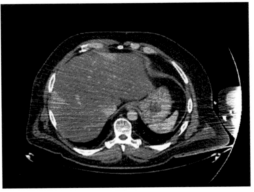

◻ **Fig. 6.11**   Photon starvation artefact when the patient's left arm cannot be elevated

6.8.5   Hardening Artefact

This artefact is caused by hardening of the radiation as it passes through excessively dense tissue. It occurs, among other things, when examining the rock bones and causes artefacts in the adjacent brain tissue (◻ Fig. 6.9). This artefact can be reduced by thinner collimation.

6.8.6   Measuring Field Overrun

Objects that protrude beyond the measuring field lead to artefacts in the edge area and cannot be assessed beyond this (◻ Fig. 6.10).

6.8.7   Photon Starvation Artefact

This occurs when the amount of radiation is too small and can lead to fringe artefacts (◻ Fig. 6.11). It often occurs in patients who cannot raise their arms above their head. When the arms are positioned next to the body, these artefacts occur at the liver. This form of positioning results in an increased demand for dose in the lateral beam path. Positioning the arms on the patient's abdomen counteracts this and the liver can be imaged almost artifact-free.

6.8.8 Ring Artefact

If individual detector rings deviate, ring-shaped artifacts will appear in the image. If a calibration does not solve this problem, the examination with the device must be stopped and the service technician must be contacted.

6.8.9 Line Artifact

Failure of individual detector elements and/or channels will cause black lines to appear across the acquired image. The acquisition must be stopped immediately and the manufacturer notified.

6.9 Radiation Protection Measures and Dose Reduction

Before performing a CT scan, the indication should first be reviewed. If an examination is justified, it must be considered whether alternative imaging with comparable informative value is possible without radiation exposure and how radiation exposure can be minimized. This is particularly true when examining infants, toddlers, and adolescents. Radiation reduction can be achieved by preset programs on the CT:

6.9.1 Dosage Modulation

First, a dose adjustment to the anatomy, shape and size of the patient can be made. During the acquisition of the topogram with the patient in isocentric position and during the acquisition, the required dose is determined. The measured values are compared with the target values of the average patient of 70/75 kg and the mAs are adjusted simultaneously. Thus, the radiation is individually adjusted. The application of lead covers e.g. on thyroid gland and eye lenses can lead to an increased dose exposure depending on the type of dose modulation.

6.9.2 Adaptive ECG Pulsing

ECG pulsing is used in cardio-CT and also in CT angiographies of the ascending aorta. Here, the patient is connected to an ECG. The examination always takes place in the same cardiac phase. In this phase, the acquisition takes place with 100% dose, outside of which a reduction down to approx. 4% takes place. The image quality and the spatial resolution are thus maintained. Unnecessary repetitions are avoided.

6.9.3 Avoidance of Overranging

For the calculations in spiral acquisitions, it is usually necessary to include half a revolution before and after the examination field. With asymmetric collimators, which close before and after the actual scan, this excess radiation is eliminated. This leads to a dose reduction of up to 25%.

6.9.4 Iterative Reconstruction

For some years now, iterative reconstruction has been used in image calculation in addition to or as an alternative to filtered back projection, by means of which image noise can be "calculated away". This reduces the necessary dose of a CT examination considerably by up to 70%. Iterative reconstruction is somewhat reminiscent of Sudoku for advanced students. Ultimately, through repeated trial and error, the computer calculates until it has the best value for each voxel in the image to achieve the attenuation measured at the detector.

Practice Questions

1. What kind of artifacts do you know that affect image assessability?
2. What is the difference between sequence CT and spiral CT?
3. Which detector types in multislice CT do you know? How do they differ?

Solutions ▶ Chap. 27

Magnetic Resonance Imaging (MRI)

Carla M. Kremers

Contents

© Springer-Verlag GmbH Germany, part of Springer Nature 2023
M. Kahl-Scholz, C. Vockelmann (eds.), *Basic Knowledge Radiology*,
https://doi.org/10.1007/978-3-662-66351-6_7

Magnetic resonance imaging is an elegant method for imaging soft tissue in particular with high contrast. A significant advantage is that MRI does not require ionizing radiation; a disadvantage, on the other hand, is the time required for some of these examinations. In this chapter, the structure and function of such an MRI scanner are explained and some frequently used sequences are presented. The difficulties associated with the application are also discussed.

7.1 Which Core Is Actually Spinning Here and What Does It Have to Do with Magnets?

The "nucleus" primarily refers to the **hydrogen protons** (i.e. the central part of a hydrogen atom) of the body under investigation, which are constantly in motion. Each hydrogen proton can be thought of as a small magnetic particle or even a compass needle. Under normal conditions, these small compass needles rotate purely randomly within our body and the rotation is called **spin**. They spin both on their axis and in a circle—similar to a spinning top about to tip over (■ Fig. 7.1a). This type of motion is called **precession.**

The speed of the precession motion (i.e. the number of rotations per unit time) depends on the strength of the surrounding magnetic field and on the type of nucleus (in our case hydrogen). It is called the **Lamor frequency** and has the unit megahertz (MHz), which corresponds to the number of revolutions per second.

In the Earth's magnetic field, hydrogen protons precess at a frequency of 2 kHz, in a 1.5 Tesla device at 62 MHz, and at 3 Tesla at 128 MHz.

The Lamor frequency can be calculated using the Lamor relation for different magnetic field strengths and core types:

$$\varpi = \gamma \times B$$

Here ϖ = corresponds to the lamor frequency, γ = to the gyromagnetic constant (it describes the rotational properties of the respective proton) and B = to the magnetic field strength of the MR tomograph in Tesla.

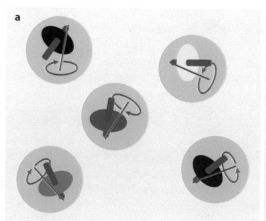
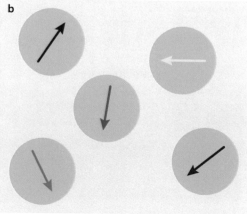

■ **Fig. 7.1** **a, b** Free precession of the hydrogen proton gyroscopes in the body. For the sake of simplicity, the precession direction of the individual spins or the rotating hydrogen proton gyros are shown in the following text as an arrow in the precession axis **b**

7.2   Longitudinal Magnetization

It becomes exciting when the compass needles are brought into a magnetic field. They then still rotate, but in the axis of the magnetic field, This is the task of the main magnet, which in most cases (exception e.g. in the so-called open MRIs) is constructed in the form of a large wire coil as an electromagnet (◘ Fig. 7.2).

In longitudinal magnetization, not all hydrogen protons align in the direction of the magnetic field. Some spins align antiparallel, i.e. in the opposite direction. For imaging, however, only the sum vector, i.e. in this case the difference between parallel and antiparallel spins, comes into play. In the image example (◘ Fig. 7.3), therefore, only one excess hydrogen proton of the original five remains for the formation of the image.

However, the orders of magnitude in the real patient are distributed differently: here, only about 6 ppm (parts per million) form the decisive amount to the image. That is, if 10,00,006 protons align themselves parallel to the magnetic field, 10,00,000 align themselves antiparallel, and six of these 20,00,000 hydrogen protons can later be used for the formation of the image. They decide the alignment of the sum vector. Fortunately, we are made up of an unmanageable amount of hydrogen atoms. The amount of the image

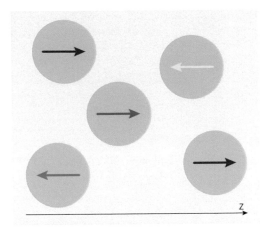

◘ **Fig. 7.3**   Within a homogeneous magnetic field, the spins (i.e. the rotating hydrogen protons within the patient body) align themselves either parallel or antiparallel to the axis of the magnetic field. This is referred to as longitudinal magnetization

responsible "excess protons" in the magnetic field direction in turn depends on the strength of the magnetic field.

> ❯ The stronger the magnetic field, the stronger the longitudinal magnetization, the more spins align parallel to the magnetic field.

7.3   MR Signal

The longitudinal magnetization alone does not yet produce an image. For this, the protons must first be excited.

In order for an image to be created, the tissue must first be excited. In the simplest case, the longitudinal magnetization is directed into a transverse magnetization by a 90° pulse radiated into the examined tissue. This so-called high-frequency pulse is a pulse of radio waves which (in the case of the 90° pulse) are aligned perpendicular to the external magnetic field and coincide with the precession frequency (Lamor frequency) of the material under investigation. This causes the sum vector of the spins to be deflected by 90° from its axis: it now no lon-

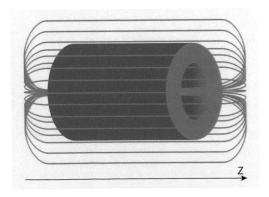

◘ **Fig. 7.2**   The main magnet with its field lines. In the magnet itself there is a homogeneous field in the direction of the patient's position (z)

ger rotates in the z-direction in an imaginary coordinate system, but in the xy-plane.

As an analogy, one can imagine a plate juggler whose rod in the hand corresponds to the z-direction. The plate, in turn, rotates after being deflected by a 90° impulse in the yx-plane.

The rotating spin vector in xy-plane now generates a voltage in a receiving coil.

> ❯ The stronger the transverse magnetization, the more spins align in the xy-plane and the stronger the signal.

In the course of time, however, there is a rapid drop in the signal. There are two reasons for this.

7.3.1 T1 Relaxation Time

After the 90° pulse has flipped the spin vectors into the xy-plane, they gradually seek their way back into the z-axis of the main magnetic field (◘ Figs. 7.4 and 7.5). Once most of the spins have left the plane of

transverse magnetization again, no signal remains for the coil.

The T1 time is the time interval in which 63% of the longitudinal magnetization of a tissue is rebuilt. It depends on the type or composition of the tissue and on the strength

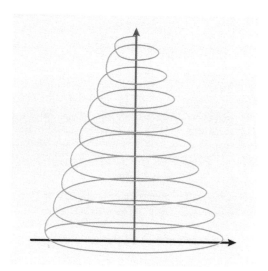

◘ **Fig. 7.4** Schematic illustration of T1 relaxation. After the 90° impulse, the spin vector wobbles back to its initial position: the z-axis

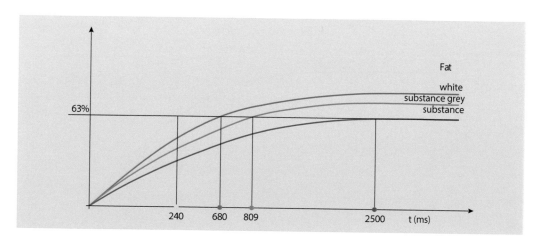

◘ **Fig. 7.5** The reconstruction of longitudinal magnetization over time. Since different types of tissues take different times to T1-relax, their spin vectors emit signals of different strengths. T1 time is the time it takes for a tissue to rebuild 63% of its longitudinal magnetization

of the magnetic field. A tissue with a short T1 relaxation time is fat. Water, on the other hand, has a long T1 relaxation time.

This results in a signal difference between the different tissue types depending on the tissue type and the "readout time": this is how the T1 contrast is created.

7.3.2 T2 Relaxation Time

For this, it first makes sense to understand the term "phase". Here, the direction of the spin vector in the xy-plane is meant. If we imagine the dial of a clock representing the xy-plane, then the clock times correspond to different phases to which the spin vectors can be directed (□ Fig. 7.6).

So now the spins start to rotate within this dial. Since each hydrogen atom in the main vector rotates at a minimally different frequency, they no longer point in the same direction over time.

The orientation of the spin vectors in the dial is called phase. In the context of **transverse relaxation,** they lose the original same direction: they dephase (□ Fig. 7.7). This effect is called T2 relaxation. The T2 time

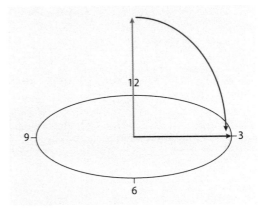

□ **Fig. 7.6**   The 90° pulse directs the spin vector from the z-axis into the xy-plane, which lies there like a clock face

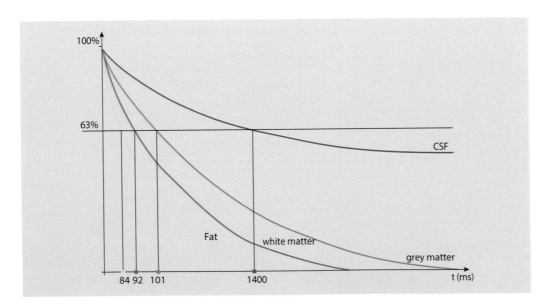

□ **Fig. 7.7**   The signal decay during T2 relaxation over time. As with T1 relaxation, the signal decay varies with tissue type and is described by the constant T2 time. The strength of the magnetic field has no significant influence on the T2 time

does not depend on the magnetic field strength of the MR scanner, but it does depend on the type and composition of the tissue. Fat has a short T2 time, the T2 time of water is long.

With the aid of the different relaxation forms and times, correspondingly different tissue contrasts can be achieved. Both relaxation forms begin simultaneously after the proton spins have been deflected from their original gyroscopic motion in the axis of the magnetic field. In this process, the protons lose their phase coherence faster than they can restore longitudinal magnetization.

❯ By aligning the hydrogen protons in a strong external magnetic field and pulse-controlled "pushing" of the magnetic field vectors, a tissue-specific signal can be generated due to the tissue-specific reaction to these alignment pulses, which MR tomography takes advantage of for imaging different types of tissue.

7.4 Location Coding

How does the MR tomograph know from which part of the patient which signal is coming? This requires several steps and a few more components in addition to the main magnet and the high-frequency coil: the **gradient coils**.

7.4.1 Layer Selection

The Lamor frequency (i.e. the rotation frequency of the hydrogen proton gyroscopes) depends on the strength of the magnetic field. Thus, if we do not make the magnetic field completely homogeneous, but slightly stronger at the head end than at the foot end of the patient, the hydrogen protons rotate with a minimally different frequency in each part of the body: faster at the head, slower at the feet. In order to generate this align-

ment of the magnetic field, additional gradient coils are attached in all three spatial directions.

Since the high-frequency pulse for deflecting the spins must exactly match their rotation frequency, it is possible not to excite the entire patient body with a corresponding pulse, but only a single layer, from which signals are then received.

❯ The steeper the layer selection gradient is chosen, the stronger is also the local difference of the rotation velocities and the thinner are the excited "body disks".

7.4.2 Phase Coding

The key to the next level is again a gradient coil: in order to deduce from which region a received signal comes in y-plane, the magnetic field is again brought out of equilibrium via a gradient. This time, however, only briefly, so that the spin vectors are brought into other phases by short-term rotation at different speeds. To visualize how this works, the dial again helps. By briefly turning on the phase-encoding gradient, the spins in the dial rotate faster as the magnetic field strength increases. If the gradient is switched off again, all spins of the excited layer run again as fast as before—but in different phases—in other words: with different starting clock times. Based on the phase of the derived signal, a conclusion can then be drawn about the position on the y-axis in the excited layer.

7.4.3 Frequency Coding

A gradient coil is also present for the third spatial plane, the x-direction, in order to make the spins rotate at different speeds depending on their position on the y-axis. Based on these different rotation frequencies, when the signal is read out, it is deduced from which position of the x-direction the signal comes. To visualize this, the analogy to music helps: there, frequencies form different pitches. If we imagine that our layer rotates with the frequency of the concert pitch A, the added gradient will cause the higher layer parts to emit higher tones than the lower ones. The pitch then reveals the x-position in the excited layer.

7.4.4 K-space and Fourier Transformation

The data now received is "stored" in the so-called **K-space.** The K-space designates a virtual data matrix in which the acquired raw data are stored in order to process them further afterwards. Accordingly, however, a gray value is not stored here pixel by pixel—it is more complicated.

The K-space is filled step by step and pixel by pixel. Each K-space line corresponds to a data acquisition in the phase encoding direction. Each K-space pixel in turn does not simply contain a gray value, but information about the entire image. The information about the image contrast is stored in the K-space center. The location information is stored in the edge regions.

With the aid of the **Fourier transformation**, the data obtained is decoded and processed into an image. This is a computational model that is used to decode the jumble of phases, frequencies, location and contrast information. This is done by an extremely powerful computer.

To obtain an image, the Fourier transform must be performed individually for each K-space row, or in our image example for each phase column, in order to decode the different frequencies from this column. For a common image matrix of 256×256 pixels, this means 256 times. The different spatial frequencies are then decoded from each phase column.

7.5 Proton Thrusting and Gradient Ballet: the Interplay of High-Frequency Pulses and Spatial Coding

Now we know how the signal is generated in the MRI and how the tomograph detects the origin of the received signal. But how does it all work together?

The moment the patient is placed in the center of the scanner, his hydrogen protons begin to align themselves in the direction of the magnetic field and, in this alignment, to circle around their axis somewhat faster than usual: Longitudinal magnetization happens even before the actual examination.

In order to select the examination layer, a layer selection gradient is now switched and at the same time a matching high-frequency pulse, which now deflects the protons from a body layer by 90° to the side: into the transverse magnetization. The receiving coil already receives a signal at this point, but it is still identical from the entire layer and does not produce an image. Now the phase-encoding gradient is switched on and off again to enable the spatial encoding in the y-direction. After an intermediate step—refocusing (▶ Sect. 7.5.1)—the frequency encoding gradient is switched on and the signal is read out, which can now also be assigned in the x-direction. This is how an axial **spin-echo sequence** works.

7.5.1 Refocusing

Since, as already mentioned, the T2 relaxation happens very quickly within a few milliseconds, the signal also goes out again just as quickly. In order to still get enough signal for an image, we get it again with a 180° pulse. The signal generated again in this way in the opposite direction is called a (spin) echo (◘ Fig. 7.8). To ensure that the protons of

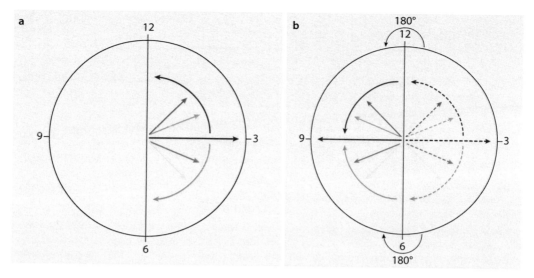

Fig. 7.8 **a, b** With the refocusing pulse, the spins that dephase in the xy-plane are "flipped" by 180° and converge again on the other side of the dial: they thus come back into phase and in this way generate a signal again—now in the opposite direction within the xy-plane

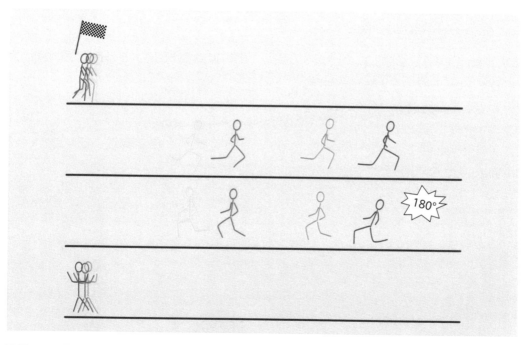

Fig. 7.9 The refocusing impulse using the example of a group of runners: if all runners remain constant in their pace, they will arrive together at the start again when they turn around at the same time, e.g. 30 s later

the layer just examined are excited to an echo, a layer selection gradient is again switched.

A popular analogy for a better understanding of refocusing is a group of runners (**Fig. 7.9**) who start a race—each constantly at his personal maximum speed. After a short time, all runners are asked to turn 180° immediately. If all runners maintain their speed constantly, they will arrive back at the starting point at the same time.

7.5.2 Echo and Repetition Time or T1 and T2 Contrast

Important parameters of an MR examination sequence are the echo time and the repetition time—both are decisive for the contrast in the resulting image, i.e. they determine which tissue types are imaged brightly (=hyperintensely) and which are imaged darkly (=hypointensely).

Let us imagine again the structure of a spin-echo sequence with the help of a diagram (■ Fig. 7.10).

The **echo time** (TE = Time to **Echo**) refers to the time span between the excitation of the protons and the reception of the signal. It determines how much **T2 contrast** is ultimately seen in the resulting images or how much an image is T2-weighted. If the TE is short, the contrast between the differ-

ent types of tissue is low and the image has little T2 weighting. A long echo time results in a heavily T2-weighted image.

The **repetition time** (TR = Time to repeat) is the time selected between two excitation pulses. It is responsible for the **T1 contrast of** the image. The longer the TR, the more time the protons had for T1 relaxation. If we recall that the time taken for T1 relaxation or for the reconstruction of longitudinal magnetization varies, it also stands to reason that a 90° pulse will cause little signal difference between different tissue compositions if T1 relaxation is again complete at the time of excitation. If the TR is chosen to be short, not all protons will be aligned along the axis of the main magnet at the time of re-excitation—accordingly, a 90° pulse will not "flip" them all into the *xy*-plane. The signal differences generated in this way correspond to a T1 weighting.

> A short repetition time TR produces a T1-weighted image. A long echo time TE produces a T2-weighted image.

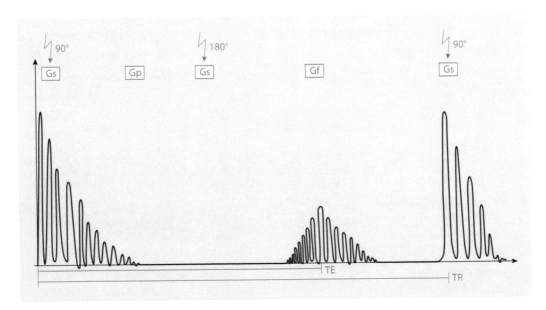

■ **Fig. 7.10**   Schematic drawing of the sequence of a spin-echo sequence

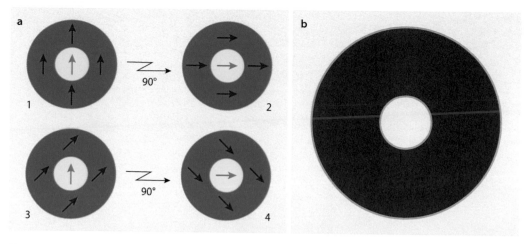

Fig. 7.11 **a, b** Schematic representation of the formation of the T1 contrast with a drop of fat in the middle of a glass of water. Since the fat drop gener- ates a lot of signal, it appears bright in the MR image, the water gives little signal, so it is dark in the MR image

T1 Weighting

Let's imagine a scenario with a drop of fat in a glass of water and remember: fat has a short T1 relaxation time, the T1 relaxation time of water is long.

After the first excitation, the protons in the fat droplet are already aligned in the plane of the main magnet, while the pro- tons of the water are still on their way back to the z-axis (■ Fig. 7.11). Thus, when a 90° pulse hits the water glass again at this point in time, the protons of the fat drop align themselves completely in the xy-plane again and emit a lot of signal. The water protons, on the other hand, are not yet completely relaxed and most of them do not circle either transversely or longitudi- nally, but obliquely to the magnetic field— so after the 90° pulse they are not folded into the xy-plane and accordingly do not emit any signal.

T2 Weighting

Decisive for the T2 weighting are the long echo time and the recurring refocusing pulses. In our example, a piece of tissue, e.g.

gray matter, is surrounded by water. Due to the recurring refocusing pulses, an almost identical echo is generated—but depending on T2 effects, the signal decreases from echo to echo, and at different rates: the T2 time of water is long—so dephasing is hardly notice- able and the signal remains strong for longer (water is imaged brightly). The T2 relax- ation of gray matter follows more quickly, the signal of the brain tissue decreases more rapidly and is imaged darkly in the image (■ Fig. 7.12).

> In order to distinguish on an image whether it is T1- or T2-weighted, it helps to look for an image location with aque- ous fluid (e.g. cerebrospinal fluid): Water is shown dark in T1 weighting and light in T2 weighting.

Characteristics of Different Weightings

In addition to T1 and T2 weighting, there is also proton weighting (PD). This is the name given to the contrast obtained by a

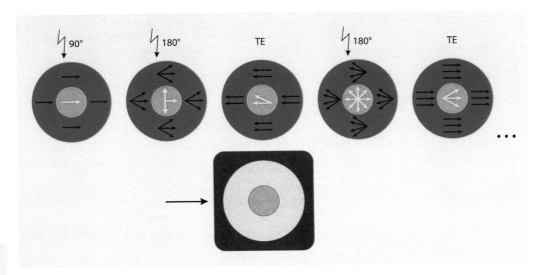

◻ Fig. 7.12 Schematic representation of the formation of a T2-weighted image with gray matter in a water glass

◻ **Table 7.1** Characteristics of the weightings

Weighting	TR	TE
T1	Briefly Approx. 500 ms	Briefly Approx. 15 ms
T2	Long Approx. 2500 ms	Briefly Approx. 15 ms
PD	Long 2500 ms	Long Approx. 90 ms

TR Time to repeat (repetition time), *TE* Time to echo (echo time)

long repetition time and a short echo time (◻ Table 7.1).

❯ Since the gray values in the images of an MRI correspond to different signal intensities, brightly imaged structures are called signal-rich or hyperintense areas, and darkly imaged lesions are called signal attenuation or hypointense areas.

7.6   Sequence Theory

What else can the device do? At least some important, widely available and common sequences should be briefly explained here.

7.6.1 Gradient Echo Sequences

In addition to the pulse or spin echo sequences described above, it is also possible, instead of high-frequency pulses, to set the spin vectors in motion by rapidly switching strong gradients with the aid of the gradient coils and to generate signals in this way. T1 as well as T2 and PD contrasts can be obtained. The gradient echo sequences can also generate smaller excitation angles than the 90° and 180° known to us so far. This can save time, for example, to avoid motion artifacts, but it also makes vessel imaging and diffusion imaging possible. On the other hand, such sequences are also susceptible to artifacts and they generate less signal, which is why they have not replaced spin echo sequences to date.

7.6.2 Fat Saturation

Fat is mapped hyperintensely in both T1 and T2 weighting. In the T2 weighting, it is therefore difficult to distinguish edema (water = hyperintense) from fatty tissue. In order to make the pathological structures (e.g. fluid or edema) more visible, the signal of the fat can be suppressed. There are various methods for this.

Inversion Recovery

For this purpose, a 180° pulse is applied before the actual examination sequence. It changes the initial position of the spins. The 90° pulse follows at the moment when the vectors of the tissue contrast to be suppressed precede in the xy-plane. Thus, they are flipped out of the 90° plane and give no signal.

This principle works for the suppression of fatty tissue, e.g. to make edema in the fatty bone marrow visible. In the same way, the signal from free fluid (cerebrospinal fluid) in the brain can be suppressed to make delicate edema in the brain tissue more visible. Sequences that function in this way are usually identified by an "IR" in their name, e.g. STIR, FLAIR or TIRM.

Frequency Selective Saturation or Spectral Saturation

Here, too, a pre-pulse is used. In this case, however, it should not reach all protons of a layer, but only the tissue to be saturated. This works because the precession frequency differs minimally in different types of tissue. Therefore, it is possible to switch a pre-pulse that specifically matches only the frequency of the spins bound in the fat tissue. The fat-bound spins are deflected from the plane of longitudinal magnetization by this highly frequency-selective pulse, thus eliminating their signal from the image.

Chemical Shift or Dixon Method

This method of fat saturation also makes use of the minimal differences in precession frequency between fat- and water-bound protons. It is particularly useful for visualizing microscopic lipids that are present in equal proportions along with water-bound protons within a voxel. Since the spins within the voxel precess at different rates, there are always brief times when the spin vectors of both tissue portions are pointed in the same direction (i.e., they are "in phase") and give off a lot of signal accordingly. Similarly, there are times when the vectors are pointing in the opposite direction, this is known as the opposite phase or "opposed phase"—as the differently aligned vectors cancel each other out, the signal at this measurement time is weak. The images obtained at the different measurement times can then be compared: If the tissue contains fat and water, it is imaged hypointense in the opposed phase compared to the in phase image.

7.6.3 Vessel Mapping

With magnetic resonance imaging is also possible to image blood vessels. There are also various methods for this, including those that do not require the administration of a contrast agent.

Angiography Time-of-Flight

This imaging is often used to image the large cerebral arteries. This again requires pre-pulses, which ensure that the tissue whose vessels are to be examined no longer emits a signal itself. The spins flowing in through the blood in the opposite direction are also saturated. Since the freshly inflowing blood does not receive such prepulses, it emits a strong signal.

Phase Constrastangiography

This type of vessel imaging is particularly suitable for slow, i.e. venous, blood flow, e.g. to exclude sinus vein thrombosis. For this purpose, effects of gradient echo sequences are used: When spins move in the direction of a switched gradient, their phase changes, which distinguishes them from the surrounding tissue. This phase difference allows them to be made visible.

Angiography Contrast-Enhanced

If longer arterial vessel sections are to be imaged, contrast-enhanced angiography is suitable. For this purpose, images of the examination volume are first taken without contrast medium. Then contrast medium is injected intravenously and images are taken again while the contrasted blood flows through the arterial vessels to be imaged. The two series are then subtracted from each other—this allows the section of vessel to be imaged to be isolated.

7.6.4 Diffusion Imaging

With diffusion imaging it is possible, for example, to image the cytotoxic edema of a stroke. To do this, several gradients are first switched in opposite directions in quick succession in order to dephase the spins within a voxel (■ Fig. 7.13). If the tissue under study is healthy, some of the dephased spins diffuse the voxel through Braun's molecular motion. If the molecular motion is disturbed, e.g., in the context of such edema, the spins remain in place. Now a rephasing pulse is generated. Then the spins remaining in their voxel generate a signal: the diffusion-disrupted areas are imaged hyperintensely. Since T2 effects also influence the image in this imaging, a so-called **ADC map** is also produced in addition to the diffusion images, in which the T2 effects are eliminated. The diffusion-disturbed

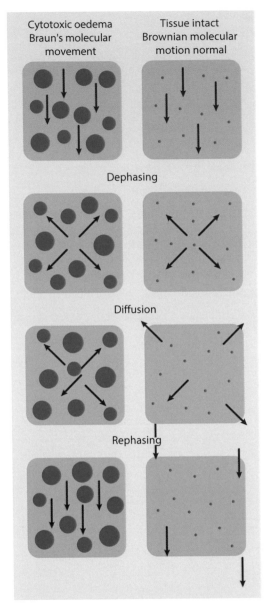

■ **Fig. 7.13** Schematic drawing of the diffusion measurement procedure

areas are imaged hypointense here—so in order to reliably distinguish a diffusion disturbance from a hyperintense lesion of a different type, these two parts of the sequence must be compared with each other.

7.7 Contrast Agent

(See also ▶ Chap. 9) In addition to contrast-enhanced MR angiography, there are other applications for MR contrast agents, such as the search for inflammation or tumors. The currently approved preparations are all based on **gadolinum**, a rare earth which, where it accumulates, shortens the T1 relaxation time and leads to signal enhancement there through T1 weighting.

As with all medications, intolerances in all forms are also possible with gadolinium-containing contrast media—even if they are rare. Nevertheless, the patient must be informed of the possible risks before any contrast medium is administered. Although most MR contrast media are eliminated renally, they do not worsen preexisting renal impairment. Nevertheless, knowledge of renal function prior to contrast administration is important because administration of gadolinium-containing contrast agents may result in skin and connective tissue disease in the setting of markedly reduced renal function. Nephrogenic systemic fibrosis means a considerable reduction in quality of life for the affected patients, but also in their life expectancy. In addition to the "normal" contrast medium with renal elimination, there are also so-called liver-specific contrast media, which are absorbed into the hepatocytes and at least partially eliminated via the bile ducts. They are particularly suitable for the evaluation of liver tumors.

7.8 Security

Although there is no X-ray radiation in MRI—and therefore no ionizing radiation that could endanger the patient being examined—there are still some aspects that need to be clarified before an MRI examination.

7.8.1 Attraction of the Magnet

Many noteworthy points are based on the strength of the main magnet. The most commonly used magnetic field strengths in medicine are in the range of 1–3 Tesla—a multiple of the Earth's gravitational pull (1.5 Tesla is approximately 30,000 times the Earth's gravitational pull).

Magnetic materials (e.g. iron) are accordingly strongly attracted by such a magnet. Metallic objects therefore have no place in the MRI scanner—unless they are explicitly suitable and intended for this purpose. If they come too close to the device, they are drawn into the main magnetic field at high speed. Thus, a stethoscope dangling harmlessly around the neck of a concerned colleague, or even a ballpoint pen, can become a projectile that endangers the life of the patient in or the staff in front of "the tunnel". The magnet's attraction does not even stop at wheelchairs, oxygen cylinders, defibrillators and patient beds!

In the event of an incident where a patient or staff member needs to be "bailed out" and the solenoid needs to be shut down, the most commonly used superconducting solenoids have a quench option. In a **quench**, all the helium (which is used to cool the magnet) is discharged through an outer tube. When the quench button—which is usually secured by a flap or similar and specially marked—is pressed, the magnetic field goes out. Once the helium has evaporated, the device is inoperable until the next refill. A helium filling is expensive—therefore this variant should only be used in an emergency, when there is immediate danger to a person.

7.8.2 Implants

Precautions must also be taken with metallic material inserted into the patient's body. **Osteosynthesis** and **joint prostheses** of the last 20 years are mostly harmless—here the magnetic attraction is less the problem than possible heating of the material—which the patient should report as soon as he notices it so that a burn does not occur.

There are also so-called "MR-compatible" models for **pacemakers**, **neurostimulators** and the like. However, this does not mean that all these patients can be examined in MRI without any worries. It must first be clarified whether both probes and aggregate are suitable and also in the implanted combination. If so, the materials may not be approved for the examination of all body regions and not for every magnetic field strength. Since, for example, pacemaker settings can be adjusted during the examination, it is important to know whether the patient is pacemaker-dependent, i.e. whether his heart beats reliably without the motivation of the small external assist device. And then such a patient must also be competently monitored during the examination.

Particular attention should be paid to **vascular clips** when inserted within the head for cerebral artery aneurysm therapy. The delicate vessels of the head are fragile and movement of such a clip can cause life-threatening bleeding. Here, too, it must be clarified beforehand whether or not the clip is suitable for MRI.

As a rule, **shrapnel** is not suitable, which can occur in older patients and in patients who have migrated from war zones.

> ❯ As a general rule, you can tolerate a lot of foreign material—but you have to be sure whether it is suitable in general and also for the planned examination.

You can get information from the manufacturer or from good sites on the net like ▶ mrisafety.com.

7.8.3 Volume

Another—manageable—danger is the noise generated during an MR examination: especially the rapid switching back and forth of gradient coils leads to mechanical stresses in the device, which are loudly noticeable. There are so-called "whisper sequences" which cause less noise by certain settings on the device, but on most devices you will not get along without loud noises. It is therefore essential to use hearing protection on and in the running device.

7.8.4 Tissue Stimulation

Due to the movements that are triggered at the molecular level during an examination, **tissue heating** can occur. To prevent the movement from becoming a burn, the energy radiated into the patient's body is measured as the **specific absorption rate (SAR)**. The device warns the examiner if the limit value is exceeded.

Rapid switching of gradient fields can cause **nerve stimulation** with **involuntary twitching** or **electrifying sensations**.

In the case of skin-to-skin contact, the development of small eddy currents is possible, which lead to **local burns.** Therefore, it is important that, for example, the calves do not lie directly next to or on top of each other and that the hands are not folded over the chest or abdomen during the examination. A thin layer of paper or cloth is already sufficient to avoid this reaction.

7.8.5 Emergency Bell

Since the patient is usually alone in the closed room, he must have the opportunity to make himself heard—if he calls for help, no one will hear him behind the soundproof wall with accompanying noise from the device. For this purpose, the patient must be given an

emergency bell, which is available on every device, before the examination begins.

Practice Questions

1. How can you tell in an MRI image its weighting?
2. Which sequence do you choose to visualize edema, e.g. in the context of inflammation?
3. Are there any contraindications for an MRI examination?
4. Is contrast medium required for vascular imaging in MRI?
5. There is an emergency in the MRI: Your patient is no longer breathing. As a radiologist, what do you have to watch out for now as well?

Solutions ▶ Chap. 27

Sonography

Christel Vockelmann and Martina Kahl-Scholz

Contents

© Springer-Verlag GmbH Germany, part of Springer Nature 2023
M. Kahl-Scholz, C. Vockelmann (eds.), *Basic Knowledge Radiology*,
https://doi.org/10.1007/978-3-662-66351-6_8

In this chapter, you will learn how ultrasound waves are generated for use in sonography and how sonographic examinations can be technically controlled.

In addition, you will learn about the areas of application, possibilities and limitations of this procedure and in which cases it can be used as a radiation-free alternative examination in imaging diagnostics.

8.1   Physical Basics of Sonography

8.1.1   Ultrasonic Waves

Sonography uses ultrasound waves to produce cross-sectional images of the human body.

> ❯ Ultrasound is the term used to describe sound waves with frequencies above the range of human hearing.

The ultrasonic waves in sonography devices are generated via the so-called **reciprocal piezoelectric effect** on a quartz crystal. The solid body serves as the transmitter and receiver of the sound waves. The piezoelectric effect is created by the contraction and elongation—i.e. compression and expansion—of the crystal (◻ Fig. 8.1a). An applied external electrical voltage causes the vibrations, i.e. the sound waves, to be emitted (= **sound wave emission**).

If the sound waves encounter an impedance jump (wave resistance) on their way, e.g. at the boundary between fatty tissue and water, they are reflected and received as an echo or resonance on the quartz crystal. The resulting sound pressure deforms the crystal and the electrical charge is shifted. This piezo effect (◻ Fig. 8.1b) produces a measurable electrical voltage which is recorded by the connected electronics and displayed as an image.

Ultrasound waves are harmless to the human body. Only a slight increase in body temperature is conceivable during an intensive examination.

The speed of propagation of the sound waves depends on the medium through which they pass and its elasticity and molecular density (◻ Table 8.1).

The ultrasound image is created by waves that are reflected, scattered and refracted at tissue junctions. This effect is caused by impedance jumps, e.g. at organ boundaries or vessel walls. Impedance (z) stands for the transition resistance, which is a product of the speed of sound (c) in the medium and the density (ρ) of the medium:

$$z = c \times \rho$$

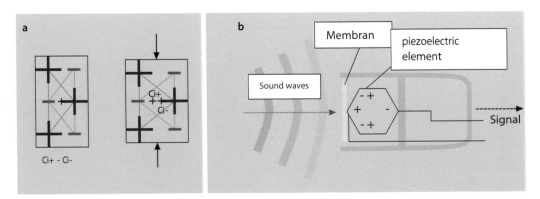

◻ **Fig. 8.1** In the resting state, the centers of the positive and negative charges lie on top of each other, the charges neutralize each other. When the crystal is compressed, the centers of the charges shift towards each other, a measurable electric voltage is produced **a**. Piezoelectric effect **b**. (From Hartmann et al. 2014)

■ Table 8.1 Speed of ultrasound waves as a function of the medium	
Air	340 m/s
Water/grease	1450 m/s
Soft tissue	1540 m/s
Bones	2700–4100 m/s

■ Table 8.2 Frequency-dependent penetration depth of sound waves into tissue		
Frequency	Resolution axial/ lateral	Depth of field
3.5	1 mm/2 mm	160 mm
5	0.6 mm/1.2 mm	100 mm
7.5	0.4 mm/0.8 mm	50 mm

❯ No border crossings, no ultrasound!

■ **What Happens to the Ultrasound Waves in the Body?**

1. **Absorption**

A large part of the ultrasound waves is absorbed, i.e. completely absorbed into a medium (lat. absorptio = absorption).

❯ The absorption increases exponentially with increasing image depth and increases linearly with the applied frequency.

The absorbed energy is converted into heat. Therefore, there are different transducers that emit different frequencies. Typically, frequencies of 3.5 MHz are used for abdominal imaging; for superficial structures, high-frequency transducers of up to 20 MHz can be used, which can produce an image extending only a few cm into the depth (■ Table 8.2).

2. **Reflection and Scattering**

If the boundary surfaces are considerably larger than the wavelength, reflection occurs.

❯ Reflection means that the angle of incidence and the angle of reflection are equal.

The sound waves are therefore reflected back, like the billiard balls on the rail. With small structures, the sound waves are increasingly scattered. Scattering is non-directional, comparable to sugar falling on the kitchen table.

3. **Refraction (Refraction)**

Refraction **deflects ultra**sound waves as they enter another medium. The effect is amplified by a more acute angle and by a higher resistance between the two media. The same effect refracts sunlight in rain and creates the rainbow.

4. **Diffraction (Diffraction)**

❯ Diffraction describes the deflection of waves at an obstacle, which leads to the creation of new waves at the obstacle and their interference (superposition).

8.1.2 Procedure

A-Mode

The A-mode is the oldest method. "A" stands for amplitude modulation. Today, the method is still used for distance determination in ENT, ophthalmology and neurology. In the early days, before the development of computer tomography, this method could be used, for example, to detect a midline shift in a brain tumor.

M-Mode

The M-mode (from "motion") can be used to map the temporal behavior of a tissue. It is used in particular in cardiology (■ Fig. 8.2). A typical example is the imaging of the movement of a heart valve or the myocardium.

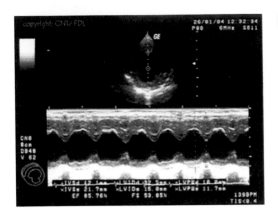

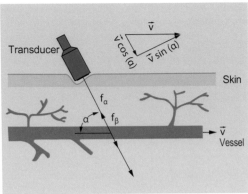

Fig. 8.2 Examination of a heart valve. (From Hartmann et al. 2014)

Fig. 8.3 Angular ratios in the determination of the Doppler shift. (From Hartmann et al. 2014)

B-Mode

The B-mode (for "brightness") is the most frequently used method. In the 2D image, the different pixels are detected with different brightness grey dots, depending on the strength of the reflected signal.

A further development of the method is 3D ultrasound, which generates spatial still images. For this purpose, in addition to the scan in one plane, the angle of the sound is swiveled in order to obtain image information in the 3rd plane. If not only a still image is generated, but the examination is performed in real time, a 4D ultrasound is created with time as the 4th dimension.

Sonography Doppler

In 1842, the physicist Christian Johann Doppler described the **Doppler effect** named after him. When the sound source and reflector move towards each other, the sound waves are bundled and reach the receiver at a higher frequency. You already know the principle: you can hear whether the sirens of an ambulance are coming towards you or moving away! This effect is used for Doppler sonography.

The effect is strongly angle-dependent (■ Fig. 8.3). If the angle between the sound source and the reflector is 90°, no signal can be obtained. The smaller the angle between sound source and reflector, the smaller the error!

Doppler sonography is used to determine flow velocities. From these, stenoses of vessels can be quantified. The classic field of application is the examination of the carotid arteries.

Sonography Color Doppler and Power Doppler

Color Doppler (synonyms: color-coded Doppler sonography; color-coded duplex sonography; FKDS) is a further development of Doppler sonography. The image is color-coded with the measured flow velocities and flow directions. The following applies by definition:

> Blood flow toward the transducer is coded red; blood flowing away from the transducer is coded blue. Faster blood flow is shown lighter than slower flow. In the image on the right, a corresponding coding is shown with an indication of the measured flow velocity.

For example, it is important to detect the direction of flow in subclavian-steel syndrome, in which flow reversal of the associated vertebral artery occurs due to stenosis of the subclavian artery (■ Fig. 8.4). Clinically, affected patients usually have dizziness, especially during physical exertion and strain of the corresponding arm.

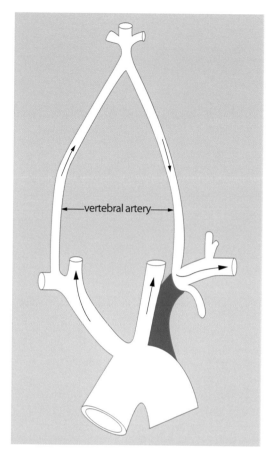

□ **Fig. 8.4** Flow reversal in subclavian steal syndrome. (From Hartmann et al. 2014)

Power Doppler is an amplitude-coded Doppler method. In contrast to FKDS, it does not detect flow velocities, but the quantity of moving particles. The power Doppler can therefore also detect much slower flows.

The use of ultrasound contrast agents can enhance the visualization of blood flow. The field of application of contrast-enhanced sonography is primarily the dignity assessment of space-occupying lesions, in particular of the liver, or during cardiac ultrasound for the detection of an open foramen ovale, i.e. a pathological connection between the right and left atrium.

8.2 Design and Operation of a Sonography Device

A modern ultrasound scanner (□ Fig. 8.5) consists of the following components:
- Control computer
- Monitor
- Keyboard
- Transducers
- Printer or connection to the PACS for image documentation

The most important elements are the various transducers, which are sensitive and should therefore not be dropped or handled with aggressive cleaning agents. Depending on the device class, the prices for such transducers can correspond to a small car. Therefore, in case of doubt, it is also worth taking a look at the operating instructions.

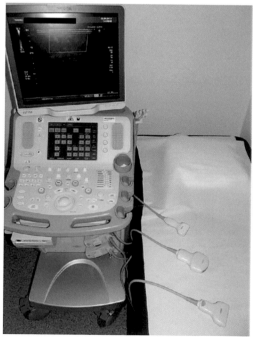

□ **Fig. 8.5** Ultrasound device. (From Hartmann et al. 2014)

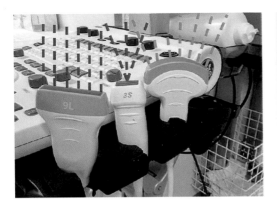

Fig. 8.6 Transducer variants. (From Hartmann et al. 2014)

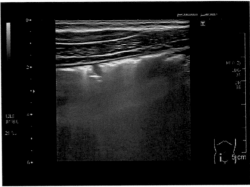

Fig. 8.7 Reverberation

8.2.1 Transducers

The transducers (■ Fig. 8.6) are subdivided according to the propagation of the sound waves into

- **Linear transducers**: The sound waves propagate in parallel, which has the advantage of geometrically accurate imaging.
- **Convex transducers** (curved array): The sound waves spread out like a fan. A larger area can be imaged.
- **Sector transducers**: The sound wave propagation is fan-shaped and radial. Typical application is cardiac ultrasound with a transcostal access path between the ribs.

Sonography Pocket Doppler

A special form is the so-called pocket Doppler, in which the ultrasound probe looks like a thick pen. It is mainly used in vascular diagnostics to measure occlusion pressure. Here, for example, the blood flow over the dorsalis pedis artery is derived from the foot and at the same time a blood pressure cuff is inflated on the lower leg. As soon as the sound of pulsating blood disappears, the blood pressure cuff is slowly released again. The blood pressure reading at which the sound reappears is the occlusion pressure. The value is lowered in the event of stenosis or occlusion of the leg arteries.

Good coupling between the transducer and the skin is important for ultrasound examinations. An insufficient coupling leads to artefacts, the so-called reverberations and an insufficient image quality. For this reason, ultrasound gel is applied to the transducer and also the patient's skin, which improves the connection between the transducer and the skin.

By the way: Reverberations (■ Fig. 8.7) also occur with intestinal air or with pathological air accumulations intraabdominal.

If the ultrasound is used in a sterile environment, e.g. during an operation, gel must also be filled into the sterile cover used for the transducer (in the case of pocket Doppler, sometimes also a sterile glove). In these cases, the sterile tube is coupled to the patient using saline solution or skin disinfectant spray, for example.

For **endosonography,** there are other special transducers that are designed for the corresponding application. These include endosonography of the pancreas, the heart, the prostate and the internal female genitals.

8.2.2 Where to Press...

Each sonography device is designed slightly differently depending on the manufacturer. Nevertheless, we would like to introduce you to the most important operating elements, which are actually always present:

- Before starting the examination: Enter the **patient's name**, usually on the top right of the keyboard, often marked with "ID". In radiology, the devices are usually linked to the RIS, so in these cases you select the patient's name from a work list.
- The selection keys for the **various organ programs are** usually located in the upper row of the keyboard and are marked "Preset".
- If multiple transducers are available, they can be changed by pressing a button, often labeled **"Probe"**.
- A button shows the **outline of a body**. This displays the so-called **body marker** in the image, which is used to document the section plane in the image.
- The often somewhat larger **"Freeze"** or **"FRZ"** button (usually on the bottom right of the device) is used to freeze the image for saving.
- In the lower part of the keyboard there is usually a knob labeled **"Gain"** or **"Depth"** which is used to adjust the overall gain.
- The **depth compensation** has a similar function, but it controls the gain for the different image depths separately. The depth control is a slider that is placed in several rows, usually in the upper right corner.
- Often the **focus** can be shifted with a **toggle switch.** This achieves an optimal image at a certain depth.
- The **trackball is** used to move markers or measuring points. You can find these via buttons, which are usually marked with crosses or dots.
- Devices with color duplex function have a (rotary) knob, usually marked with colored dots, or a **"Color"** or **"CDI"** button, which can be used to set the color duplex or to amplify it by rotation.

- The **power mode** is often marked with "PW" and is also designed as a rotary knob.
- New and especially larger devices often also have a **touchscreen** for operation.

8.3   Possibilities and Limits of Ultrasound Diagnostics

Ultrasound diagnostics is the primary diagnostic imaging method for abdominal complaints, vascular diseases and for diagnosing cardiac function. Exceptions are highly acute diseases, e.g. polytrauma patients. In these cases, a computer tomography can provide an accurate diagnosis in a very short time, while sonographic clarification requires sufficient time, depending on the experience of the examiner. For an ultrasound diagnosis of the entire abdomen without significant peculiarities, even the experienced examiner needs 10–15 min. In principle, one can examine almost everything with ultrasound, especially when it comes to children. Thus, fractures can also be detected with sonography (◘ Fig. 8.8).

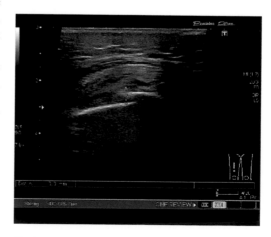

◘ **Fig. 8.8**   Fracture in the child on sonography

❯ However, the result is more dependent on what the examiner sees and documents as an image than with any other procedure.

Practice Questions
1. What is the piezoelectric effect?
2. Please briefly explain the meaning of A-, M- and B-mode.
3. What is the meaning of the red and blue coding in color Doppler or a lighter or darker display?
4. What is the pocket Doppler and where is it used?
5. In which clinical situations is sonography mainly used?

Solutions ▶ Chap. 27

8

Contrast Agent

Martina Kahl-Scholz

Contents

© Springer-Verlag GmbH Germany, part of Springer Nature 2023
M. Kahl-Scholz, C. Vockelmann (eds.), *Basic Knowledge Radiology*,
https://doi.org/10.1007/978-3-662-66351-6_9

Contrast media (CM) are important in X-ray diagnostics in order to make certain tissues, but also pathological processes, e.g. tumors, visible and to be able to assess them better. They are divided into different classes (positive/negative, water-soluble/insoluble, ionic/non-ionic, monomer/dimer) and used for different examinations. In addition to this aspect, however, the chapter also deals with the most common side effects that can be triggered by CM.

9.1   X-ray Contrast Medium

Contrast media (CM) are used in radiology to better highlight tissue structures and thus make them assessable. Since certain organs (e.g. the abdominal organs) have a similar density, they would be difficult to distinguish in imaging without CM.

In addition, the aim of using X-ray contrast media is to achieve better imaging while at the same time being well tolerated by the patient.

Good imaging is dependent on
— a high contrast,
— a detailed representation,
— a long enough contrast display depending on the examination.

Good tolerance of the contrast agent means that the CM
— does not negatively affect any physiological processes/functions,
— does not penetrate the blood-brain barrier or cell membranes,
— can be quickly and completely excreted again,
— does not result in any undesirable side effects.

The **enhancement**, i.e. the accumulation of CM in the organs or tissues, is dependent on the respective organ or tissue structure and in part allows conclusions to be drawn about a specific structure in the body (e.g. in the

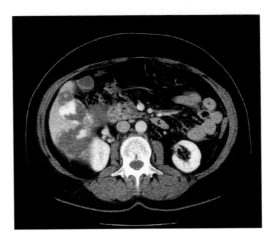

□ **Fig. 9.1**   Hemangioma of the liver with contrast enhancement

case of the hemangioma by the so-called rosette phenomenon, □ Fig. 9.1).

❯ Tasks of contrast agents
 — Contrast enhancement in fabrics that otherwise differ little or not at all in density
  – Improvement of the assessability of functional processes (e.g. blood flow, excretion, etc.)

9.1.1   Classification of X-ray CMs

Contrast media can reduce the absorption of X-rays (so-called negative X-ray contrast media) in order to differentiate from the surrounding tissue, or increase it (so-called positive X-ray contrast media).

X-ray contrast media are therefore divided into **two main groups:**
1. Substances with **lower density** than the environment to be imaged = **negative contrast media** (gases, water, methyl cellulose, sorbitol, mannitol)
2. Substances with a **higher density** than the environment to be depicted = **positive contrast media** (differentiation into water-soluble, water-insoluble and oil-containing)

Contrast Media Negative

Negative contrast agents (■ Fig. 9.2) used in X-ray diagnostics include gases, i.e. carbon dioxide (CO_2), nitrogen dioxide (NO_2), noble gas and simply: air (e.g. for imaging the stomach and intestines). But also water (or water-mannitol solutions), methyl cellulose, paraffin suspensions and sorbitol (sugar alcohol, sugar substitute) or mannitol belong to the negative CM.

❯ Sorbitol intolerance should be clarified before using Sorbitol!

Side effects of Mannitol may include:
— Disturbances of the fluid and electrolyte balance
— Hypotension
— Allergic reactions
— Cardiac arrhythmias
— Vertigo

Similar to methyl cellulose, carbon dioxide is used, for example, in gastrointestinal diagnostics, e.g. for double-contrast examination of the stomach and for imaging in virtual colonoscopy (■ Fig. 9.3a, b). It is generally better absorbed in the intestine than room air and thus, as studies have shown, better tolerated by the patient.

CO_2 can also be used in intra-arterial angiography of the kidneys, the lower extremity and in the diagnosis of dialysis shunts as a contrast medium with very few side effects. Patients with an intolerance to

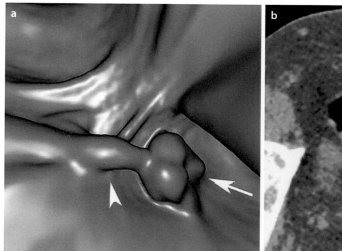

■ **Fig. 9.2** Negative contrast agents. (From Hartmann et. al 2014)

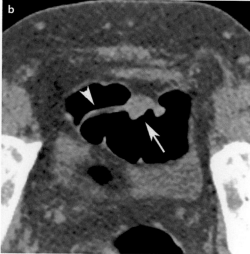

■ **Fig. 9.3** Virtual colonoscopy in 3D **a** and 2D **b** reconstruction. A pedunculated polyp was seen (arrow). (From Mang et al. 2008)

iodine-containing contrast media and patients with renal insufficiency are of particular benefit. However, CO_2 must not be used in angiography of the thorax, upper extremities or supraaortally, as this can trigger serious neurological complications, in the worst case accompanied by strokes.

Double Contrast—What Does that Mean?

Double contrast means performing fluoroscopy with a positive CM (usually barium, section water-insoluble contrast media) and a negative CM (e.g. cellulose, water, CO_2). The negative CM provides better distension (widening, expansion) of the bowel and distribution of the positive CM, resulting in better contrast of the bowel folds. This technique (the best known method is the enteroclysma, i.e. the contrast enema according to Sellink) is no longer frequently performed, as other imaging methods (especially magnetic resonance imaging) are now preferred for the desired visualization.

Room air is used (partly supplementary) for imaging the gastrointestinal tract (e.g. colon double contrast examination) and for arthrographies (contrast medium-supported radiological joint examination).

Contrast Media Positive Water-Soluble Contrast Media Containing Iodine (◻ Fig. 9.4)

Iodine-containing, water-soluble contrast media are used for the imaging of
- Vessels (angiography, phlebography),
- Renal pelvic calices and urinary tract (e.g. MCU, cystography),
- Gastrointestinal tract (oral),
- Bile ducts (e.g. ERCP, PTCD).

Especially in computed tomography (specifically: CT angiography, CT coronary angiography) they are often used. They are also used in myelography.

▪ **Why Iodine?**
Iodine-containing CMMs are used because iodine as a chemical element has a high contrast density as well as a relatively low toxicity and forms a strong bond with the other chemical structures of the contrast agent complex.

▪ **Triiodobenzoic Acid (Renal)**
These are contrast media that are largely excreted through the kidney by glomerular

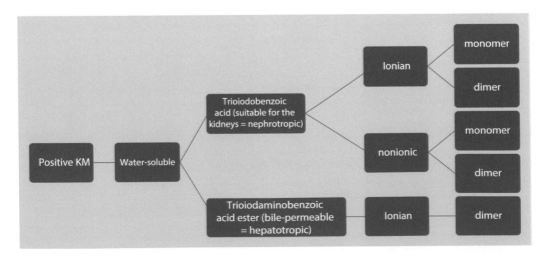

◻ **Fig. 9.4**   Positive, water-soluble contrast agents. (From Hartmann et. al 2014)

filtration (therefore renal = nephrotop). A small part is also excreted via the liver-biliary system and the intestine.

Triiodobenzenes produce a well-contrasted representation and are classified into ionic and non-ionic CMs, whereby ionic CMs are no longer used in practice because they have a higher side-effect potential (■ Table 9.1).

❯ If the limit is exceeded or if liver function is impaired, the CM is excreted via the kidneys (renal insufficiency)!

In the case of a pathological restriction of liver metabolism, special attention should be paid to a particularly gentle slow infusion.

■ **Table 9.1** Comparison of ionic and non-ionic contrast media[a]

	Ionian	**Nonionic**
Osmo-lality	High (hence also "high osmolality CM"; the osmolality largely determines the side effect spectrum)	Low (hence "low osmolar CM")
Load-ing	Electrically charged	Not electrically charged
Solubil-ity	Only sufficiently soluble as salt (meglumine salts > sodium salts)	Water soluble due to hydro-philic side chain groups
Protein Binding	Approx. 10	Approx. 1.5
Side effects[a]	Total: 12.66	Total: 3.13
	Heavy: 0.22	Heavy: 0.04
	Very heavy: 0.04	Very heavy: 0.004%

[a]Modified after Katayama study, Japan, 1986–1988

■ **Contrast Media Ionic**

Ionic contrast agents carry a salt group in their chemical structure, which gives them an ionic charge. They have a high osmolality (number of osmotically active particles in a solution) and a higher plasma protein binding. This also makes them less well tolerated, in contrast to non-ionic CM (■ Table 9.1). The BfArM (Federal Institute for Drugs and Medical Devices) declared in 2000 on the i.v. application of certain ionic contrast media:

❯ Ionic high-osmolar contrast media exhibit a higher chemotoxicity and a higher osmotoxicity than the low-osmolar non-ionic contrast media preferred today. Chemotoxicity and osmotoxicity cause a variety of undesirable effects on different organs and organ systems, respectively. The intravascular application of ionic contrast media is associated with a significantly higher risk of triggering a contrast medium side effect in all patient groups compared to the application of non-ionic monomeric contrast media.

Ionic CMMs are hardly ever used in X-ray diagnostics, especially as i.v. CMs (■ Fig. 9.5)—their use should be well weighed up with regard to possible risks and pre-existing underlying diseases (morbidities) of the patients.

■ **Contrast Media Non-Ionic**

As the name suggests, non-ionic CMs have no ionizing group, but a hydrophilic (i.e. water-loving) group that ensures solubility. Since they have a lower osmolality than ionic CM (but still twice as high as that of plasma), they are also referred to as low-osmolar CM (■ Table 9.1). Because of this property, they are also associated with side effects much less frequently.

Intravenous iodine-containing contrast media are eliminated renally. Only a small proportion is excreted hepatically via the bile. This proportion may cause you to see

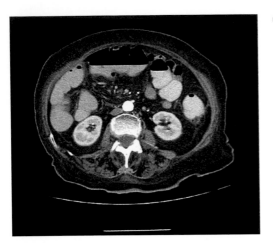

Fig. 9.5 More strongly contrasted colon (right) after rectal filling with diluted contrast medium, orally given CM (loops of small intestine) is more diluted due to fluid retention in the intestine in case of bridenileus in the right lower abdomen

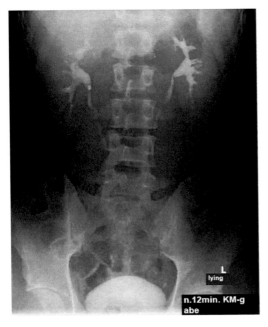

Fig. 9.6 Intravenous pyelogram (IVP) 12 min after CM administration

contrast of the gallbladder one or two days after intravenous contrast administration (☐ Fig. 9.6).

■ **Monomers and Dimers**

Both ionic and nonionic contrast agents have monomeric and dimeric variants. The difference lies in the chemical structure: the number of benzene rings in dimeric nonionic CMMs is two, in monomeric nonionic CMMs only one—due to the more complex structure, dimeric nonionic CMMs are also more viscous, i.e. more viscous, and must therefore be warmed up before application, as the viscosity decreases with increasing temperature.

❯ CM are before their use in a heat cabinet to reduce the viscosity. Due to the viscosity, the CM can only be injected with increased force. Therefore, errors can occur with CM pumps when they are cold. Therefore, care must be taken to ensure that a heat sleeve is used.

Dimeric ionic contrast agents, on the other hand, have two acid groups, for example.

Water-Insoluble Contrast Media

■ **Barium Sulphate**

Barium sulphate ($BaSO_4$) is used in the diagnosis of the gastrointestinal tract as an orally administered CM (☐ Fig. 9.7). However, today it is only used in very rare cases.

Since barium sulfate is hypotonic to blood plasma, it can cause dehydration in the intestine.

It must not be used in cases of suspected ileus (intestinal obstruction), perforation or suture insufficiency, dysphagia (risk of aspiration!) or other serious illnesses.

Contrast Media Containing Oil

■ **Oils**

Oils that have been iodized are used in lymphography. However, they are difficult to degrade in the body and produce by-products, and are therefore associated with many disadvantages and side effects. Since

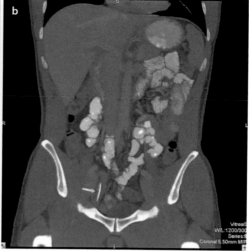

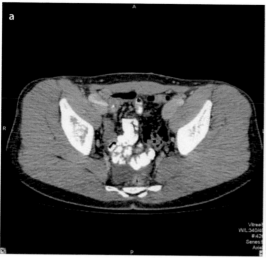

Fig. 9.7 Coronary reconstruction with elongated foreign body in the terminal ileum (arrow); in the selected bone window, the foreign body stands out better from the **diluted barium sulfate** in the other intestinal loops due to its higher density. (From Fabel 2006)

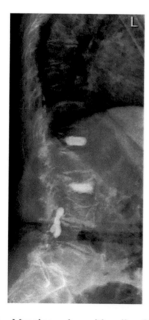

Fig. 9.8 Myeolography with oily CM. (From Hartmann et al. 2014)

water-soluble contrast media would diffuse too quickly in the lymphatic system, and thus no good imaging of the lymphatic vessels is possible, there is no alternative. In the past, iodinated oils were also used in myelog-raphy (**Fig. 9.8**), but due to the severe side effects, this is now only performed with water-soluble non-ionic contrast media.

> The amount of CM to be administered depends on the examination, the weight of the patient and the iodine concentration of the CM. In CT, concentrations of 400 mg iodine/ml are often administered. Thus, if a patient is injected with 100 mL of CM, he or she will receive 40 g of iodine! The daily requirement of an adult is 180–200 µg per day.

9.2 MR Contrast Medium

The functioning of MRI is related to relaxation times as already shown. The signal strength of the tissue is significantly influenced by the T1 and T2 relaxation time. The use of contrast agents increases the signal difference between the tissues and thus the image contrast.

To achieve this, substances with a large magnetic moment (many unpaired electrons on the outermost shell) are used, which accelerates the ambient relaxation (decay of magnetizations) in the environment. Gadolinum complexes are commonly used MR contrast agents in this context.

❯ The amount of relaxation time reduction is called relaxivity. It is a measure of the effectiveness of an MR contrast agent.

Since the effect is stronger in T1 measurements, CM are mainly used in such sequences.

MR-CM can be used as positive ("whiteners") and negative ("blackers") depending on the measurement in which they are used. Since they shorten the relaxation times in both T1 and T2 time, they can lead to different image effects.

— The shortening of the T1 time leads to a faster reconstruction of the longitudinal magnetization and thus to a signal amplification (white).
— The shortening of the T2 time leads to a faster decay of the transverse magnetization and thus to a signal drop (black) (❑ Fig. 9.9).

9.2.1 Gadolinum

Gadolinum is the "all-rounder" among the MR contrast agents, has seven unpaired electrons and greatly reduces the relaxation time (in T1-weighted sequences with signal enhancement). However, the free paramagnetic ions are very toxic. Therefore, the MR contrast agents used are derivatives of gadolinum (❑ Fig. 9.10). These include:

- **Non-Specific Gadolinum Complexes**
  — Are excreted via the kidney,
  — distribute only in the extracellular space (no penetration of the blood-brain barrier),
  — have an HWZ of 90 min,
  — are not metabolized or bound to proteins,
  — have a high stability.

❯ The accumulation of gadolinium in a tissue depends on the general condition of the patient (fever), the waiting time after

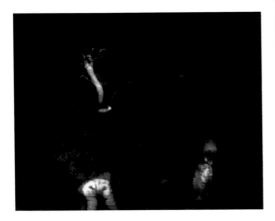

❑ **Fig. 9.9** Magnetic resonance cholangiopancreaticography (MRCP) with negative contrast of the stomach with 100 mL of pineapple juice immediately before the examination. Note the signal-elevated distal loops of small bowel and the pineapple juice signal-extinguished stomach. The contrast is due to the high manganese and iron content of the pineapple juice

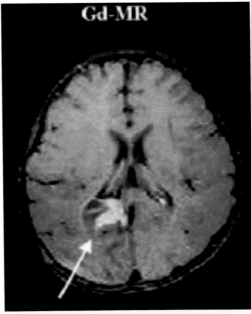

❑ **Fig. 9.10** Imaging of a neuroectodermal tumor in a 5-year-old girl using gadolinum MR. (From Choi 2005)

the injection and the dose ("much helps much"). The contrast medium may "behave differently" in a patient with fever than in patients without fever. This may play a role in the findings.

MR contrast media are generally well tolerated. Side effects occur in only 1–2% of examinations, mainly affecting the kidney. In a few cases, allergic reactions have also been reported.

❯ The edema signal in STIR or TIRM sequences is masked by CM administration, so these sequences must be performed before contrast administration.

9.3 Sonographic Contrast Agent

Contrast agents used in sonography perform their function by increasing the reflection of ultrasound waves—this results in a stronger signal response, which can be read on the ultrasound screen as higher contrast.

The imaging of contrast microbubbles in diagnostic sonography is based on excitation of the microbubbles in the sound field, whereby the microbubbles start to oscillate.

❯ The higher the intensity of the irradiated ultrasonic waves, the stronger the reaction of the microbubbles (up to bubble destruction).

9.4 Contraindications

The most important contraindications are given in the following overview:

- **Contraindications for CM Application**
Absolute Contraindications
- Severe kidney dysfunction not previously requiring dialysis
- Manifest hyperthyroidism

- Anaphylactoid reaction to the iodine-containing CM to be used
- Certain thyroid carcinomas

Relative Contraindications
- Heart failure
- Severe hepatic dysfunction
- Hematological diseases (Waldenström's disease)

❯ After CM injection, thyroid scintigraphy is not informative!

9.5 Side Effects

Adverse reactions caused by CM may be dose-dependent or dose-independent (◻ Table 9.2).

Among other things, vasodilatation may occur, which causes a drop in blood pressure (hypotension). Histamines released from mast cells are responsible for an immediate allergic reaction and in turn lead to vasodilation of the small peripheral vessels. This is the cause of a possible circulatory shock. Furthermore, an involvement of the coagulation system and the CNS is discussed.

◻ **Table 9.2** Undesirable direct side effects/reactions to CM

	Dose-dependent response	**Dose-independent response**
Response type	Direct (local) effect on organs and tissues as well as organ systems	Systemic response
Pathological process	Chemotoxic	Anaphylactic
Symptoms	Sensation of warmth/cold, reddening of the skin, headache	Nausea, vomiting, urticaria, itching

Many patients assume that a CM reaction is accompanied by an iodine allergy—but an iodine allergy would not be compatible with life, since we need iodine as an indispensable component of our human metabolism.

❯ An adverse CM reaction is not based on an iodine allergy, but is due to an intolerance of the CM complex.

Locally, especially with iodine-containing contrast media, pain, damage to the vessel walls, vasodilatation (→ drop in blood pressure) may occur.

❯ Low osmolar CMs are generally better tolerated than high osmolar ones, non-ionic ones better than ionic ones.

Special caution and **close scrutiny of** the **use of** CM is required in patients with:
— Status after severe CM reaction
— Allergies
— Bronchial asthma
— Kidney disease
— Thyroid disorders

9.6   Pregnancy and Breastfeeding

Pregnancy is a relative contraindication for an X-ray examination. The radiation exposure is relatively high for the unprotected child, depending on the planned examination. In certain emergency situations, it is nevertheless unavoidable to perform an examination on a pregnant patient. There are no precise data on the extent to which CM is transferred to the fetus and exposes it in this case.

About 1% CM is found in the mother's milk. That this amount has a harmful effect on the infant has not yet been proven. The current recommendation does not call for any special measures. Nevertheless, a 24-hour breastfeeding break can be considered.

Practice Questions
1. Which negative and positive contrast media are used in radiology?
2. What factors influence the accumulation of gadolinum in tissues?
3. What is meant by "double contrast"?
4. What are absolute, what are relative contraindications for the administration of CM?
5. What should be considered during breastfeeding with regard to the administration of CM?

Solutions ▶ Chap. 27

Radiotherapy

Guido Heilsberg

Contents

© Springer-Verlag GmbH Germany, part of Springer Nature 2023
M. Kahl-Scholz, C. Vockelmann (eds.), *Basic Knowledge Radiology*,
https://doi.org/10.1007/978-3-662-66351-6_10

Radiation therapy, also known as radioon-cology or radiotherapy, is a medical specialty that deals primarily with the treatment of malignant tumors with the aid of ionizing radiation.

10.1 Possibilities and Principles of Radiooncology

10.1.1 Brachytherapy

In contrast to "teletherapy", in which the radiation hits the body externally and over a distance, the distance between the radiation source and the body in brachytherapy is less than 10 cm.

Application: **Intracavitary** (the radionu-clide is placed in a body cavity for a short time), **interstitial** (the radionuclide is placed temporarily or permanently in the tissue), **contact therapy** (radionuclide is placed in a carrier that remains on superficial tissue for a certain time).

Indication for **intracavitary brachyther-apy** is the vaginal application for irradiation of the vaginal stump in corpus carcinoma. However, it is also possible for small superficial carcinomas in the esophagus or other cavities. The transport of the radioactive substance to the target site is carried out remotely from a lead-resorber in the so-called **afterloading** procedure. For this purpose, the lead resor is connected via one or more tubes to the applicator, which in turn is introduced into the body cavity. For the temporary method of **interstitial therapy,** more or less flexible plastic tubes several millimeters thick are pulled through the tissue intra-operatively with a sharp metal needle. Over a period of several days, these cavities are filled several times with radioactive material, usually 192 iridium by afterloading. The technique is used for ENT tumors, large soft tissue tumors or as an interstitial boost for anal carcinoma and breast-conserving breast carcinoma.

10.1.2 Particle Therapy

In particle therapy, the **Linear Energy Transfer (LET)**, i.e. the energy transfer of a particle, plays a decisive role. The radiation quality and the relative biological effectiveness (RBE) depend on the LET of the respective radiation. A distinction is made between loosely ionizing radiation (low LET) and densely ionizing radiation (high LET); a high LET therefore has a higher biological effectiveness than a low LET.

Protons belong to the low-LET radiation group and their relative biological effectiveness is 1.1, which is approximately the same as that of photons and gamma rays, whose RBE is 1. Heavy ions with a high LET have a RBE of 2–4. The dose is expressed in **Gray equivalent (GyE)** or in RBE (relative biologic effectiveness).

Acceleration takes place via the cyclotron and the synchrotron.

10.1.3 Therapy Concepts in Radiooncology

Radiation is also used to treat benign diseases, but it is mainly used to treat cancer with the aim of curation or palliation. It can be used as the sole form of treatment or in combination with chemotherapy, antibody therapy or hormones ("**primary**" or "**definitive**") and in combination with surgery (**pre- or post- or intra-operative radiotherapy**).

■ Radiotherapy Alone
Radiotherapy alone is more often used in palliative situations. Only in smaller and radiosensitive tumors is radiotherapy a curative therapy.

Radiotherapy in Series   Radiotherapy can be given either in one series without any change in the irradiated volume or in several series.

The number of series and their target structures depend on the disease, the pre-treatment and also the individual situation.

Boost Irradiation The **boost** is applied to a macroscopic tumor or to an area with an increased risk of recurrence.

It is possible to perform the boost **sequentially**, i.e. following the irradiation series, or during the irradiation series either **concomitantly** or as a **simultaneously integrated boost (SIB)**.

Radiotherapy can also be combined with other treatments (multimodal):
— Chemotherapy: e.g. for squamous cell carcinoma
— Antibodies: e.g. for ENT tumor for which chemotherapy is contraindicated
— Hormones: e.g. for prostate carcinoma
— Surgery; preoperative ("neoadjuvant") with the aim of tumor reduction; postoperative or adjuvant; intraoperative.

10.1.4 Fractionation

The standard regimens are 5 × 2 Gy/week and 5 × 1.8 Gy/week (normofractionation).

▪ Hypofractionation
This is the reduction of fractions with a simultaneous increase in individual doses. Advantages: shorter treatment time.

▪ Hyperfractionation
This is the increase of fractions in a unit of time. It is used if, for example, a radiation session is cancelled. The single dose to be made up is often applied before the weekend, i.e. on Friday as the second session of scheduled radiotherapy. The idea is that the normal tissue will have recovered from the sublethal (almost fatal) radiation damage by Monday.

Dose-scaled, accelerated hyperfractionation is used for tumors with a high cell division rate.

▪ Palliation
For palliative treatment, a therapy regimen must be individually tailored to the patient's situation and the therapy goal.

10.2 Irradiation Planning

As soon as all important information about the cancer such as TNM stage, histology, receptor status, etc. is available, the patient is presented to the interdisciplinary tumor board and the therapy concept is determined. The radiation oncologist discusses the recommended procedure, the therapy and its side effects with the patient. In a physical examination, the doctor himself gets an idea of the extent of the tumor and, during the discussion, assesses whether the radiotherapy can be carried out on an outpatient basis, which positioning on the treatment table is possible or advisable and whether certain preparations are necessary, e.g. implantation of markers in the target organ or dental rehabilitation in the case of treatment in the mouth and throat area. In addition, it is clarified to what extent the patient is ready for the therapy.

The irradiation ordinance includes the following aspects:
— Intention (curative, palliative)
— Definition of the target volume
— Definition of organs at risk (OAR)
— Radiation type: photons or electrons
— Beam energy: Example six or 15 MV photons, fouror 18 MeV electrons
— Irradiation technique: standing field/ multi-field irradiation, IMRT, stereotherapy, brachytherapy etc.
— Single and total dose
— Fractionation
— Positioning and positioning aids for the patient
— Name, first name, date of birth and diagnosis of the patient
— Irradiating institution, name and signature of attending specialist, date

Storage is an important preliminary measure so that the irradiation can always be applied in a reproducible manner.
- It must be as comfortable as possible.
- The planned irradiation technique must also be taken into account.
- It must be possible to reproduce it exactly.

10.2.1 Further Processing

MRI and/or PET-CT slices are superimposed on the planning CT images (= fusion, matching) and thus support the determination of the contours.

The target volume results from:
- **Tumor volume:** Tumor, possibly with lymph node metastases or distant metastases.
- **Clinical tumor volume (CTV):** macroscopic tumor + the region with scattered tumor cells.
- **Planning Target Volume (PTV):** CTV.

From many years of experience, the dose values for the individual organs are known, the exceeding of which threatens a functional impairment. In so-called **dose volume histograms,** the organ volumes that receive a certain dose are represented graphically.

▶ In an emergency, extensive radiation planning is not necessary.

10.3 Design and Function of Radiooncological Irradiation Equipment

10.3.1 Linear Accelerator

The classic treatment device is the linear accelerator. It consists of an X-ray machine with an accelerating tube as an additional device that provides the rays with higher energy. It is called **ultra-hard X-rays**. It makes it possible to reach deeper tumors—in contrast to conventional X-ray therapy, which has a superficial effect (▶ Chap. 2). The accelerator arm (gantry) rotates in one plane around the treatment table. Its position is specified as the gantry angle.

The section in which the electrons are generated is called the **electron gun.** The acceleration of the electrons is achieved by a 1–2.5 m long **accelerator tube,** which the electrons have to pass through. Here an alternating voltage with high frequency prevails. The tube ends in the beam head. There, the electron beam is deflected by means of magnets in a circular motion through 270°. As a result, the previously different energy levels of the individual electrons are brought into line with each other, and the beam becomes more homogeneous.

When the accelerated electrons collide with the **target,** high-energy photons are produced and the target is strongly heated during this process. A water pipe and a copper block are integrated in the machine for cooling. The resulting photons pass through the **primary collimator,** which is used to absorb photons that are not moving in the direction of the useful beam. In this case, the primary collimator is a lead funnel, which absorbs the rays on the walls that are not directed at the patient and therefore have no therapeutic effect. In the further course of the beam there is a balancing filter made of metal (**photon balancing body**), which homogenizes the photon radiation. A further element is the electron catcher (beamstopper or **beamhardener**). It intercepts the soft (low-energy) radiation components ("hardening").

During treatment with electrons, the radiation emerges directly (without a brake target). Instead of hitting the compensating body, the electrons hit a micrometer-thick metal foil (**scattering foil**), which expands the beam to an enlarged diameter.

The two transmission ionization chambers measure the absorbed dose in monitor units (**ME**, "MU").

The field to be irradiated is projected onto the patient's surface by means of a mirror in the irradiator head using a light source. The position of the light source has the same distance to the skin or surface as the brake target. It indicates the **focus-to-skin distance (FHA)**.

Four tungsten or lead blocks (apertures) delimit the four field edges (**collimators**), their four apertures are movable, and the field lengths and field widths (*X*1, *X*2, *Y*1, *Y*2) are defined above them.

Before the first session and at certain intervals during the treatment, it is checked and documented whether or not radiation is actually administered exactly as specified in the calculated plan. If this verification recording takes place directly before the radiation and any necessary corrections are made immediately, this is known as **IGRT** (image-guided radiotherapy). Computer programs help to measure (**match**) the distance from given structures (e.g. bone contour, trachea, teeth) in advance. An additional metal clip (**marker**) in the tissue allows the target volume to be defined more clearly. Newer linear accelerators have a cone beam CT.

Respiratory Gated Radiotherapy

With respiratory control, only a narrow cranial and caudal safety margin is required for irradiation of lung tumors, since the respiratory tumor movement does not have to be taken into account. Similarly, the method spares the heart in left-sided breast cancer. It is only irradiated in inspiration.

■ Gating or Breath Hold Technique

The above-mentioned technique is called gating (gate: the gate that opens and closes). A simpler method is breath-hold radiation, which is preferably used for left-sided breast cancer to protect the heart.

10.3.2 Dose Distribution in Tissue

Deep Dose Profile

Electrons and photons both belong to particle radiation (fast-moving atoms, ions or elementary particles with rest mass), but they have different weights and behave differently as to when and to what extent they release their energy. Diagrams with so-called **depth dose curves** (◘ Fig. 10.1) characterize the dose progression in tissue.

Decisive for the depth dose curve are: the **beam modality** (high energy photons reach deeper volumes), the **beam energy** (higher energies penetrate deeper), the **field size**, the **focus-skin distance** and the **material** irradiated.

■ Photons and Electrons

When it hits the skin or surface, the **photon beam** emits about 70–80% of its dose. It penetrates further into the tissue on its path and regains energy through the secondary electrons.

❯ The higher the energy of the photon beam, the less dose the skin receives and the deeper the dose maximum lies in the tissue.

Electrons also develop their dose maximum under the skin, but they subsequently have a different behavior than photons, because after penetrating the skin they maintain the direction of their movement and penetrate deep into the tissue (one reaches deeper PTV with them).

10.3.3 Irradiation Techniques

■ Isocentric and Isocentric Irradiation at the Linear Accelerator

The isocenter is the point located on the central beam at a distance of 100 cm from the target. It is where the axes of the gantry, collimator and table meet. The patient is posi-

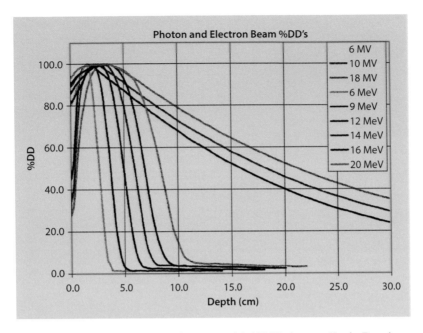

◘ Fig. 10.1 Depth dose profile for 6–18 MeV electrons and 6–18 MV photons. *Y*-axis: Dose in percent, *x*-axis: Tissue depth. (From Purdy et al. 2012)

tioned in the planning CT in such a way that the isocenter is in the middle of the target volume. If this is sometimes not successful, the planning computer calculates how far and in which directions the patient must be moved with the table during the initial setting (off-set) in order to meet the specification.

■ **Coplanar Irradiation**

Normally, the central beams of all fields are placed in a plane that is typically transverse to the patient's axis (coplanar irradiation). Stereotaxy, on the other hand, is a non-coplanar procedure (◘ Fig. 10.2), which is why the table must be partially realigned during a session.

■ **Isodoses**

Isodoses are points with the same dose (connected by lines, they are called isodose curves).

■ **Simple Techniques**

Standing Field

The simplest technique is the standing field, where the field size, the hearth depth and the energy are fixed.

Counterfields

A standing field is not suitable for target volumes located deeper in the body. Counterfields (opposing single fields) halve the radiation exposure of healthy tissue.

Multi-Field Technique—Conformal Irradiation

A common technique is the multi-field method. This brings the isodoses closer to the PTV, so that the healthy tissue can be better protected.

■ **IMRT**

IMRT (intensity-modulated radiotherapy) is another method of conformal irradiation. Here, either the **sliding window technique** (irradiation while the MLC are moving) or the **step-and-shoot technique** (with irradiation interruption) are used. This allows the dose to be varied from point to point.

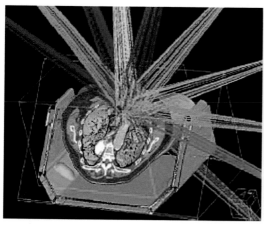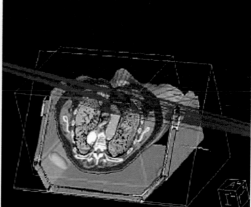

□ Fig. 10.2 Non-coplanar stereotaxy using ten fields compared to coplanar VMAT

■ **VMAT**

Volumetric Modulated Arc Therapy (VMAT) is borrowed from the IMRT technique: the number of small dose-modulated fields irradiated in gantry positions increases, the gantry moves in a circle or semicircle, and the irradiation time is shortened.

of **radiosurgery** when the dose (12–25 Gy) is applied all at once. **High targeting accuracy** is extremely important, especially for brain radiation (e.g., for acoustic neuroma, meningioma). The **Cyberknife** is used to compensate for the movements of the patient or the target volume.

10.3.4 **Irradiation Variants**

■ Tomotherapy

The tomotherapy device is a combination of linear accelerator and computer tomogram. The advantages are that several volumes can be irradiated in one procedure and that long volumes can be achieved. In addition, the adjacent tissue is optimally spared in the case of shell-shaped target volumes.

■ Stereotactic Radiotherapy

Stereotaxy is the term used to describe radiotherapy that is applied in a spatially targeted and highly precise manner. The treatment is carried out via numerous, very small radiation fields of the linear accelerator in noncoplanar arcs. In the actual **stereotaxy** (Stereotactic Radiotherapy, SRT), treatment is administered 3–5 times, each time with high individual doses. One speaks

10.3.5 **X-ray Therapy Equipment**

For radiotherapy in the kV range, a conventional X-ray apparatus is used, but with higher voltage than in diagnostics (30–200 kV).

In many forms of heel pain (achillodynia, fasciitis plantaris, heel spur) and other inflammatory degenerative diseases, such as tennis elbow (epicondylitis humeroradialis), there is an inflammation of the soft tissues (connective tissue, ligaments, tendons) with the classic features of pain, redness and swelling in addition to the (age-related) signs of wear and tear. In these cases, X-ray therapy with small individual doses between 0.5 and 1 Gy and total doses of about 6 Gy, also called stimulation radiation, is effective.

Basaliomas and spinaliomas whose surgical removal would produce cosmetically unattractive results (e.g. on the nose, lip) or would be associated with functional limitations (e.g. on the eye) can be successfully treated with conventional therapy.

Practice Questions

1. What is IMRT and VMAT?
2. What happens during stereotaxy?
3. What are the different forms of brachytherapy?
4. What is "boost therapy"?
5. Explain the terms tumor volume, clinical target volume, and planning target volume.

Solutions ▶ Chap. 27

Nuclear Medicine

Ursula Blum

Contents

© Springer-Verlag GmbH Germany, part of Springer Nature 2023
M. Kahl-Scholz, C. Vockelmann (eds.), *Basic Knowledge Radiology*,
https://doi.org/10.1007/978-3-662-66351-6_11

Nuclear medicine is like X-ray—only the other way round. In nuclear medicine, it is the patient who radiates and not the device—or, to put it more technically, the emission rays of the applied radioactive substances are used for imaging. Here, molecular metabolic processes can often be made visible.

Beta and alpha emitters are used in nuclear medicine therapy. Many therapies are very specific.

11.1 Imaging and Therapeutic Options

11.1.1 Scintillation Counter: Scanner, Gamma Camera, Gamma Probe

The principle of image generation or radioactivity detection is the same for the gamma scanners, the gamma camera and the gamma probe. With the scanner systems no longer in use today, the organ to be examined was scanned line by line, and the image was often created using a directly connected plotter. The **gamma camera** replaced the scanner. Almost all examinations are performed with the gamma camera. They are available as special shield-nozzle cameras, as single-head, two-head and three-head systems. Single images of regions (e.g. thyroid, kidney, lung) can be produced, as well as whole-body images (bone scintigraphy, inflammation scintigraphy) and 3-dimensional images using SPECT (single photon electron computed tomography, e.g. in heart or brain diagnostics).

Gamma probes are very small measuring devices that are used especially in the operating room for the detection of sentinel lymph nodes. Other possible applications are the intraoperative detection of parathyroid glands. Here, the radiation is converted into an acoustic signal.

The radioactive radiation hits a scintillation crystal (usually a thallium-enhanced sodium iodide crystal). This produces a flash of light in the crystal which strikes a photocathode. An electron is released. This is subsequently amplified by a secondary electron multiplier (SEV, or photomultiplier, PM). The voltage increases from dynode to dynode, so that a large number of electrons (amplification approx. 105–109) strike the anode. Amplification and discrimination take place, and images are generated by means of a connected EDP. To avoid stray radiation as far as possible, a collimator is usually placed in front of the crystal.

11.1.2 Semiconductor Cameras

Semiconductor cameras are currently only available as special cameras (e.g. heart, chest). The radiation is collected directly by the semiconductor (e.g. cadmium-zinc-telluride) and converted into electrical charge. The detectors are significantly smaller than those of a "normal" gamma camera, and examination times can be significantly reduced due to the good energy resolution.

11.1.3 PET

When a positron emitter decays, a positively charged antiparticle (=positron) is formed. This then meets an electron in the body. This produces the so-called annihilation radiation; a pair of γ-quanta with an energy of 511 keV is always formed. The γ-quanta are emitted at an angle of 180° to each other. Only when both γ-quanta hit the detection crystal, they are detected as true radiation by the device and further processed as true signal. This nearly simultaneous impingement of the radiation is called **coincidence**. Due to the various other factors, such as the temporal impingement of the radiation and the local registration of the radiation,

3-dimensional cross-sectional images are generated. A spatial assignment of the accumulation is sometimes difficult, since not all anatomical structures can be clearly distinguished from each other on the basis of their metabolism.

A PET device usually consists of many small detection crystals (bismuth germanate, BGO or lutetium oxyorthosilicate, LSO) arranged in a ring and in series. Several crystals are amplified via an SEV.

The examination is performed in 2D or 3D technique with attenuation correction. 2D technique means that only coincidences within one collimator row are detected; in the 3D technique, these are detected across all collimator rows. This means that the 3D technique is significantly more sensitive than the 2D technique, whereas the 2D technique provides very homogeneous images.

An attenuation correction is always necessary. Different tissues cause different attenuation of the passing radiation. In the case of pure PET systems, the attenuation correction is carried out by means of a so-called transmission measurement. An external radiation source (68 Gy rod source) is used and an exposure is started. The tomogram created in this way is then overlaid with the emission data from the PET examination. This procedure must be carried out for each bed position and thus considerably extends the time the patient is in the device. In the hybrid devices, the attenuation correction is performed by the CT or MRI data set.

11.1.4 Hybrid Systems

SPECT-CT, PET-CT, PET-MRI: Here, the nuclear medicine systems are combined with the respective radiological device. The combination allows a reliable anatomical assignment of the enrichments. Pure PET systems have become rare. The hybrid devices can always provide attenuation correction of the nuclear medicine data through the radiolog-

ical data set. In this case, all examinations can be performed. SPECT-CT is used in conventional nuclear medical diagnostics (e.g. heart, brain, bones), PET-CT or PET-MRI mainly for oncological questions.

11.1.5 Therapy Options

Almost all nuclear medicine therapies are performed on an inpatient basis for reasons of radiation protection. Exceptions to this are radiosynoviorthesis (RSO, section Radiosynoviorthesis) and palliative pain therapy for bone metastases.

Radioiodine Therapy

Usually, radioactive iodine (^{131}I-NaI) is taken in capsule form. Less frequently, it can be administered in liquid form or injected intravenously. The radioactive iodine is distributed according to the physiological iodine metabolism. It is absorbed through the gastrointestinal tract into the blood, then into the thyroid gland. Here it is absorbed into the active thyroid tissue. Depending on the disease, different doses are reached in the target tissue.

In the case of malignant diseases of the thyroid gland, radioiodine therapy can be used to eliminate the remaining tissue or to treat metastases.

The patient will be hospitalized for at least 48 h. The time of discharge depends on the legally prescribed residual activity in the body. If necessary, the patient should still comply with some radiation protection measures after discharge (e.g. restricted contact with radiation-sensitive persons, external radioactivity measurements), these will be communicated to the patient on discharge.

Radiosynoviorthesis (RSO)

RSO is a targeted treatment of chronic inflammation of the synovium (synovitis). Different substances are available for different joints. There is proven success in rheumatic joint diseases and psoriatic arthritis, among others. RSO is also used for activated arthrosis or for irritation after implantation of artificial joints. The following are used:

- ^{90}Yttrium: Knee joint
- ^{186}Rhenium: Shoulder, elbow, hip, hand and ankle joints
- ^{169}Erbium: Finger and toe joints, metacarpophalangeal and metatarsophalangeal joints

❯ The application is strictly intra-articular under X-ray control (exception: knee joint). Incorrect injection leads to tissue necrosis of the affected area.

The treated joint should be immobilized for 48 h.

Palliative Pain Therapy for Bone Metastases

Skeletal metastases that accumulate in skeletal scintigraphy can be treated with various radioactive substances. The indication is usually made interdisciplinary with all treating physicians and after exhaustion of conservative pain therapy.

Possible substances for therapy are the emitters ^{89}strontium, ^{153}samarium, ^{186}rhenium, ^{188}rhenium and ^{32}phosphorus. All substances are applied intravenously. After administration, the patient should be monitored for 2–3 h. A scintigraphy can be performed after the administration of samarium or rhenium.

The α-emitter ^{223}Ra-radadium dichloride was newly approved (November 2013) for the treatment of bone metastases in prostate cancer. This preparation is also administered intravenously.

Radioimmunotherapy

In radioimmunotherapy, antibodies (here CD20 surface antigen) are radioactively labelled. The ^{90}yttrium-labelled ibritumomab tiuxetan (Zevalin®) is approved for the treatment of B-cell lymphomas.

^{131}I-MIBG (Meta-Iodo-Benzyl-Guanidine) Therapy

Special tumors can accumulate MIBG. These tumors are then amenable to MIBG therapy. These include, for example, malignant pheochromocytoma, malignant paraganglioma, carcinoids, medullary thyroid carcinoma and neuroblastoma.

Several medications can interfere with MIBG uptake and should be suspended according to half-life. Both pheochromocytoma and paraganglioma can release catecholamines, so these patients may require medication with α- and β-blockers.

❯ The therapy is carried out via a slow intravenous infusion, during which blood pressure and heart rate should be monitored.

Peptide Therapy

Neuroendocrine tumors show an increase in somatostatin receptors. These receptors can be used to detect neuroendocrine tumors by scintigraphy. Tumors that show a corresponding accumulation are amenable to peptide therapy. Here, ^{90}Yttrium-DOTATOC or ^{177}Lu-DOTATOC are used.

Selective Internal Radiotherapy (SIRT)

SIRT can be used to treat inoperable primary liver tumors or inoperable metastases of other tumors. In this procedure, small glass or synthetic resin particles—marked with ^{90}Y—are injected intra-arterially into the liver. The microspheres have a diameter of 20–30 μm (glass microspheres) or 20–60 μm (resin microspheres).

Prior to treatment, selective liver angiography occludes all vessels leading to extrahepatic tissues (e.g. stomach, intestine) and a distribution scintigram with ^{99m}Tc-MAA is performed. This scintigraphy is used to exclude extrahepatic accumulations and to calculate the liver-lung shunt.

■ Liver-Lung Shunt

This refers to vascular connections between the lungs and liver, through which the microspheres also reach the lung tissue and lead to tissue damage (radiation pneumonitis). A shunt >20% represents a contraindication to therapy, from a shunt volume of 10% the dose is adjusted.

11.2 Radiation Protection

In a nuclear medicine practice or department, different areas are defined. There is the monitoring area (effective dose >1 mSv/year) and the control area (effective dose >6 mSv/year). There are no restricted areas (local dose rate >3 mSv/h). The controlled area may only be entered with restrictions. The controlled area usually contains the hot laboratory, the camera rooms, the decay room and a waiting area (incl. WC) for patients to whom the radioactive substance has already been applied. The control area is entered and exited via a sluice with measuring devices for the detection of radioactivity.

❯ For work in the controlled area, the "5 A's of radiation protection" apply in principle:
  — Distance: Always keep as much distance as possible from the radiation source.
  — Shielding: If possible, radioactive materials should be shielded (tungsten, lead glass, Plexiglas).
  — Length of stay: Any unnecessary stay should be avoided and any stay should be as short as possible.
  — Activity: As little as possible, as much as necessary (ALARA principle: As Low As Reasonably Achievable).
  — Avoid ingestion: Avoid incorporation of radioactive material.

11.2.1 Hot Laboratory

In the hot laboratory, the radioactive substances are stored, prepared and portioned. Usually, the highest radioactivity is to be expected here.

Generator

In each hot lab there are at least two ^{99}molybdenum generators with different activity. Each generator has its own shielding. ^{99}Mo decays with a HWZ of 65.9 h to ^{99m}technetium. This is dissolved out of the generator using sterile saline solution.

Lead Castle (Screening Wall)

The structure of a lead castle is regulated in DIN 25407. It is the direct preparation area of the radiopharmaceuticals.

A lead castle consists of individual lead bricks that can be variably combined. In part, the building blocks are encased in stainless steel to prevent liquids from seeping into the joints. In addition, a component with a lead glass pane is placed on top to protect the sensitive eye lenses from the emitted radiation. Additional spacers and shielding are used within the lead castle.

Spacers

According to the square law of distance, the dose per area decreases with the distance to the radiation source due to the divergence of the radiation. Thus, you only get a quarter of the dose if you double the distance to the radiation source. With a spacer (a kind of pliers for medicine vials), you can quickly increase the distance from 0 cm (vial in your hand) many times over.

Syringe Shields

Each drawn up syringe is clamped into a shield. For gamma emitters (^{99m}Tc etc.) these are usually made of tungsten with a lead glass insert.

For beta emitters (e.g. radiosynoviorthesis, palliative pain therapy), shields made of Plexiglas are used. Depending on the radionuclide used, the syringe in combination with nitrile gloves may also provide adequate protection (^{169}Er).

Transport Equipment

The radiopharmaceutical is usually applied in the application room. In order to keep transport distances as short as possible, the application rooms are often set up directly next to the hot lab and connected to each other by an airlock. The airlock is also shielded.

For all other routes within the department, suitable lead transport containers must be used. These come in different sizes depending on whether you need to transport a single syringe or a larger container (e.g. for waste disposal).

Waste Containers

Strict waste separation takes place in a hot lab. A distinction is made between contaminated waste (including questionable contamination) and safely non-contaminated waste.

The contaminated waste is collected and stored in special lead-lined containers.

Decay Space

In the decay room, all radioactive waste is stored until it can be disposed of in accordance with the clearance limit.

11.2.2 Investigation Area

In the examination rooms, the patient is the largest source of radiation. To protect the staff, there are mobile radiation protection walls that can be moved around the room like a screen. Protective gloves must be worn when handling blood samples (e.g. for renal scintigraphies).

If a pulmonary ventilation scintigraphy is performed, there is an increased risk due to the radioactive aerosols used. For this reason, as few staff as possible should be present in the room. Care should be taken that, if possible, the aerosols or the patient's breathing air (**"para-breathing"**) does not escape.

> In a nuclear medicine department it is mandatory that all radiopharmaceuticals are labelled and shielded (lead castle, transport containers, etc.). On each syringe it must be indicated at least which nuclide it contains, when which activity was raised.

11.2.3 Leaving the Department

Each time they leave the controlled area, employees must check that they are free of radioactive contamination. A **contamination monitor** at the entrance or exit of the controlled area is used for this purpose. This has various detectors to check not only the hands, but also shoes and clothing.

The results of the measurement must be documented and must be within specified tolerance limits. In the event of contamination, this must be detected, documented and, if possible, removed. If this is not completely possible, further measures may have to be taken.

> If the necessary radiation protection measures are observed and implemented, the occupational radiation exposure per year is about 1–3 mSv.

11.3 Detection of Radioactivity

11.3.1 Scintillation Detectors

A medium with a high atomic number Na/OZ 53 is used in the so-called scintillation detector. Scintillation detectors emit the excitation energy produced by the passage of photons or electrons in the form of light. Such a scintillation detector is the core of the gamma camera, which records the distribution of an applied activity in the patient.

Probe Measuring Station

A simple scintillation detector used in in vivo diagnostics is the so-called probe measuring station. The NaJ crystal contained here is only equipped with a single, relatively large collimator. This has the task of protecting the detector from ambient radiation. A probe measuring station is used to determine the percentage activity uptake of an applied radiopharmaceutical at different times. The up-take measurement is of particular importance, for example, for the planning of a radioiodine therapy.

Gamma Probe

The scintillation detector of the gamma probe is particularly small at 10–20 mm, which is surrounded by a lead collimator. The gamma probe is used, for example, for the preoperative or intraoperative detection of the sentinel lymph node. This can be detected with the aid of an acoustic signal or a visual display.

Borehole Logging Station

Another scintillation detector is located in a so-called borehole measuring station, which is used for the detection of low activities. Thus, allergens or hormone levels can be determined via antigen or antibody reactions (IRMA/RIA) in patient serum or urine by measuring radioactive compound components. Since very small amounts of activity are involved, the detector encloses the sample in a U-shape. The sample volume is chosen in such a way that it can be completely sunk into the central bore. This allows all outgoing quanta to reach the detector. It is encased in lead to protect it from ambient radiation. Only tracers with

low energy can be measured, because at high energy pulses of the neighboring sample flow into the measurement.

Liquid Scintillators

Low-energy beta particles cannot be measured by solid-state scintillators due to their short range. Detection is possible with the aid of liquid organic scintillators (e.g. ^{3}H, ^{14}C, ^{90}Sr). The dissolved scintillator converts the resulting electrons into light. They are measured by two PMPs.

Gas Ionization Detectors

A gas in a chamber (air, noble gases such as He, Ar, Kr, Xe) is used as a medium with a low atomic number. When a gamma ray hits the gas ionization chamber, the gas is ionized by releasing the electrons. A positively charged gas molecule remains on one side and a free electron on the other side. When high voltage is applied, these charge carriers are transported to the negatively charged cathode or the positively charged anode. A current flows which can be measured. The working range of the ionization chamber is defined depending on the high voltage applied. In the so-called recombination range, the charge carriers escape measurement because negative and positive particles recombine. In the saturation range, which follows the recombination range in terms of voltage, the applied high voltage is so high that no more recombinations can take place; every charge carrier is registered. Ionization chambers operate in this range. If the high voltage is increased further, the primary generated electrons are accelerated so strongly that they ionize further atoms. An electron avalanche is created which is proportional to the primary event (working range of the proportionality counter tubes). If the high voltage is increased further into the so-called trigger range, a single primary electron can lead to the ionization of the entire chamber volume, which is important in the detection of minute amounts of activity in radiation protection.

Activimeter

A cylindrical ionization chamber is the basic component of the so-called active meter. The activity to be applied is measured with the aid of the active meter. The activity is inserted into the chamber. Thus, the same measurement geometry is always given. The chamber should be protected from contamination. The surrounding lead shielding protects the measuring chamber from incident background radiation, which would lead to a falsification of the measurement. Activitmeters can measure different nuclides. The response is very wide in a measuring range up to 200 GBq and in an energy range from 35 KeV to 3 MeV. Daily checks of the activimeter including the zero effect and the sensitivity are carried out. In addition, semi-annual linearity checks are required. Measuring systems in radiation protection.

According to the recommendation, every employee working in the monitoring or controlled area is obliged to determine the personal dose equivalent at a representative point of the body surface.

Personal Dosimeter

The monitoring of radiation exposure can be performed, for example, by a film dosimeter when dealing with photon, electron or neutron radiation. Such a dosimeter consists of a two-part sliding shadow cassette containing absorbers of different atomic numbers (e.g. aluminum, copper, lead). The absorbers on the front and back are differently shaped and offset so that, when evaluating the blackening of the films inside, it is possible to determine with varying sensitivity from which direction the radiation exposure occurred. Due to the different density of the absorbers, when radiation passes through, its energy can be determined. The

evaluation of the personal dosimeter worn on the front of the torso is carried out once a month by the responsible central personal dosimetry office.

Ring Dosimeter

Another dosimeter used in routine nuclear medicine is the ring dosimeter, which determines the radiation exposure of the hand and is used in the hot laboratory. The ring contains a thermo-luminescence detector, a substance (e.g. calcium fluoride contaminated with manganese) which stores the absorbed radiation energy. The crystal is heated once a month by an appropriate evaluation point. This causes the stored energy to be emitted in the form of visible light. The ring is used in addition to the film dosimeter.

Electronic Dosimeters

Electronic dosimeters are immediately readable. They display the measured values digitally and give an acoustic warning when the set dose or dose rate is exceeded. They contain special photodiodes which convert the energy of the incident photons into electric current. The measured values should be documented every working day.

Whole Body Counter

Whole-body counters are used for the detection of incorporated radiation, with the aid of which the nuclide present in the body can be identified and the amount of activity present can be determined. Whole-body counters contain scintillation and also semiconductor detectors to increase the detection sensitivity. Semiconductors are crystalline substances, e.g. germanium or silicon contaminated with lithium, which insulate at low temperatures but become conductors when energy is applied. They are characterized by good energy resolution, but are less sensitive than scintillation detectors. Because of the extremely high sensitivity of a whole-body counter, shielding against ambient radiation is extremely costly.

Contamination Measuring Equipment

The contamination measuring instruments used in routine nuclear medicine are equipped with ionization detectors operating in the proportionality or trigger range. If input events are high and easily detectable, they can be recorded with the proportionality counter tube proportional to the input event (application in contamination meters and portable site dosimeters). Smaller activity contaminations are detected with the Geiger-Müller counting tubes operating in the trigger range (application in portable local and electronic personal dosimeters). Increasingly, contamination meters are also equipped with scintillation detectors. They can be used to detect contamination with alpha, beta and gamma radiation.

11.4 Image Formation Systems

11.4.1 Gamma Camera

The gamma camera is a detector system that reproduces the activity distribution in the patient as a two-dimensional image (scintigram). Depending on the tracer used, the recorded scintigram provides information about blood flow, storage, metabolism and receptor density of an organ system. Single images with constant activity distribution (static images) or dynamic image series can be acquired, in which the activity distribution changes constantly during the acquisition period.

The measuring head of the gamma camera consists of a collimator, the sodium iodide crystal used to convert the gamma quanta into light, and the photomultipliers connected to it via a light-conducting layer, which convert the light into electrical signals.

Collimators

A prerequisite for the correct spatial analysis of the incident gamma quanta is the use of a so-called collimator. It ensures that only gamma quanta of a certain flight direction are allowed to pass through and consists of many lead septa, which are separated from each other by small holes.

> ❯ The thickness of the lead septa depends on the energy of the radionuclide used.

If they are too thin, gamma quanta can penetrate the lead (**septa penetration**), if they are too thick, too many gamma quanta are absorbed, the count rate decreases. While septa that are too thin lead to a deterioration of the spatial resolution, the use of a collimator with septa that are too thick can be compensated by extending the acquisition time.

The imaging properties of a collimator depend on its geometry and its distance from the source, i.e. the patient. The geometry of a collimator depends on the ratio hole size/sept length. The divergence angle α is the reference quantity and indicates the maximum angle at which gamma quanta can still just penetrate the bores.

The following applies:
— long septa/small holes/small divergence angle/high spatial resolution,
— short septa/large holes/large divergence angle/low spatial resolution.

The spatial resolution is also dependent on the distance between the patient and the collimator. The greater the source-detector distance, the poorer the imaging quality.

> ❯ The collimator must always be moved as close as possible to the patient.

In patients suffering from claustrophobia, an optimal quality of the image can almost always be achieved by intensive education about the importance of being close to the collimator.

The sensitivity of a collimator is described by the ratio of outgoing to detected quanta. The more quanta reach the detector, the higher the sensitivity of the collimator. It is influenced by the hole size, the number of holes and the septa length.

The following applies:

- large bores/short septa/high sensitivity,
- small bores/long septa/low sensitivity.

However, the spatial resolution decreases with increasing bore size and shorter septa.

❯ Spatial resolution and sensitivity are competing properties. A collimator with good spatial resolution has low sensitivity, one with high sensitivity has poor spatial resolution.

The collimator most commonly used in routine applications is the **parallel-hole collimator**, whose septa are perpendicular to the detector plane.

With **converging** collimators, the septa diverge conically (as seen from the patient). This results in a magnification of the object.

The **diverging collimator** reduces the size of the object. It is used when the dimensions of the object are larger than the field of view of the camera. The septa converge conically (as seen from the patient).

The rarely used **Pinhole collimator** works on the principle of the pinhole camera. It has only one hole and magnifies the image to the maximum. The resolving power is excellent, the sensitivity very low because of the one hole.

❯ Collimators weigh between ten and 100 kg. If the collimator is changed, its attachment to the measuring head must be conscientiously checked to prevent any risk to the patient.

Sodium Iodide Crystal

The field of view of the thallium-doped sodium iodide crystal (UFOF, useful field of view) is 54 × 40 cm for single-head cameras and 42 × 31 cm for a three-head system. The CFOV (central field of view) is the actual imaging area, which is 75% of the UFOF. Under the influence of photon radiation, individual molecules of the crystal structure are excited. When these fall back to the ground state, the excitation energy is emitted in the form of light. The brightness of the light is proportional to the absorbed photon energy, and the amount of light is proportional to the number of events that occur. The high atomic number of NaJ implies a good absorption behavior. The crystal must be adapted to the energy of the radionuclide used. If it is too thin, many quanta leave the crystal unattenuated, the probability of detection decreases. If it is too thick, multiple absorption occurs. The thickness is 9.53 mm for the main use of ^{99m}Tc.

Photomultiplier

A number of **photomultipliers (PMP)** are coupled to the crystal without reflection via a translucent silicone layer. These have the task of converting the resulting scintillation light into electrically measurable pulses. PMPs are vacuum tubes on which a thin metal layer = cathode is vapor-deposited.

Electrons are released from it when the scintillation light hits it. The number of electrons is proportional to the amount of light emitted from the crystal. By applying a high voltage, the released electrons are accelerated onto sheets (dynodes) and release secondary electrons, each of which is accelerated again onto the next dynode. The partial voltage is applied to the dynodes in such a way that from cathode to anode each dynode is positive to the previous one. The high voltage between each dynode must remain the same to maintain proportionality to the incident scintillation light. An avalanche of electrons finally arrives at the anode located at the end of the accelerating path. Each PMP is associated with a preamplifier which converts the incoming charge pulses into voltage pulses, the magnitude of which is in turn proportional to the absorbed quantum energy.

The linear amplifier connected to it linearly exponentiates the voltage pulses. The shape of the signal duration is shortened in order to be able to receive further signals as quickly as possible.

Gamma Spectrum

If we now assume ^{99m}Tc, all measured pulses would have to be registered with the energy of 141 KeV, given proportionality. Due to voltage fluctuations, inhomogeneities of the crystal, scattering of the incoming photons etc., a relatively broad energy distribution around 141 KeV arises. Scattered quanta release a pulse of lower energy than those absorbed via a photoelectric effect, a pulse spectrum is obtained. Radionuclides can have one or more energy peaks, e.g. ^{111}In (171 KeV and 215 KeV).

Measuring Head Electronics

The resulting signals are located in the measuring head via a special resistor network. It divides the output signal of each PMP into four location signals: x^+, x^-, y^+, y^-. The PMP closest to the absorption site registers the most light quanta and provides the highest output pulse. All PMPs further away from the absorption site register correspondingly less light, and the output pulse is lower (distance-squared law). The sum signals x^+, x^-, y^+, y^-, are supplied from the spatial signals of all existing PMPs, which generate a signal via two differential amplifiers x and y. The sum of the resulting output pulses forms the Z signal, which corresponds to the height of the absorbed energy. This is forwarded to the pulse height analyzer and only if it is within the set energy window x and y are forwarded to the connected electronics for registration and the content of the corresponding pixel of the image matrix increases by one. The more decays are detected at one and the same location, the larger the number of pixels in the associated matrix. Common matrix sizes are 64 × 64,

128 × 128, 256 × 256, 512 × 512. However, each detector needs a certain time to process the absorbed quanta. Another signal cannot be accepted during this time, it escapes the measurement (dead time). The resulting count rate losses increase as the amount of activity increases.

SPECT

SPECT (Single Photon Electron Computed Tomography) cameras usually consist of two to three measuring heads running on a ring system. To determine the three-dimensional image of the nuclide distribution in an object, two-dimensional image data are acquired with a gamma camera. The measurement is repeated at different projection angles, with the camera rotating stepwise around the object. Each of the acquired scintigrams represents a two-dimensional projection of the three-dimensional nuclide distribution. Here, all object points (3D) are reproduced in a 2D image of the object oriented parallel to the detection surface of the camera. By back-projection, a three-dimensional image of the nuclide distribution can be generated from this set of 2D images. Thus, in this type of image reconstruction, the 2D image data is back-projected onto the object volume (hence the name of the method) by mapping the intensity of each pixel as a line perpendicular to the detection surface back in the object volume. The depth information is of course lost in the process. It can be recovered by combining images taken at different angles. This type of unfiltered back projection of the raw data leads to smearing of the image, which is why filters are used to improve the image quality (filtered back projection). This method must also be considered an approximation, since the attenuation of gamma radiation due to photoelectric effect and scattering as it passes through the object is not included. These effects are taken into account in the iterative reconstruction procedures, in which measured projections are compared with projections calculated by means of correction factors. Through repetitions in which these correction factors are refined further and further, the three-dimensional nuclide distribution that would correspond to the 2D projections measured by the camera is determined. The acquired scintigrams are displayed on a monitor of the computer system, stored on hard disk, and, if desired, output via a connected documentation system. A suitable software enables the evaluation and post-processing.

When displaying the tomograms, there is a time window of about 30 min between the first and the last acquisition, so that a fast-moving change in activity in the patient cannot be recorded with a SPECT camera.

11.5 Radionucleotides in Medical Application

Various radioactive substances are used in medicine (■ Table 11.1). A distinction is made between substances used for diagnostic imaging, for therapeutic purposes and for laboratory chemical diagnostics.

In laboratory chemical diagnostics, in addition to radioactive substances (predominantly ^{125}I) in the RIA (radioimmunoassay)

■ **Table 11.1** List of some common radioisotopes. (Modified according to Nuclear Medicine, 4th edition, Kuwert)

Isotope	Application	Radiation, keV	HWZ	Production
$[^{99m}TcO_4]TcO_4$	Diagnostics	γ, 140	6.01 h	Generator
$[^{123}I]$	Diagnostics	γ, 159	13.3 h	Cyclotron
$[^{124}I]$	PET	β^+, 188	4.18 d	Cyclotron
$[^{131}I]$	Therapy	β^-, 191 γ, 364	8.02 d	Reactor
$[^{111}In]^{3+}$	Diagnostics	γ, 171, 245	2.80 d	Cyclotron
$[^{90}Y]Y^{3+}$	Therapy	β^-, 934	2.67 d	Generator
$[^{89}Sr]^{2+}$	Therapy	β^-, 583	50.5 d	Reactor
$[^{186}Re]ReO_4$	Therapy	β^-, 359 γ, 137	3.72 d	Reactor
$[^{188}Re]ReO_4$	Therapy	β^-, 795 γ, 155	17 h	Generator
$[^{88}Sm]^{3+}$	Therapy	β^-, 203, 228 γ, 103	1.93 d	Reactor
$[^{18}F]F$	PET	β^+, 242	109.8 min	Cyclotron
$[^{11}C]CO_2$	PET	β^+, 385	20.4 min	Cyclotron
$[^{13}N]NH_3$	PET	β^+, 491	10 min	Cyclotron
$H_2^{15}O$	PET	β^+, 735	2 min	Cyclotron

HWZ Half-life, *Tc* Technetium, *TcO₄* Pertechnetate, *I* Iodine, *In* Indium, *Y* Yttrium, *Sr* Strontium, *Re* Rhenium, *Sm* Samarium, *F* Fluorine, *C* Carbon, *CO₂* Carbon dioxide, *N* Nitrogen, *NH₃* Ammonia, *H₂O* Water

or IRMA (immunradiometric assay), other, non-radioactive substances are also used; in particular, enzymes in the enzyme immuno-assay (EIA) or enzyme-linked immunosorbent assay (ELISA), fluorescent or luminescent substances should be mentioned here. The laboratory chemical methods will not be discussed further here.

11.5.1 Diagnostic Imaging

The most commonly used radioactive substance in imaging is ^{99m}technetium (^{99m}Tc). It has a physical half-life of 6.01 h. It decays into ^{99}technetium, emitting γ-radiation with an energy of 140 keV.

^{99m}Technetium is produced in a generator system. In the system ^{99}molybdenum (HWZ 65.9 h) is firmly bound as sodium molybdate (Na_2 $^{99}MoO_4$). This decomposes to sodium pertechnetate (Na $^{99m}TcO_4$), which is dissolved out of the generator system using sterile physiological saline and a vacuum container.

A generator can be used for approx. one week. The yield of radioactive technetium decreases in the course of the week.

The obtained ^{99m}technetium ($^{99m}TcO_4$) can either be used directly (e.g. in thyroid diagnostics) or it is combined with inactive substances in labelling kits.

Other generator systems include the ^{188}tungsten/^{188}rhenium generator, the ^{68}germanium/^{66}gallium generator, or the ^{90}strontium/^{90}yttrium generator.

Positron emitters are required in PET diagnostics. These have different half-lives. ^{18}F-compounds such as the ^{18}F-FDG are available from commercial suppliers.

11.6 Radiopharmacology

In routine diagnostics, the $^{99m}TcO_4^-$ labelled radiopharmaceuticals in particular play a major role. The use of ^{99m}Tc is simple. Either the eluate can be injected immediately (e. g. thyroid examination) or it is processed by means of commercially available labelling kits mainly by chemical reduction to complex compounds.

The marking devices are usually supplied as powder in a small sealed glass vial. They are stored according to the manufacturer's instructions. They consist of a small proportion of a reducing agent (tin[II] salts) and an excess of the complexing agent (chelating ligand). The complexing agent has been developed for the respective examination, e.g. the phosphonate compounds for bone scintigraphy. The ligands are freeze-dried (lyophilized) and packed in a protective atmosphere (nitrogen or argon). All kits are sterile and pyrogen-free.

Radioactive labelling with the eluate is carried out according to the manufacturer's instructions. Often the labelling can be carried out at room temperature within a few minutes. The resulting radiopharmaceutical can be used within the specified expiry time.

11.7 Quality Assurance Measures of Radiopharmaceuticals

Radiopharmaceuticals are subject to various quality criteria. These are laid down in the European Pharmacopoeia (Ph. Eur.) and the German Medicines Act. These include:

— Radioisotope purity,
— Chemical purity and identity,
— Radiochemical purity,
— Specific activity,
— Stability,
— Microbiological purity.

The quality criteria must always be fulfilled. The responsibility for the individual sub-items differs in some cases.

— **Ready-to-use   radiopharmaceuticals**: These are not modified by the user, but only applied (e.g. injection solutions, capsules). Quality assurance is the sole responsibility of the manufacturer. The user should check the information on the supplied product with the accompanying note as well as the activity.

- **Kit preparations**. The manufacturers are responsible for the ingredients of the kits. The ingredients are guaranteed sterile and pyrogen-free. In addition, controls of the preparation are carried out by means of sample generators and sample kits.

In the respective department, the manufacturer, according to the law the doctor, is responsible for the preparation of the radiopharmaceutical and its properties. Errors can occur during all preparation steps. The main disturbing factors are free pertechnetate and reduced Tc colloid.

- **Self-produced radiopharmaceuticals**: the entire responsibility lies with the manufacturer. These radiopharmaceuticals are e.g. self-produced cyclotron products or radioactively labelled patient parts (e.g. platelets, erythrocytes).

11.7.1 Radioisotope Purity

In practice, this includes testing the so-called molybdenum breakthrough. Each ^{99}Mo/^{99m}Tc generator must be tested before the first application in order to exclude any possible invisible leakage (e.g. due to transport damage) of ^{99}Mo into the eluate.

Here the generator is eluted normally. Afterwards, the eluate is measured without shielding and with an appropriate lead sheathing on all sides (6 mm lead) in the activimeter in the technetium window. The lead sheath shields the low-energy radiation of the ^{99m}Tc (141 keV) and only 65% of the higher-energy ^{99}Mo (739 keV). The quotient Q must be <0.04%.

$$Q = \frac{Eluatmessung\,mit\,Abschirmung\,(MBq)}{Eluatmessung\,ohne\,Abschirmung\,(MBq)} \times 100$$

❯ The activimeter, formerly also called curiemeter, is a measuring device that indicates the activity of a measured sample.

11.7.2 Chemical Purity

This refers to the proportion of the desired substance in the total substance mixture. In the monographs on radioactive medicinal products, the requirements for chemical purity are laid down by specifying limits for the chemical impurities.

Chemical purity must be guaranteed by the manufacturer.

11.7.3 Radiochemical Purity

The ratio, expressed as a percentage, of the radioactivity of the radionuclide in the desired chemical form to the total radioactivity of the radionuclide in the radiopharmaceutical is referred to as radiochemical purity.

The main causes of contamination lie in the **preparation**. In addition to an undesirable oxygen supply (e.g. leaky stopper, aeration cannula), an excessively high amount of radioactivity can also lead to poor labelling yield (a lot does not always help a lot). Also "old" eluates or the first eluate after a longer elution break (e.g. weekend, holidays) have an influence on the radiochemical purity. Other causes of contamination are technical, such as chemical instabilities or autoradiolysis.

To determine the radiochemical purity, the individual components are separated chromatographically and measured. Another possibility is a solid phase extraction in cartridge form.

11.7.4 Specific Activity

The specific activity is characteristic for each isotope and results from the measure the ratio of the activity to the mass.

11.7.5 Stability

The stability of the radiopharmaceutical depends on various factors. Particularly in the case of high-energy therapeutic substances, changes can occur as a result of the radiation, so that these substances must be consumed relatively quickly after production.

11.7.6 Microbiological Purity

Every radiopharmaceutical should be free of bacteria if possible. Due to the sometimes only short half-lives of various substances, the exact status can sometimes only be determined after the radioactivity has subsided. A rapid test, the so-called Limulus amoebocyte lysate test (LAL test), is prescribed for the ^{18}FDG, for example. In this test, the sample is combined with the lysate. If endotoxins are present in the sample, this becomes visible by means of various methods. Only after receipt of the result may the injection solution be released for consumption. The release is to be checked by the applying physician.

11.8 Contamination and Decontamination Measures

11.8.1 Contamination

This refers to (unintentional) contamination of the environment (including the air), objects or persons with radioactive substances.

Contamination is not necessarily directly detectable, since radioactivity cannot be perceived by the human senses. The handling of all open radioactive substances must therefore be done very carefully.

Contamination hazards exist in all work steps, starting with the elution of the generator, kit preparations, preparation of the patient dose up to the application.

The **patient** is also a **possible source of contamination**. These include, in particular, incorrect inhalation of radioactive substances (e.g. lung ventilation examination), uncontrolled excretion of substances in the case of various incontinence diseases with possible contamination of objects (chairs, toilet, door handles) as well as due to contact with all excretions of the patient (e.g. urine, stool, saliva, stomach contents, blood).

Contamination checks must be carried out at each workplace at least once a day when handling open radioactive substances, and immediately if contamination is suspected. The corresponding results must be recorded.

When leaving the controlled area, the personnel must carry out a **contamination check**, e.g. by means of a hand-foot clothing monitor or hand monitor in the personnel airlock. The measurement results are to be recorded.

Items leaving the controlled area (e.g. cleaning utensils, litter, wheelchair) must also be checked and the results recorded.

11.8.2 Decontamination

This refers to the removal of (hazardous) impurities, in this case radioactive substances.

The primary goal is to reduce radiation exposure to the body; other goals are to prevent the spread of contamination and to prevent incorporation.

- Contamination: What to Do?
- Blocking the contamination area
- Contact another person. If this is not possible, clearly mark the contamination area, avoid carry-over
- In case of possible personal contamination: decontamination as quickly as possible
- Remove contaminated work clothing without further contamination of other areas
- Localization of contaminated skin areas as precise as possible
- Multiple dry decontamination of the skin by means of adhesive film, this leads to a removal of >90% of the activity
- Wash with plenty of lukewarm water and decontaminant, dry with disposable towels
- Success control by means of monitor, if contamination is still detectable → wash thoroughly again using a soft brush
- **Lack of decontamination success**: Repeat all points. If the effect is <10% and the contamination <10 Bq/cm^2, further measures can be dispensed with. Otherwise, the radiation protection officer must initiate further measures
- **Special measures appropriate to** the **situation**: e.g. hair washing; eye and mouth rinsing, if necessary venous stasis and wound rinsing in the case of skin injury
- Only after personal contamination has been ruled out should the **area** be approached:
  - Determination of the location and extent of contamination of surfaces and objects: Any decontamination should not increase the risk of contamination and incorporation of personnel, therefore appropriate protective clothing is mandatory
  - Absorbing liquids with absorbent material from the outside to the inside
  - Wet wipe if necessary (from the outside to the inside)
  - If necessary, further physical measures (scraping, grinding, brushing)
  - Non-removable contaminations are covered (adhesive foil) and marked
  - In case of contamination of work equipment with short-lived substances, wait for decay time (in decay room, marked)
- Clarification of the cause of contamination
- Documentation of contamination

Practice Questions

1. Name the 5 As of radiation protection.
2. What do you do in case of contamination with ^{99m}Tc?
3. Name the major components of a gamma camera.
4. Name the most important (most common) nuclear medicine therapy—naming benign as well as malignant diseases.
5. What is the difference between X-ray examinations and nuclear medicine examinations?
6. Which radioactive radiation do you know? Name one possible application in each case.
7. What do you mean by coincidence?
8. What is a SPECT examination?

Solutions ▶ Chap. 27

Emergencies and Extreme Situations

Christel Vockelmann and Martina Kahl-Scholz

Contents

© Springer-Verlag GmbH Germany, part of Springer Nature 2023
M. Kahl-Scholz, C. Vockelmann (eds.), *Basic Knowledge Radiology*,
https://doi.org/10.1007/978-3-662-66351-6_12

In this chapter, some extreme situations that can be encountered in everyday clinical practice will be briefly addressed and presented. These include, of course, emergencies, such as those that can occur in the form of a KM intolerance or a seizure.

12.1 Extreme Situations

In everyday professional life, one often encounters extreme situations. For some, this starts with the oncological patient having a tracheostoma or discovering only one leg when "uncovering" a patient lying in bed, and for others with small babies suffering from cancer or patients covered in blood being admitted after a traffic accident. The extreme situations are individual to each examiner and can be psychologically stressful. However, it is very important to distance oneself mentally as much as possible in order to be able to do the best possible for the patient quickly and effectively. Here we go into a few examples:

12.1.1 Polytrauma

The definition of a polytrauma is a multiple, life-threatening injury caused by an accident. Here, very good interdisciplinary cooperation and organization is essential for the patient. The procedures and protocols differ depending on the hospital. It is always important to have a clear organization. In any emergency, it must be clear who is "in charge" in order to treat quickly and effectively. And in the case of an emergency on the street or at the airport, this can also be you as a PJ'ler or radiologist, who then has to give clear instructions to bystanders and passers-by so that the patient is well cared for as quickly as possible. In the hospital, the initial measures are well organized in the shock room, then the patients are usually

examined in the CT. Bony injuries, organ and vascular injuries can be detected and assessed very quickly so that further measures can be initiated immediately.

12.1.2 Anaphylactoid Reaction

You are a few years in the profession and have performed at least 5000 CT examinations with contrast agent. A few patients have complained of a few spots at most after the examination. Then comes the next CT. An outpatient in whom you have performed a CT angiography of the pelvic-leg vessels. You look at the images while the patient sits in the waiting room. The MTRA notices that the patient is relatively pale. She calls her. The patient is already cold sweaty and shows red pustules and dyspnea. They recognize that there is an allergic reaction and call the anesthetist from the intensive care unit. He now quickly injects the medication against the anaphylactoid reaction.

Fortunately, the rapid intervention helped. The next day you can already see the patient again in front of the hospital.

12.1.3 CT-Guided Puncture

Mr. Müller has a pulmonary nodule. This is to be punctured in the CT. You routinely run through your program. The needle is placed and a sample obtained. However, the patient was relatively restless, so that the access route was difficult. You note: A pleural effusion has formed. Probably an intercostal artery is injured. You ask the MTRA to connect KM and run an angio in the aortic program over the area. CT shows the findings—there is bleeding from the intercostal artery and the patient gets a haemothorax (◘ Fig 12.1). You call the surgeon. Fortunately, the patient is stable until the surgeon takes him to the OR.

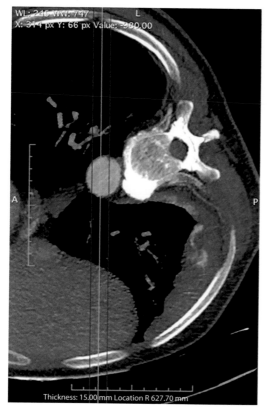

Fig. 12.1 CT angiographic evidence of arterial bleeding from the intercostal artery into the pleural space

12.1.4 Seizure During Stent Angioplasty

(See also section on seizures).

A patient has a high-grade restenosis of the carotid artery. As almost every day in angiography, a stent angioplasty is to be performed in this patient. Everything is going as usual. The wire has successfully passed the stenosis, and the initial dilatation went smoothly. Blood pressure is rather high throughout the procedure, up to blood pressure values of about 180 mmHg systolic. But the patient says that's always the case. Then the stent is released, angiographically the stenosis is completely eliminated. At that point, the patient starts seizing. You ask for

Rivotril to treat the seizure and instruct to let CT know. The fears are confirmed. The patient presents with a large ICB (intracerebral hemorrhage). The neurosurgical colleagues are called in, but surgical therapy does not seem advisable. In the next few hours the patient is in intensive care. His condition does not improve, however, and he dies a few days after the operation.

12.2 Contrast Agent Incident and Emergency Medication

12.2.1 Side Effects

Adverse reactions caused by KM may be dose-dependent or dose-independent (□ Table 12.1).

Among other things, vasodilatation may occur, which causes a drop in blood pressure (hypotension). Histamines released from mast cells are responsible for an immediate allergic reaction and in turn lead to vasodilation of the small peripheral vessels. This is the cause of a possible circulatory shock.

□ Table 12.1 Adverse direct side effects/reactions to KM

	Dose-dependent response	Dose-independent response
Response type	Direct (local) effect on organs and tissues as well as organ systems	Systemic response
Pathological process	Chemotoxic	Anaphylactic
Symptoms	Sensation of warmth/cold, reddening of the skin, headache	Nausea, vomiting, urticaria, itching

Furthermore, an involvement of the coagulation system and the CNS is discussed.

Many patients assume that a KM reaction is accompanied by an iodine allergy—but an iodine allergy would not be compatible with life, since we need iodine as an indispensable component of our human metabolism.

> ❯ An adverse KM reaction is not based on an iodine allergy, but is due to an intolerance of the KM complex.

Locally, especially with iodine-containing contrast media, pain, damage to the vessel walls, vasodilatation (→ drop in blood pressure) may occur.

> ❯ Low osmolar CMs are generally better tolerated than high osmolar ones, nonionic ones better than ionic ones.

Contrast Induced Nephropathy (CIN)

Contrast-induced nephropathy is defined as a deterioration of renal function (symptomatic by pathological creatinine values 3–10 days after the application of KM) after the administration of iodine-containing, intravasally applied contrast media. It occurs in 7–10% of patients, with patients with pre-existing renal insufficiency or diabetes mellitus with renal insufficiency being particularly at risk. In this group of patients, contrast media should not be administered if possible. However, if it cannot be avoided for compelling diagnostic reasons, the following aspects should be taken into account:

- Before the examination, the patient should be sufficiently hydrated, i.e. supplied with fluid (i.v. hydration with isotonic NaCl solution is optimal).
- Nephrotoxic substances should be avoided as concomitant therapies or discontinued if necessary.
- During the investigation:

- Use of a low osmolar and viscous KM
- Use as little KM as possible!
- Repeated KM administration should be avoided at all costs!

Hyperthyroidism and Thyrotoxic Crisis

If iodine-containing contrast medium is used (e.g. in the course of an angiography), the iodine plasma level is increased due to cleavage of the iodine nucleotide. A normal healthy thyroid gland can adapt to the increased iodine load. However, if autonomous production or an immune disease of the thyroid gland is already present, hyperthyroidism and even a thyrotoxic crisis may occur.

The frequency with which hyperthyroidism occurs depends on several factors:
- Severity of iodine deficiency prior to iodine exposure,
- Extent of exposure to iodine,
- Frequency of functionally autonomous cells in the thyroid gland,
- Age of patients.

■ Symptoms of Hyperthyroidism Include
- Weight loss (despite sufficient food intake)
- Accelerated pulse
- Sweating
- Hypertension
- Nervousness, restlessness
- Sleep disorders
- Possible goiter

■ Symptoms of Thyrotoxic Crisis Include
- Stage 1 (lethality less than 10%): Extreme sinus tachycardia (>150/min) or tachyarrhythmia with existing atrial fibrillation, heart failure; high fever; gastrointestinal and neurological symptoms, exsiccosis, dehydration
- Stage 2: Clouding of consciousness
- Stage 3 (lethality: over 30%): Unconsciousness

In patients at risk, perchlorate (irenate) is used prophylactically before and 1–2 weeks after the examination with a thyrostatic. Perchlorate decreases iodine uptake into the thyroid gland.

- Prophylaxis with Perchlorate

Example of Prophylactic Treatment of Iodine-Induced Hyperthyroidism

- 2–4 h before KM administration 25 drops of Irenate (perchlorate)
- 3 × 15 drops of Irenat/day for one week
- Check TSH basal, T4, T4 after three and six weeks

Example of Treatment in Manifest Hyperthyroidism and Vital Indication

- 2–4 h before KM administration 25 drops of Irenate (perchlorate)
- 3 × 15 drops of Irenat/day for two weeks
- 20 mg/day Favistan (thiamazole) for two weeks

Nephrogenic Systemic Fibrosis (NSF)

This form of fibrosis can occur (very rarely) in patients who already have stage 4 or 5 renal failure and are undergoing testing with gadolinum. Why it occurs is not yet fully understood. It may become symptomatic in the period from 2 days to 18 months after exposure to gadolinum-containing BM. There are prophylactic measures that can be taken to reduce the risk of NSF. These include:

- If KM administration is diagnostically essential in high-risk patients, then cyclic gadolinum KM or KM with a low risk classification should be used (□ Table 12.2).
- The lowest possible dose should be aimed for and repeated administration should be avoided at all costs.

Circulatory Arrest

- Symptoms
- Lack of (carotid) pulse
- Respiratory arrest, gasping possibly after 15–40 s

□ **Table 12.2** Risk classification of gadolinum contrast agents in relation to the development of NSF. (According to EMEA)

Risk class	Contrast agent
High risk	Optimark, Omniscan, Magnevist, Gado-MRT-Ratiopharm
Medium risk	Vasovist, Primovist, Multihance
Low risk	Gadovist, ProHance, Dotarem

- Cerebral seizures possible after 15–45 s
- Pupil dilation and loss of light reaction after 30–60 s

- Resuscitation
- Cardiac massage: Find a hard surface, if not already available → pressure point in the middle of the chest (lower half of the sternum) → compression depth approx. 4–5 cm → 100 compressions
- Ventilation: after the first 30 compressions (frequency 100–120/min) → first ventilation cycle of approx. 1 s with ventilation twice
- Continue as above in the ratio **30 (cardiac compressions):2 (ventilations)**
- **Special features:**
  - in pregnant women from the 20th week of pregnancy, lift the pelvis to the right and move the uterus to the left during positioning before chest compressions
  - for children, five ventilations initially; if only one caregiver is present, 30 (cardiac compressions):2 (ventilations); for the 2-helper method, 15 (cardiac compressions):2 (ventilations)

- Emergency Medication
- Suprarenin® (adrenalin 1:1000): dilute 1 mL (1 mg) with 9 mL physiological saline solution
- Glucocorticoids (e.g. dexamethasone 40–100 mg, prednisolone 200–500 mg)

- H_1 and H_2 antagonists
- Atropine 0.5 mg
- Midazolam 5 mg
- i.v. narcotics
- Crystalloid solutions
- Colloidal volume substitutes

Seizures

A seizure does not have to occur as a side effect, but it can occur at any time due to an existing underlying disease (epilepsy, brain tumors, metastases, scarring in the brain, etc.), e.g. also in the MRI or CT during the examination procedure.

There are various forms of seizures, of which the grand mal seizure and status epilepticus are the most relevant in emergency medicine.

▪ Grand Mal Seizure

This type of seizure is divided into different phases:
- Preconvulsive phase with general symptoms such as headache, fatigue, hallucinations
- Convulsive phase (tonic stage) with fall, loss of consciousness, apnoea, tongue bite, extensor tonus
- Convulsive phase (clonic stage) with rhythmic contractions of the musculature, enuresis, tongue biting, cyanosis
- Postconvulsive/postictal phase followed by a brief comatose state, twilight, confusion.

This is the most common type of seizure you will encounter. The most important treatment measure here is to prevent injury to the patient, e.g. by falling off the examination table. A biting wedge or similar is no longer used today. In the case of a short-lasting seizure, acute drug therapy is not usually necessary. It is important that you get support from the doctor in charge.

▪ Status Epilepticus

- If a tonic-clonic seizure lasts longer than five minutes or if an entire series of seizures occurs without the patient regaining consciousness in the meantime, this is referred to as status epilepticus. The danger here is an undersupply of oxygen (hypoxia) and dangerous cardiovascular stress.

▪▪ Acute Therapy for Status Epilepticus

- Oxygen supply, blood pressure control, if possible ECG and blood sugar control
- Benzodiazepines i.v., e.g. 2–4 mg lorazepam (alternatively diazepam 10–20 mg or clonazepam 1–2 mg)
- If there is no effect after five minutes, the administration is repeated
- Phenytoin and valproate are reserve drugs that are only given if the status epilepticus cannot be terminated even by administration of benzodiazepines.

Practice Questions

1. A patient suddenly becomes cold sweaty and develops dyspnea after a CT scan with KM. What is your first thought?
2. What can extreme sinus tachycardia, high fever; gastrointestinal and neurological symptoms indicate?
3. What can be done prophylactically to prevent hyperthyroidism from iodine-containing KM?
4. What are the resuscitative measures in case of circulatory arrest?
5. How is status epilepticus defined and what is dangerous about it?

Solutions ▶ Chap. 27

Legislation

Christel Vockelmann

Contents

© Springer-Verlag GmbH Germany, part of Springer Nature 2023
M. Kahl-Scholz, C. Vockelmann (eds.), *Basic Knowledge Radiology*,
https://doi.org/10.1007/978-3-662-66351-6_13

Due to the manifold dangers of ionizing radiation, several laws and regulations play an important role. In addition to the national requirements, European and international requirements must also be observed. The laws that are important for the application of ionizing radiation to humans are arranged hierarchically. In the Federal Republic of Germany, the Basic Law (Constitution, GG) is the supreme law (▶ Sect. 13.1). The Atomic Energy Act (AtG) (▶ Sect. 13.4) is subordinate to the Basic Law. As of 2016, the Radiation Protection Ordinance (StrSchV) (▶ Sect. 13.6) and the X-ray Ordinance (RöV) (▶ Sect. 13.5) are subordinate to the Atomic Energy Act. The Radiation Protection Act (StrlSchG) will probably enter into force in 2018, replacing the X-ray Ordinance and the Radiation Protection Ordinance, but will ultimately correspond to a large extent to the content of the X-ray Ordinance and the StrlSchV.

Due to the manifold dangers of ionizing radiation, several laws and regulations play an important role. In addition to national requirements, European and international regulations must also be observed. First of all, however, it is important to differentiate between the various terms.

- **Laws** are binding on everyone and are established by the parliamentary legislature. The Basic Law can serve as an example.
- **Legal ordinances** are also binding on everyone, the obvious example for us being the X-ray ordinance. They are issued by the executive, i.e. the government, on the basis of laws. An amendment, e.g. adaptation to changed conditions, is possible more quickly than with laws.
- **Guidelines do** not represent binding requirements, but are applied for concrete implementation.

- **Standards** or **rules of** technology are not binding. They serve as proof of safety.

The laws that are important for the application of ionizing radiation to humans are arranged hierarchically. In the Federal Republic of Germany, the Basic Law (GG) is the supreme law (▶ Sect. 13.1). The Atomic Energy Act (AtG) (▶ Sect. 13.4) is subordinate to the Basic Law. The Radiation Protection Ordinance (StrSchV) (▶ Sect. 13.6) and the X-Ray Ordinance (RöV) (▶ Sect. 13.5) are subordinate to the Atomic Energy Act. In order to transpose the Euratom Directive 2013/59/Euratom into German law, the Radiation Protection Act (StrlSchG) is expected to enter into force in 2018 and replace RöV and StrSchV. In terms of content, both ordinances will be largely reflected in the new law.

13.1 Basic Law (GG)

Articles 1 to 19 of the Basic Law set out the fundamental rights that every person, and in particular every citizen, has.

》 Article 2 Basic Law

1. Everyone has the right to the free development of his personality, provided that he does not infringe the rights of others and does not offend against the constitutional order or the moral law.
2. Everyone has the right to life and physical integrity. The freedom of the person is inviolable. These rights may be interfered with only on the basis of a law.

This means that medical treatment or a diagnostic measure is only permissible with the patient's consent. The patient may revoke the consent at any time.

❯ Treatment without consent is an interference with the physical integrity of the patient.

This is where the Criminal Code (StGB) comes into play:

» § 223 Criminal Code bodily injury

1. Whoever physically abuses another person or damages his or her health shall be punished by imprisonment for not more than five years or a fine.
2. The attempt is punishable.

13.2 Patients' Rights Act

The Patients' Rights Act is part of the German Civil Code (BGB). The law came into force on 20 February 2013 and is intended to create transparent regulations for patients and doctors, particularly in the areas of information, documentation and rights of access. For imaging procedures, the necessary documentation was already stipulated in detail in RöV and StrSchV before the Patients' Rights Act came into force. For practice, the Patients' Rights Act results in a number of important requirements, in particular for information.

13.2.1 Reconnaissance

Informing patients is a medical activity and cannot be delegated to non-medical staff. The physician providing the information must have a corresponding level of knowledge about the intervention or measure about which he is providing the information. In practice, this means that a physician can explain an appendectomy if he has at least assisted in the procedure and has experience with possible complications and their treatment. The extent of the explanation depends on the urgency and danger of the intervention. In the case of an emergency CT scan for a suspected perforated aortic aneurysm, the patient does not need to be informed in detail in writing about possible complica-

tions of the contrast medium. Nevertheless, the physician should discuss the examination with the patient, provided the patient is responsive, in order to learn about possible contraindications.

❯ In the case of patients for whom information is not feasible due to their physical or mental situation, the legal representative must be informed of the planned measures.

Here, too, the urgency and danger of the planned measures must be taken into account and, if necessary, a telephone explanation, if possible with fax confirmation by the caregiver, is also possible.

Duties/Rights During the Practical Year

A recent ruling by the Karlsruhe Higher Regional Court has declared the provision of information by PJ students to be legal under certain conditions. They must be familiar with the examination or intervention and be able to assess the risks. The participation in clarification discussions and, in the next step, the clarification under the supervision of the training physician is the prerequisite for PJ'ler to be allowed to clarify independently, provided that they can call a doctor for this at any time and should also point out to the patient that he or she can always speak to a doctor as well.

The patient must be offered a copy of the written copies of the information and should confirm receipt or refusal of the copy, preferably in writing. The patient's signature confirming receipt of the copy must not, of course, already be on the copy.

❯ The patient may revoke his or her consent at any time; an intervention or examination against the patient's express will is not permitted.

What Must Be Disclosed?

The patient should be informed about the planned measures in such a way that he/she can decide for him/herself whether the planned procedure makes sense for him/her (self-determination information). To this end, the patient must be informed about the risks of the planned treatment, but also about the risks that may arise if the measure is not carried out.

The actual treatment information includes the specific treatment (e.g. computer tomography) with possible risks (e.g. contrast agent incident with anaphylactic shock). In the end, it is not the frequency of risks that is important, but the consequences. Thus, possible lethal complications should be mentioned, even if their probability of occurrence is very rare but possible.

Information should also be provided on possible alternatives to the proposed procedure, especially if there are in fact approximately equivalent procedures.

Information Requirements

The doctor is obliged to inform the patient about the disease, the planned therapy and also the probable development of the state of health.

If the doctor recognizes that the treatment costs are not fully covered by the health insurance, the patient must be informed in writing about the costs incurred. A typical example of this are IGel services (individual health services) or also a planned dental prosthesis.

13.3 Data Protection

Information about a person's state of health is very sensitive data that must be handled responsibly. Even as a medical student, you, as well as the nursing staff and medical technical assistants (MTA), are subject to **medical confidentiality.** Therefore, you must not leave information about patients lying around openly or pass it on. Electronic documents such as patient files or X-ray images must not be freely accessible, but must be password-protected. As a doctor, you are only allowed to see information about patients you are treating. The patient decides to whom information about his or her state of health may be disclosed. Without the patient's consent, the X-ray results of an examination, for example, may not be passed on to the referring physician or general practitioner. In order to make it possible to work sensibly here, this passing on of information to the referring physician is often regulated in the treatment contract that the patient concludes with the hospital. The consultation of other specialist groups also requires the patient's consent. In the case of emergency consultations, such as the consultation of a neurosurgeon in the event of intracerebral hemorrhage, you may, however, act in the presumed interests of the patient.

The same applies to the information of relatives. The spouse does not generally have a right to information, but in an emergency you may assume that the patient agrees to his or her spouse being informed about the state of health.

The storage of external X-ray examinations also falls within the scope of data protection. Here, too, you need the patient's consent.

Electronic data transmission must be encrypted. An example of such encrypted sending of X-ray images is the operation of teleradiology home offices. Here, there must be a secure connection between the teleradiologist's home computer and the hospital so that the images cannot be intercepted and the information misused.

13.4 Atomic Energy Act (AtG)

The content of the X-ray and Radiation Protection Ordinances is based on the regulations of the EURATOM Directives and the Atomic Energy Act, which regulates the peaceful use of nuclear energy and protection against the dangers of nuclear energy. As you can guess from the name, EURATOM stands for an organization in Europe. The European Atomic Energy Community (Euratom) was founded in 1957 by the Treaty of Rome at the same time as the European Economic Community, now renamed the European Community (EU), by France, Italy, the Benelux countries and the Federal Republic of Germany.

13.5 X-ray Ordinance (RöV)

The Ordinance on Protection against Damage Caused by X-rays, the full title of the X-ray Ordinance, came into force in its original version in 1973. The last amendment has been valid since 01 November 2012. A core statement of the X-ray Ordinance is the requirement to avoid any unnecessary exposure to radiation for humans and the environment. It also regulates quality requirements and necessary quality controls by users and medical authorities. The medical authorities are institutions located at the respective state medical associations that monitor the quality assurance of medical radiation applications. Comparable institutions exist as dental authorities for the dental field. The X-ray Ordinance regulates areas with X-ray radiation with a limit energy of more than 5 keV and less than 1 MeV. The handling of radioactive substances and ionizing radiation not covered by the X-ray Ordinance is regulated by the Radiation Protection Ordinance.

13.6 Radiation Protection Ordinance (StrSchV)

The Ordinance on Protection against Damage Caused by Ionizing Radiation, abbreviated to Radiation Protection

Ordinance (StrSchV), is an ordinance within nuclear law. The legal basis for it is § 54 of the Atomic Energy Act. The StrSchV was last amended in 2011; the original version dates from 1976.1 The purpose of the ordinance is described in § 1:

》 The purpose of this Regulation is to lay down the principles and requirements for precautionary and protective measures applicable to the use and exposure to radioactive substances and ionizing radiation of civil and natural origin in order to protect man and the environment against the harmful effects of ionizing radiation.

The StrSchV applies in areas in which radioactive substances are worked with. In addition to nuclear medicine in the field of medicine, this also affects, for example, the personnel of nuclear facilities.

Medical personnel are partly subject to both the X-ray Ordinance and the Radiation Protection Ordinance.

13.7 Radiation Protection Areas

The radiation protection areas (■ Fig. 13.1, ■ Table 13.1) are regulated in § 19 RöV. These areas describe the working areas

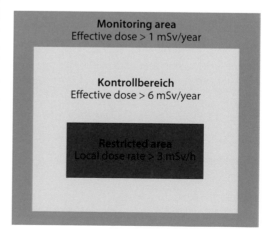

■ **Fig. 13.1** Radiation protection areas. (From Hartmann et al. 2014)

| **Table 13.1** Radiation protection areas ||
Radiation protection area	**Dose**
Restricted area	>3 mSv/h
Control area	>6 mSv/a
Monitoring area	>1 mSv/a

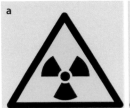
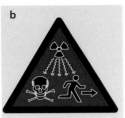

Fig. 13.2 Radiation warning sign. **a** Currently used and **b** future internationally used radiation warning sign. (From Hartmann et al. 2014)

in which ionizing radiation may occur. A residence time of 40 h in a week and 50 weeks in a calendar year serves as the basis for defining the areas.

This classification is not relevant for patients.

■ **Restricted Areas**

These exist in radiation therapy and in nuclear facilities. In radiotherapy, the radiation bunker or the after-loading room is a restricted area when the linear accelerator is radiating or the radiators are extended in after-loading. Only the patient may be in the room at this time. Persons holding or assisting the patient as well as medical personnel are not allowed to be there and the area must be marked with a light signal (restricted area—no access). Outside the actual irradiation, the restricted area becomes a controlled area.

■ **Control Areas and Supervised Areas**

These are available in every X-ray, radiotherapy or nuclear medicine department.

If you enter a **controlled area** for occupational reasons, you belong to the group of occupationally exposed persons. Persons under the age of 18 are only permitted access for training purposes. For pregnant employees, it must be ensured that the uterine dose is less than 1 mSv until the end of the pregnancy.

Control areas must be marked. This marking must contain at least the words "No access—X-ray" or, in nuclear medicine, "Controlled area". In addition, you will

often encounter the radiation warning sign. The sign currently used in Germany, the black propeller on a yellow triangle (■ Fig. 13.2a), will be replaced internationally in the future by a red triangle with a deterrent symbol. Here, a skull and crossbones and a departing human are found below the propeller (■ Fig. 13.2b).

Before you are allowed to work in the controlled area, you must be instructed by the radiation protection officer. This instruction must be repeated annually. You must tolerate this instruction. Only if you are prevented from doing so, the instruction can be given in writing in exceptional cases.

X-ray rooms belong to the controlled areas during admission or fluoroscopy, otherwise to the monitoring area. In the case of X-ray equipment in intensive care units or mobile C-arms, there is of course no spatially identifiable controlled area. Here, a controlled area of 1.5 m applies by definition for mobile X-ray exposure devices or 3 m or 4 m for C-arms, depending on the image converter size. Marking is not required for this, provided that it is ensured that uninvolved persons do not enter the area unintentionally.

If you work in the controlled area, you are required to determine your **body dose.** For this purpose, you must wear an appropriate **X-ray badge.** You are also obliged to wear appropriate protective clothing (lead apron, thyroid protection) in the controlled area. This obligation does not apply in

13

nuclear medicine, as here a **lead apron** would make the radiation longer-wave and thus absorbable.

However, the obligation for **protective clothing** and **personal dosimetry** with determination of the body dose does not only concern employees. The body dose must also be determined immediately for persons who are "in the controlled area for reasons other than their (…) examination or treatment". For this purpose, for example, rod dosimeters are used which can be read after the examination. This dose must also be documented.

The **monitored area** is characterized by a dose rate of more than 1 mSv/year. Persons who permanently stay in these areas also belong to the group of occupationally exposed persons.

13.8 Occupationally Exposed Persons

In addition to medical personnel, occupationally exposed persons also include personnel of nuclear facilities and, in the meantime, airline personnel who are regularly on board aircraft. Two categories are distinguished, depending on the potential radiation exposure. The dose limits are to be understood as an "or" rule, i.e. it is sufficient, for example, to reach the organ dose of the eye lens in order to belong to category A (◘ Table 13.2).

The results of the Federal Office for Radiation Protection show that the radiation exposure of the vast majority of medical personnel is less than 1 mSv/year. For flying personnel, on the other hand, the average radiation exposure is 2–3 mSv/year.

If there is actually a radiation exposure of more than 20 mSv/year, an official permit can be issued in individual cases allowing a radiation exposure of up to 50 mSv/year.

> However, according to Directive 96/29/EURATOM, the radiation exposure may not exceed 100 mSv in five consecutive years.

In Germany, approx. 360,000 persons are currently monitored. In 2007, there was a radiation exposure of more than 20 mSv effective dose in 11 cases.

◘ **Table 13.2** Persons exposed to radiation		
	Category A	**Category B**
Medical examination	Annual	By order of the Authority
Effective dose	>6 mSv/calendar year	>1 mSv/calendar year
Organ dose eye lens	>45 mSv/calendar year	>15 mSv/calendar year
Organdosis skin, hands, forearms, feet, ankles	>150 mSv/calendar year	>50 mSv/calendar year

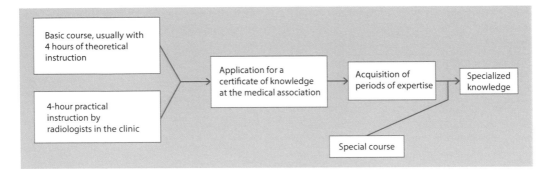

◘ Fig. 13.3 The path to expertise. (From Hartmann et al. 2014)

13.9 **Technical Knowledge**

The X-ray and Radiation Protection Ordinances stipulate that the medical use of X-rays may only be ordered or carried out by doctors who have the appropriate specialist qualifications. For this purpose, you must attend radiation protection courses and perform a specified number of examinations under supervision. In addition to the overall specialist qualification in X-ray diagnostics, there are also specialist qualifications in CT, skeletal diagnostics, emergency diagnostics, interventions and much more (◘ Fig. 13.3). In order to retain your specialist knowledge, you must attend an update course in accordance with RöV and possibly also StrlSchV (for nuclear medicine and radiotherapy as well as MTRA) every five years at the latest.

13.10 **Justifying Indication**

Examinations may only be performed if a competent physician has provided the "justifying indication" according to § 23 RöV or § 80 StrlSchV. It must be assessed whether the benefit of the planned examination outweighs the risk of radiation exposure and whether the question cannot be answered by another examination with lower radiation exposure.

In order to be able to establish the justifying indication, the physician must be in possession of the corresponding specialist knowledge. For example, a doctor with emergency specialist knowledge may order an X-ray of a patient's ankle following supination trauma. However, he may not order an X-ray of the lung with the question of metastases in a tumor disease. This requires a thoracic specialist qualification or a general specialist qualification.

> ❯ Questions such as progress monitoring are not sufficient to establish a justifiable indication.

13.11 **Medical Devices Act (MPG)**

You will encounter the MPG in your work every day. It stipulates that only appropriately tested medical devices may be used. X-ray devices also fall under this regulation, as do perfusers or pressure syringes. In order to be allowed to operate these, you must be instructed in the respective device.

13.12 Maternity Protection Act (MuSchG)

The Maternity Protection Act is intended to protect the health of mother and child. This includes, among other things, that pregnant women are not allowed to work at night. Working in the controlled area is possible under certain conditions, as mentioned above. Contact with potentially infectious material must be avoided. Therefore, you must not draw blood or place venous accesses during pregnancy.

13.13 Working Time Act

This regulates occupational health and safety under public law. Among other things, there are limits on the maximum permissible daily working time, minimum rest breaks and protective regulations on night work. The law is binding for employers and employees. There are regulations on working hours on weekdays, weekly working hours and on-call duty.

Practice Questions
1. What must the doctor explain?
2. What is regulated by the X-ray Ordinance and what by the Radiation Protection Ordinance?
3. What is meant by "justifiable indication"?
4. Does pregnancy under the Maternity Protection Act preclude working in the radiological field?

Solutions Chap. 27

Disease Patterns

Contents

Neurology

Christel Vockelmann, Ursula Blum, Martina Kahl-Scholz and Guido Heilsberg

Contents

© Springer-Verlag GmbH Germany, part of Springer Nature 2023
M. Kahl-Scholz, C. Vockelmann (eds.), *Basic Knowledge Radiology*,
https://doi.org/10.1007/978-3-662-66351-6_14

The brain controls all important functions, from motor skills and sensory perception to vital processes such as breathing, heartbeat and digestion. It is a complicated system of neurotransmitters and neuroreceptors. The spinal cord is, so to speak, the connection between the central switching station "brain" and the other parts of the body such as the neck, trunk and extremities.

14.1 Anatomical Structures

Christel Vockelmann

The anatomical structures of the neurological system include the neurocranium with its various parts, the myelon as well as the cranial nerves (central nervous system, CNS) and the peripheral ganglia and nerves (peripheral nervous system, PNS).

The imaging of the CNS plays a major role, therefore we will limit ourselves here to the brief imaging of the brain (encephalon) and spinal cord (medulla spinalis).

The **cerebrum** (telencephalon) forms the largest part of the brain and is structurally characterized by the two hemispheres, several furrows (sulci) and convolutions (gyri). Other parts are the **diencephalon** with thalamus, subthalamus, hypothalamus, pituitary gland and epiphysis as well as the **mesencephalum**, **cerebellum**, **pons** and the **medulla oblangata**, which merges into the myelon. The boundary between the latter two structures is at about the level of the **foramen magnum**. Important in the context of imaging are the basal ganglia (also called the truncal ganglia), which include the putamen and pallidum (together Nucl. lentiformis) and Nucl. caudatus. between the aforementioned nuclei is found the capsula interna, laterally to it the capsula externa, the striatum and the capsula extrema, in each of which important pathways run.

The brain is supplied by numerous blood vessels. The four **main arteries** are the left and right internal carotid arteries and the right and left vertebral arteries. The vertebral arteries form the basilar artery, which in turn feeds the cerebral arterial circle (also known as the circle of Willis) inside the skull (frequent location of aneurysms, etc.). The term carotid T for the intracranial part of the internal carotid artery with its branching into the middle cerebral artery and anterior cerebral artery is commonly used in clinical practice and is particularly important in the acute diagnosis of stroke. The intracranial vessels are divided into segments M1 to M4 for the middle cerebral artery or P1 to P4 for the posterior cerebral artery (each to the next vessel division), and A1 (to the anterior communicating ramus) and A2 for the anterior cerebral artery.

Brain and spinal cord are surrounded by cerebrospinal fluid, which is formed by the choroid plexus.

The spinal cord is about 45 cm long and extends to the 1st/2nd LWK. Like the cerebrum, it is divided into the grey and white matter, which carry different nerve fibers. The spinal nerves, which are responsible for the nervous supply of the neck, trunk and the arms and legs, branch off from the spinal cord.

14.2 Disease Patterns

Christel Vockelmann

14.2.1 Intracranial and Spinal Hemorrhages

Intracranial and intraspinal hemorrhages are described according to their localization. **Epidural hemorrhages** can be localized both intraspinally and intracranially between the cranial bone or vertebral body and the dura mater. In the skull in particular, the cause is often a calvaria fracture, which leads to a rupture of the meningeal artery and can thus progress rapidly.

14

❯ Because of its space-occupying nature and potentially rapid progression, epidural hematoma is a neurologic or neurosurgical emergency.

Subdural hemorrhages (SDH = subdural hematoma) often occur post-traumatically between the dura mater and the arachnoid with any necessary relief. In older people in particular, even a trivial trauma is sufficient to lead to rupture of the bridging veins (◘ Fig. 14.1).
   Subarachnoid hemorrhage (◘ Fig. 14.2) can occur with aneurysm rupture.

❯ A history of falls should not deter one from looking for an aneurysm in the basal cisterns in a SAB, as the patient may have fallen due to the aneurysm rupture.

An important sign is the accumulation of blood in the basal cisterns with punctum maximum around the aneurysm. Another cause is a post-traumatic SAB, which is then not localized basally.

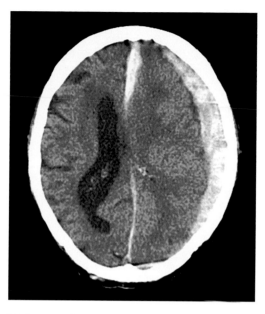

◘ **Fig. 14.2**   Subarachnoid hemorrhage on CT scan

Intracerebral hemorrhage (ICB), when localized in the basal ganglia (◘ Fig. 14.3) or pons, is usually hypertensive in origin; when localized elsewhere, reasons for ICB must be sought. Possible causes are:
- Arteriovenous malformations,
- Cavernomas,
- Intracerebral tumors or metastases,
- Sinus vein thrombosis (bleeding in the neighborhood of the thrombosed sinus).

◘ Table 14.1 shows the main distinguishing features.

■ Clinic

Epidural and subdural hematomas become clinically obvious mainly because of increasing headache; a history of trauma and possibly medication with anticoagulants or antiplatelet agents suggest hemorrhage. SAB is characterized by a thunderclap headache of unknown severity. Typically, aneurysm ruptures affect younger people who report physical exertion before symptom onset. ICB results in neurological deficits similar to ischemic stroke, matching the affected portion of the neurocranium.

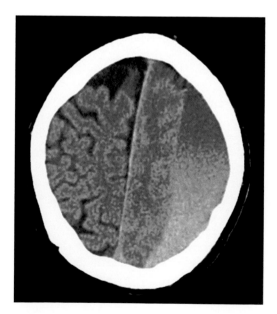

◘ **Fig. 14.1**   Subdural hematoma on multiple CT scans

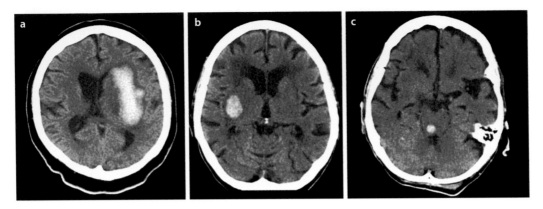

□ Fig. 14.3   Intracerebral hemorrhage on CT. **a** Basal ganglia on left. **b** Basal ganglia on right. **c** Pons

□ Table 14.1   Differentiation of hematoma localization

	Epidural Hematoma	Subdural Hematoma	Subarachnoid Hemorrhage
Anamnesis	Acute trauma	Often insidious onset with trauma that has already occurred some time ago	Thunderclap headache after physical exertion
Patients concerned	Any age	Rather older patients	Often younger patients
Localization	Often temporoparietal	Frontoparietal, often along the falx or tentorium	Basal cisterns → aneurysm rupture, parietal/occipital → rather traumatic
Form	Biconvex, does not exceed the cranial sutures, does not respect the falx	Concave crescent-shaped, exceeds the cranial sutures	Along the gyri and sulci of the brain surface

14

■ **Diagnostics**

CT

The method of first choice is the cranial CT, with which an acute hemorrhage can be sensitively detected or excluded. In case of SAB in the basal ganglia, CT angiography should be performed immediately to detect an aneurysm. With increasing duration of SAB, vascular spasms occur, which make aneurysm detection difficult or impossible.

MRI

MRI is necessary in the further work-up of atypical ICB with then blood-sensitive sequences and angiographic procedures. It is important to detect **CSF congestion**, e.g., due to dilatation of the temporal horns by entrapment or hemorrhage infiltration into the ventricular system. In these cases, neurosurgical relief must be performed.

Spinal hemorrhages are usually poorly recognizable on CT; in this case, MRI is necessary at an early stage with appropriate sequence selection (hemorrhage-sensitive sequences, T1s fat-saturated).

Intracranial hemorrhages change their characteristics on imaging over the course of days and weeks (□ Table 14.2). Because of the changes with T1-weighted signal enhancement on MRI, an MRI should be performed within a maximum of three days for atypical intracerebral hemorrhages to detect contrast enhancement.

◻ Table 14.2 Temporal changes in imaging

	CT	MRI Compared to White Matter		
		T1w	**T2w**	**T2*w**
Peracute (0–24 h)	Hyperdens (cA. 50 HU)	Isointens	Slightly hyperintense	Slightly hypointense
Acute (1–3 days)	Hyperdens (cA. 50 HU)	Slightly hypointense	Greatly hypointense	Hypointens
Early subacute (3–7 days)	Slowly deflating	Strongly hyperintensive	Strongly hyperintensive	Hypointens
Late subacute (7–14 days)	Increasingly isodens	Strongly hyperintensive	Strongly hyperintensive	Hypointens
Chronic (>14 days)	Hypodense to liquorisodense. If applicable calcifications	Central isointense, slightly hypointense rim	Central slightly hyperintense, margins strongly hypointense	Greatly hypointense

14.2.2 Ischemic Diseases

A lack of blood supply to the brain is the most frequent cause of **stroke**, accounting for about 70%. The incidence is 130/1,00,000 inhabitants. After myocardial infarction and tumor disease, stroke is the third most frequent cause of death. The cause is often arteriosclerotic vascular disease of the extracranial vessels supplying the brain, followed by embolic occlusions. In younger patients, inflammatory changes of the vessels or sinus vein thrombosis may lead to stroke.

Ischemic myelon infarction is rare overall. A typical cause may be aortic dissection. Myelon infarction is feared as a complication after surgical or interventional procedures on the aorta.

▪ Clinic

A classic symptom is brachiofacial hemiparesis of the contralateral half of the body. Dizziness and visual disturbances or cranial nerve failures may also be symptoms of an acute stroke. Prodromes are, for example, amaurosis fugax or TIA symptoms, i.e. a transient ischemic attack.

▪ Diagnostics
CT

An acute stroke is, comparable to a heart attack, an absolute emergency that requires immediate imaging. In this case, the native cranial CT is the first elementary component due to its speed and high availability. If there is no hemorrhage (hyperdens with density values around cA. 50 HU) and no demarcated infarct (hypodense, missing gray-white differentiation, edema), an intravenous lysis therapy is started directly in the appropriate clinic. Time is brain! Every minute saved improves the patient's prognosis.

Perfusion Imaging

The native CT is usually supplemented by perfusion imaging (section computed tomography) with which large infarct areas that can no longer be saved even by immediate therapy and areas that are threatened but can still be saved can be detected, even if no infarct is yet demarcated in the native image.

CT Angiography

The third pillar is CT angiography to find intra- or extracranial occlusions. Acute thrombotic occlusion of the middle cerebral artery or internal carotid artery is recanalized by interventional techniques similar to those used in myocardial infarction (Sect. 14.4.1).

MRI

Diagnosis of ischemic diseases of the neurocranium and myelon is performed in MRI. The classic constellation here is **signal enhancement in diffusion weighting** with **signal depression in ADC**, which is already present in the peracute stage. With increasing time, **edema with signal enhancement in T2w sequences** then develops (◻ Fig. 14.4).

This edema has its peak approximately between the 3rd to 5th day. In the further course, the necrosis zone is organized with glioses and cystic formations. This process can be well traced on imaging with a regressing diffusion disorder and increasing glioses (CT: hypodense to the parenchyma; MRI: hyperintense in the FLAIR, T1 hypointense) and cystic formations (CT and MRI liquorisodense and -isointense, respectively, ◻ Fig. 14.4).

The localization and extent of an infarct allow conclusions to be drawn about its genesis. Thus, territorial (embolic) infarcts are assigned to the supply area of the intracranial vessels. Border zone infarcts are localized in the transition zones between the supply areas and are hemodynamically caused. Lacunar infarcts are of microangiopathic origin (◻ Fig. 14.5).

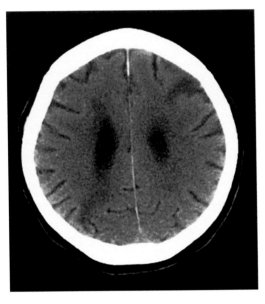

◻ **Fig. 14.5** Anterior border zone infarct on the left and posterior border zone infarct on the right in the native CT scan

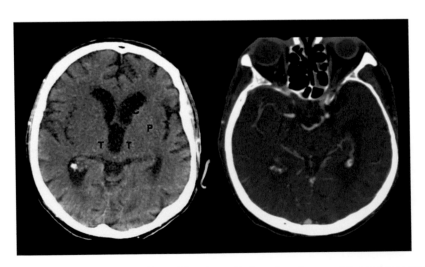

◻ **Fig. 14.4** CT-native and CT-A with blunted basal ganglia (caput nucleus caudatus and putamen/pallidum on the left with occlusion of the middle cerebral artery in the M1 segment—arrow)

14.2.3 Intracerebral Tumors

The classification of brain tumors is based on the WHO classification (■ Table 14.3). This reflects the degree of malignancy of the tumors.

In addition, there are other tumors, some of which have typical localizations and age peaks. In the end, the clear image-morphological assignment is often not successful.

In adults, **metastases** occur more frequently than brain tumors (■ Fig. 14.7). Here, in addition to intracerebral metastasis, **meningeal carcinomatosis** or **intramedullary metastasis** is increasingly common. Characteristic imaging shows melanoma metastases and frequently also metastases of renal cell carcinoma, both of which can be delineated **hyperdense** on **CT** and **native T1-weighted hyperintense** on **MRI**.

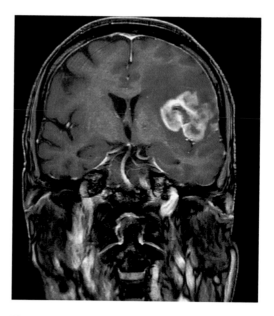

■ **Fig. 14.6** Glioblastoma (coronary T1, contrast enhanced)

■ **Table 14.3** Classification of brain tumors according to WHO

Grade	Description	Example
I	Benign tumors that can potentially be cured by surgical removal	Craniopharyngeoma, pilocytic astrocytoma or neurinomas and schwannomas
II	Infiltrative tumors, histologically benign, frequently recurrent	Oligodendroglioma, diffuse growing astrocytoma
III	Malignant tumors with reduction of survival time	Anaplastic astrocytoma, plexus carcinoma
IV	Very malignant tumors with a significant reduction in survival time	Glioblastoma (■ Fig. 14.6), medulloblastoma

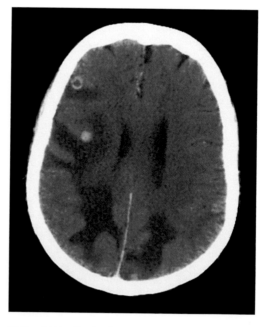

■ **Fig. 14.7** Cerebral metastases bds. with annular enhancement and finger-shaped edema in contrast-enhanced CT

■ Clinic

The symptomatology of cerebral masses depends on the localization of the finding.

For example, a mass in the frontal brain may be accompanied by a change in the patient's personality. Other symptoms are stroke-like symptoms or a seizure.

Cerebral metastasis can also be the first symptomatic manifestation of a tumor, and the first look should then be at the lung as the most common organ of origin.

In contrast, in the absence of a tumor history, a primary tumor is more likely to be assumed in the case of a myelon mass; if myelon metastases occur, the tumor is usually already known.

■ Diagnostics
CT

Often the first diagnosis is a cranial CT scan due to stroke-like symptoms or a seizure. Here, a **hypodense "finger-shaped" edema** can be detected, which mostly respects the cortex. The space-occupying character can be delimited by a **constriction of the cerebrospinal fluid spaces.**

MRI

Further imaging then requires the administration of a contrast agent, although this can also be performed as part of a complementary MRI diagnosis. The **finger-shaped edema** can also be delineated on MRI. To allow contrast passage through the blood-brain barrier, imaging should be performed no earlier than 5 min after contrast administration. On the basis of the localization, the age of the patient, any calcifications in the CT and the contrast medium accumulation, a tentative diagnosis of the type of mass can be made. If necessary, this can be reinforced by MR spectroscopy, but ultimately a definite statement about the type of tumor is not always possible. Cerebral metastasis is indicated by the presence of several contrast-enhancing lesions.

An important differential diagnosis (◻ Table 14.4) to intracerebral tumor is **abscess**, which is classically characterized by marked **hyperintense signaling** in the diffusion.

❯ Signal enhancement of a space involvement in the diffusion weighting is indicative of an intracerebral abscess!

14

▣ **Table 14.4** DD of selected brain tumors

	Frequent localization	Frequency of all primary brain tumors	Age and gender distribution	Tumor grading	Imaging
Astrocytoma	Supratentorial	9%	30–60 LJ M > w	II + III	With increasing de-differentiation, increasing KM enhancement, surrounding finger-shaped edema
Glioblastoma multiforme (=astrocytoma grade IV)	Cerebral hemispheres, bars (butterfly glioblastoma)	20%	50TH–70TH LJ M > w	IV	Severe KM enhancement, garland-shaped, extensive necrosis and hemorrhage
Oligodendroglioma	Frontal brain, basal ganglia	4%	40TH–60TH LJ M > w	II + III	In 2/3 of the cases, extensive scaly calcifications, little surrounding edema, KM uptake depending on the grading (II or III)
Ependymoma	Proximity to the ventricular system	<0.5%	Children and adolescents, 30–40 LJ	Variable	Inhomogeneous KM enhancement, no perifocal edema; caution: drip metastases
Primary CNS lymphoma	–	Rarely	For immunocompetence 50–60th year, for immuno-incompetence earlier		On CT often hyperdense due to cell richness, on MRI isocense in T1w and T2w with homogeneous KM enhancement
Pilocytic astrocytoma	Infratentorial	0.3%	1st–2nd cent of life; m > w		Large cystic tumor portion with vigorous KM-absorbing node
Medulloblastoma	Infratentorial	Rarely	1st decade of life	IV	Inhomogeneous tumor of the cerebellum, hemorrhages, frequent infiltration of the ventricular system, drip metastases
Colloid cyst	Third ventricle, foramen monroi…	<2%	Mostly between 20 and 40 LJ, m > w	Benign	CT: Hyperdense, smooth bordered in 3rd ventricle; variable on MR, T1w usually hyperintense, usually no enhancement

14.2.4 Cerebrospinal Fluid Circulation Disorder

Common to all cerebral space-occupying lesions is the risk of cerebrospinal fluid circulation disturbance, i.e. congestion of the ventricular system. This can be caused supra as well as infratentorially by an entrapment of the parenchyma at the tentorium, falx or foramen magnum. Obstruction of interventricular foramen or aqueduct in hemorrhage also results in CSF circulatory obstruction.

■ Clinic

The classic symptom is headache. Often the examination of the fundus of the eye reveals a congestion papilla.

■ Diagnostics

CT/MRI

The most important imaging procedure is the CT. Further clarification takes place in the MRI. In both procedures, the **widening of the cerebrospinal fluid spaces** and, if necessary, the cause for this can be detected.

> ❯ An early sign of a cerebrospinal fluid circulation disorder is a widening (>3 mm) of the temporal horns.

14.2.5 Intracranial Extraaxial Tumors

In addition to cerebral tumors (synonym: intraaxial tumor), meningioma is a frequent finding in neurocranial imaging. This usually benign tumor originates from the meninges and displaces the adjacent brain parenchyma.

Other extraaxial rare tumors are the epidermoid, schwannomas especially of the vestibulocochlear nerve ("acoustic neuroma") or tumors of the pituitary gland.

■ Clinic

Mostly incidental finding. Symptoms usually occur only with very large meningiomas. Acoustic neuroma is characterized by tinnitus, dizziness and a disturbance in sound perception.

■ Diagnostics

CT

Classical is besides the convex contour to the cranial dome with a protrusion to the dura, the so-called **dural tail**, a very strong, early and homogeneous contrast enhancement. The blood supply of a meningioma is via branches of the external carotid artery, and the contrast enhancement does not have to cross the blood-brain barrier. In addition, meningiomas are frequently calcified.

Meningiomas can occur anywhere on the meninges, although spinal meningiomas are very rare (◘ Fig. 14.8).

A special case of meningioma is malignant meningioma, which exerts pressure on the adjacent brain parenchyma and becomes symptomatic accordingly.

Acoustic neuromas show a strong contrast enhancement of the partly very small tumors. Larger findings may lead to a widening of the internal acoustic meatus with an "ice cream cone"-like configuration of the tumor.

> ❯ In the case of space occupying lesions in the cerebellopontine angle, three diagnoses must be considered: meningioma, acoustic neuroma (=wannoma) and epidermoid tumor. The differential diagnosis is made in MRI with KM sequences and diffusion weighting (the epidermoid shows a strong diffusion restriction with signal enhancement).

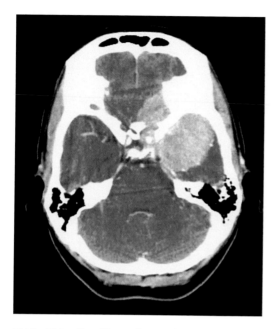

Fig. 14.8 Cuneiform wing meningioma on the left with strong contrast enhancement on CT

14.2.6 Cystic Intracranial Lesions

As with tumors, it must first be decided whether the finding is intrecerebral or intracranial but not originating in the brain. The most common lesion is the **arachnoid cyst**, a cyst often in the middle cranial fossa that displaces the brain but is not space-occupying. More rarely, cysts are intracerebral, such as a **neuroepithelial cyst**. In this case, the presence of a cystic mass or a cerebral infection must always be considered in the differential diagnosis. **Virchow-Robin spaces** are protrusions of the subarachnoid space around vessels, which appear as intracranial cysts. The most frequent localization is the basal ganglia, where the cysts develop along the lenticulostriatal branches of the middle cerebral artery. Differential diagnosis is a lacunar infarction in the basal ganglia.

■ Clinic

Most often it is an asymptomatic incidental finding. Large arachnoid cysts may occasionally cause intracranial pressure symptoms.

■ Diagnostics
CT/MRI

CT and MRI with liquorisodense and -isointense imaging, respectively. The arachnoid cyst displaces the adjacent brain parenchyma without signal alterations. No contrast enhancement.

Neuroepithelial cysts are often located supratentorially adjacent to the lateral ventricles.

14.2.7 Chronic Inflammatory CNS Processes: Multiple Sclerosis

The most common chronic inflammatory CNS disease is multiple sclerosis (MS). Often optic neuritis is the first symptom with no pathological findings on imaging. MS is a demyelinating disease in which MS plaque forms with destruction of myelin due to etiologically unclear inflammation. The disease mostly affects younger patients between 20 and 40 years of age. In most cases, the disease progresses in relapses. Glucocorticoids are used as therapy during the relapse.

■ Clinic

In about 1/4 of the cases, optic neuritis ("The patient sees nothing, the doctor sees nothing!") is the initial symptom. Sensory disturbances, weakness of the extremities or even a loss of sensitivity in the supply area of the trigeminal nerve are further symptoms.

■■ Diagnostics
CT

In addition to imaging, CSF puncture is obligatory in the suspected diagnosis of MS. The CT shows **hypodense areas of** the white matter only in advanced disease, which are not distinguishable from a pronounced microangiopathic damage of the brain.

MRI

MRI of the neuroaxis shows typical changes, but imaging alone cannot prove MS. Typical findings are **highly oval T2w**

hyperintense demyelinating foci periventricu-
larly, which then show a cockscomb-like
appearance in the sagittal image. Other typical findings include juxtacortically located
lesions and distribution supra- and infratentorially (this includes a spinal manifestation). The lesions are T1w frequently
hypointense (so-called "black holes")
(◻ Fig. 14.9). Temporal dissemination (corresponding to the relapsing course of the disease) can be evidenced by KM-receiving
lesions (typically not completely annular but
horseshoe-shaped) or new lesions at least one
month after symptomatology (◻ Table 14.5).

An important differential diagnosis in a
clinic similar to MS is acute disseminated
encephalomyelitis (ADEM), which causes
similar lesions in the CNS, but here all
lesions have the same stage.

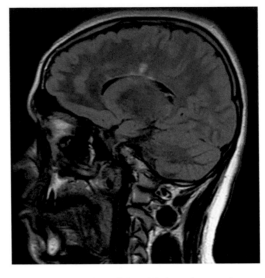

◻ **Fig. 14.9** Sagittal flair with hyperintense demyelinating foci around the corpus callosum

◻ **Table 14.5** McDonald criteria for spatial dissemination (at least three criteria for radiological diagnosis)

At least nine 2w hyperintense lesions	At least one infratentorial lesion (also located in the myelon)	At least one juxtacortical lesion	At least three periventricular lesions and evidence of temporal dissemination
Dissemination over time			
KM-absorbing focus at least three months after initial symptoms		Evidence of a new lesion T2w, at least 30 days after symptomatology	

14.2.8 Acute Inflammatory CNS Processes

This includes the following processes:
- **ADEM**: Rare disease with symptoms typical of MS, but monophasic.
- **Encephalitis**: Infection of the brain with various pathogens. Occurs frequently as meningoencephalitis derived from inflammatory processes, e.g. of the sinuses or mastoids. Typical manifestation in herpes encephalitis (type I, herpes simplex) in the temporal lobes and the limbic system. Important differential diagnosis for this is paraneoplastic limbic encephalitis with a similar pattern of distribution. This occurs most frequently in bronchial carcinoma as the primary tumor.
- **Abscess**: circumscribed melting inflammatory process, often derived from sinusitis or due to hematogenous dissemination. Common in immunocompromised patients.

Ultimately, almost all pathogens can also affect the CNS. These include, for example, **neurocysticercosis** due to infestation with the pork tapeworm, **toxoplasmosis** and **tuberculosis**. It is important to assess all clinical and imaging findings in order to arrive at the correct diagnosis.

- Clinic

The classic symptom of meningitis is neck stiffness combined with headache. Other symptoms depend on the severity and localization of the disease. Immunocompromised patients in particular are more frequently affected by encephalitis.

- Diagnostics

MRI (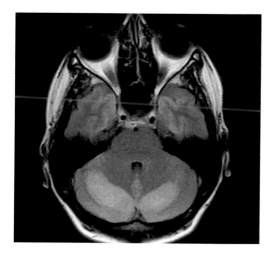 **Fig. 14.10)**

In the case of encephalitis or meningoencephalitis, the cerebrospinal fluid (CSF) puncture is a very important diagnostic tool for detecting cells and possibly also a germ

□ **Fig. 14.10** Cerebellitis with hyperintense, relatively symmetrical signal elevations in the flair in the cerebellum bds

in the CSF. Imaging often shows normal findings on MRI in encephalitis. If changes are detectable, it is often **edema with signal elevations T2w** and possibly **KM enhancement**. If there are corresponding changes in the limbic system, herpes simplex encephalitis or limbic encephalitis must be considered. Parasitic infections often show **calcifications** in later stages. A cerebral abscess shows a **marginal KM enhancement** with **central fluid**. For the differential diagnostic differentiation from a tumor the diffusion is important, which shows a strong diffusion restriction with a strongly hyperintense signal.

14.2.9 Epilepsy

Epilepsy is characterized by the repeated occurrence of seizures. If these seizures are primarily generalized and affect the whole brain, there are often genetic causes. In the case of focally initiated seizures, there is often local damage to the brain. Therefore, it is important to know the possible localization of the damage during imaging.

Tumors, infarcts or bleeding can be the cause of epilepsy. More difficult to detect are anlage disorders. The most common are **heterotopia**, i.e. scattered grey matter that has not migrated to the cortex, and **focal dysplasia**, a developmental disorder with a blurring of the medullary-cortical boundary or disturbances in the grey matter. Another disorder in the setting of epilepsy is **hippocampal sclerosis** (also known as ammonic horn sclerosis). Etiologically unclear, the disease leads to nerve cell destruction of the hippocampus.

■ Clinic

Depending on the location of the damage, the picture of epilepsy is very diverse. From the classic seizure with twitching of extremities to sensory disturbances and absences, other symptoms can also occur in the course of a seizure.

■ Diagnostics

CT

CT is the rapidly available method for the first seizure that can rule out bleeding or a tumor as the cause.

MRI

Further imaging takes place in the MRI. Causes, such as old infarcts or tumors, are often already clear after computed tomography. In the case of malformations such as heterotopia or focal dysplasia, thin-slice sequences are required both T1w and as flair sequences in order to be able to detect the malformation here.

Hippocampal sclerosis can be well delineated in coronal images as a **reduction in volume of a hippocampus** with **enlargement of the adjacent temporal horn. In** addition, there is a **signal enhancement in T2w or better flair sequences**.

14.2.10 Phacomatoses

Phacomatoses are neurocutaneous syndromes, i.e. diseases involving the skin and nervous system. They are based on certain genetic defects, which are often inherited in an autosomal-dominant manner. The most common is neurofibromatosis type 1 Recklinghausen's disease). Typical are café-au-lait spots of the skin and neurofibromas, especially optic gliomas. In neurofibromatosis type 2, the leading feature is acousticus schwannomas. Bilateral acoustic schwannomas are sufficient to establish a diagnosis of neurofibromatosis type 2. Tuberous sclerosis (Bourneville-Pringle disease) also belongs to the phacomatoses. Classically, subependymal nodules, cortical tuberosities, hypomelanotic patches of the skin as well as angiomyolipomas of the kidney and also rhabdomyomas of the heart as well as giant cell astrocytomas are found. These are mostly located in the area of the foramina monroi and belong to WHO grade I tumors. Sturge-Weber syndrome is an angiomatosis, mainly in the supply area of the trigeminal nerve. Such angiomas are also found intracerebrally. Another phacomatosis is Von Hippel-Lindau disease. The disease is characterized by cerebral hemangioblastomas. In addition, renal cell carcinomas, but also renal cysts, pheochromocytomas and cystadenomas of the testis occur frequently in these patients.

■ Clinic

Neurofibromatosis type 1 and also Sturge-Weber syndrome and tuberous sclerosis are usually manifested in childhood. Neurofibromatosis type 2 and Von Hippel-Lindau disease are often diagnosed in young adulthood. The clinic is characterized by the skin changes and the corresponding affected structures of the nervous system.

■ Diagnostics

MRI

Neurofibromas, which include optic gliomas and acoustic schwannomas, can be **homogeneously** delineated on MRI **with a strong KM enhancement.** Large acoustic neuromas lead to a **dilatation of the internal** acoustic meatus. The image occasionally resembles an ice cream cone in large acoustic neuromas.

14.2.11 Neurodegenerative Diseases

The brain is subject to a natural aging process with a degradation of brain substance as well as iron deposition in the basal ganglia. However, certain neurodegenerative diseases present a relatively typical pattern of findings on MRI, so that MRI is performed as standard for the clarification of neurodegenerative diseases (■ Fig. 14.11). Important differential diagnostic criteria are shown in ■ Table 14.6.

> Every dementia should be clarified once with a sectional image diagnosis of the neurocranium, in order to exclude e.g. tumors or a normal pressure hydrocephalus as a cause.

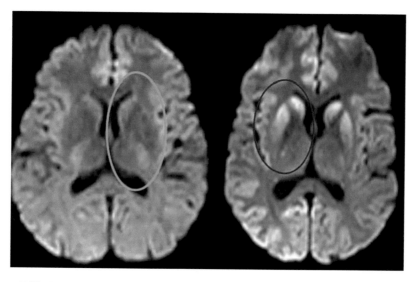

■ **Fig. 14.11** Diffusion enhancement (right image) in the basal ganglia in Creutzfeldt-Jakob disease, for comparison normal findings on the left

■ **Table 14.6** Differential diagnosis of different neurodegenerative diseases

	Clinic	Diagnostics
M. Alzheimer	Short-term memory impairment, no delirium, existing > six months, onset at mean 70th year	Temporally accentuated atrophy, atrophy of the hippocampus
Vascular dementia	Abrupt onset, history of stroke, other neurological deficits	Pronounced microangiopathy, infarcts with involvement of both thalami and/or temporomesial structures
Multisystem atrophy	Parkinson-like symptoms, additional e.g. orthostatic dysregulation, micturition disorder, impotence	Atrophy putamen and/or olivopontocerebellar, hot cross bun sign (hyperintense cross figure in bridge foot in T2w)
Frontotemporal lobar degeneration	Behavioral problems, change of character	Unilateral frontotemporal atrophy

(continued)

◾ Table 14.6 (continued)

	Clinic	Diagnostics
Normal pressure hydrocephalus	Triad of gait disorder, dementia and urinary incontinence	Dilatation of the ventricular system; sample liquor puncture
M. Parkinson	Onset with unilateral rigor, tremor and hypokinesia	Mostly normal findings; possibly changes in the iron content of the substantia nigra, atrophy of the hippocampus
Creutzfeld-Jakob disease	Rapid dementia, myoclonia...	Flair and diffusion with signal enhancement of the basal ganglia and/or cortex
Progressive supranuclear paralysis	Parkinson's-like symptoms	Mesencephalic atopy (Mickey mouse character)
Huntington's chorea	Excessive movements (choreatic hyperkinesia)	Bilateral atrophy of the nucl. caudatus (coronary T1w), also putamen and globus pallidus
Wernicke's encephalopathy	Brain-organic psychosyndrome, unsteadiness of gait and stance, eye movement disorders	Atrophy or KM uptake of the corpora mamillaria

14.3 Diagnostics

14.3.1 Diagnostic Radiology

Sonography

Sonography is used in newborns as the primary diagnostic tool for assessing the neurocranium. In adults, access for the sound waves through the cranial dome is very limited. Here, sonography is used as transcranial Doppler sonography for the assessment of the intracranial vessels, often supplemented by CT or MR angiography.

Conventional X-ray Diagnostics

Conventional X-ray diagnostics of the brain skull are no longer performed. One of the last indications is the position control of a valve in certain VP shunts before or after MRI examinations.

Fluoroscopy/Angiography

Angiographic examinations are used to clarify intracerebral vascular processes such as AV malformations or aneurysms and, increasingly, to treat these interventions. Coils, i.e. small metal spirals, are used to fill aneurysms.

Computed Tomography (CT)

CT is the method of choice for almost all emergency indications for imaging of the neurocranium. CT can reliably detect or rule out hemorrhage. Also, most tumors that have become symptomatic can already be detected with a CT. Since the lenses of the eye are very sensitive to radiation, the layers in the CT of the head are angulated at the base of the skull. This ensures that the lenses of the eye are not in the direct radiation field.

In acute stroke, a so-called lysis protocol is generally used today. First, a native CT of the head is performed. After exclusion of hemorrhage, intravenous lysis therapy can be initiated if indicated. In addition, a CT perfusion and a CT angiography of the supra-aortic vessels are performed. In the case of large infarctions, the CT perfusion can be used to estimate how much infarction is imminent and how much tissue can still be saved. This is achieved by evaluating repeated images of the brain during a contrast medium run, which allows parameters such as blood volume and blood flow in the various parts of the brain to be calculated. CT angiography then reveals stenoses or occlusions of the vessels so that, if necessary, therapy can also be initiated immediately with interventional reopening of the vessels.

Magnetic Resonance Imaging (MRI)

MRI with its high soft tissue contrast is ideally suited for clarifying the neurocranium. Here, the examination protocol, which always consists of several sequences, must be adapted to the question. When asking for fresh infarcts, a diffusion measurement must be performed. For the question of old infarctions, T2w sequences are performed, which are susceptible to susceptibility artifacts (T2* or SWI). Sagittal flair sequences, with which the configuration of the demyelinating foci can be well delineated, are helpful in the clarification of MS. Contrast medium, which is detectable in T1w sequences, is required for the clarification of tumors and metastases, but also inflammatory processes.

14.3.2 Nuclear Medicine

Ursula Blum

Brain

Blood Flow, Regional Cerebral Blood Flow (RCBF)

Regional cerebral blood flow (rCBF) can be visualized using various tracers. The questions range from focal imaging in epilepsy, psychiatric diseases, a statement about the perfusion reserve of the brain in previous TIA's to brain death diagnostics.

Different areas of the brain are of particular interest for different questions, e.g.

the search for a focus in epileptic seizures or the identification of the speech or visual center before a planned operation.

There are ^{99m}Tc-ECD (ethyl cysteinate dimer) and ^{99m}Tc-HMPAO (hexamethylpropenylene aminooxime) available. Both substances are almost equivalent.

ECD is used in questions about surviving brain tissue after a cerebral infarction because it does not accumulate in brain cells that are still perfused but dead. Another domain of ECD is inflammation diagnostics. In addition, the contrast between gray and white brain matter, especially in the temporal lobe, is better than with HMPAO.

Other possibilities for the determination and visualization of rCBF lie in PET.

For this purpose, ^{15}O labelled water ($H_2^{15}O$) or ^{15}O-butanol can be used. However, these products have a very short half-life of 2 min, so that a cyclotron must be available in the immediate vicinity.

Since rCBF is associated with regional sugar metabolism, ^{18}F-FDG can also be used.

Normal findings depend on the age of the patient. Normally, the accumulation in the gray matter is 2–3 times higher than in the white matter.

In **epilepsy diagnostics,** the radiopharmaceutical is injected during the seizure (under EEG monitoring, if possible within 10 s), and the image is then recorded in the phase after the seizure. During the seizure, the focus is stronger than the surrounding brain tissue (hyperperfused), while in the seizure-free interval it is usually weakened (hypoperfused).

In the case of **reduced** cerebral perfusion in the context of a TIA (transient ischemic attack) or a PRIND (prolonged reversible ischemic neurological deficit), there are usually no conspicuous findings in cross-sectional imaging. In the perfusion examination, a reduction in cerebral perfusion in the affected section of the brain can already be detected.

If vasoconstriction in the brain is suspected, the examination can be performed with additional application of Diamox (1000 mg over 5 min i. v.). This reveals the so-called perfusion reserve of the brain. Diamox dilates the arterioles, and perfusion therefore increases significantly in a healthy state of the vessels. If vasoconstriction is present, the vessels are already maximally dilated, so that increased perfusion cannot occur in these regions. The examination should be performed at the earliest 24 h after a basic scintigraphy.

Dementia is characterized by reduced blood flow in different regions of the brain.

▪ ▪ Forms of Dementia, Localization in the Cerebrum

– Alzheimer's dementia:	Bitemporal and/or biparietal
– Lewy body dementia:	Similar to Alzheimer's disease, additional visual cortex
– Fronto-temporal dementia:	Frontotemporal
– Vascular dementia:	Multiple circumscribed defects

In **brain death diagnostics** (▪ Fig. 14.12), the patient is placed directly on the camera and injected. This is followed by the creation

▪ Fig. 14.12 Brain death diagnosis

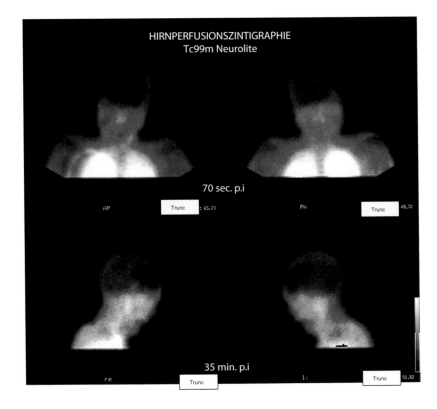

of a dynamic sequence, as well as static images of the skull, thorax (including thyroid and stomach) and, if necessary, a SPECT.

In these patients, the blood-brain barrier is non-functional. There is no accumulation in the brain at all.

The marking must be checked for quality. This check should be carried out according to the kit manufacturer's specifications (e.g. thin layer chromatography).

The images of the thorax must not show any major accumulations in the thyroid gland or stomach. These images also serve as a quality control, but are not sufficient as the sole quality control.

Neurodegenerative Diseases

■ Receptor Scintigraphy

Receptor scintigraphy is used in the diagnosis of Parkinson's disease. Especially in the early stages of the disease, clinical differentiation from other diseases may be difficult. Receptor scintigraphy can be used to distinguish idiopathic Parkinson's disease (PD) from atypical PD syndromes such as multisystem atrophy (MSA), progressive supranuclear gaze palsy (PSP), and corticobasal degeneration (CBD). This distinction is important for the treatment of the disease and the prognosis of the patient.

SPECT tracers such as ^{123}I-benzamide (IBZM) and ^{123}I-ioflupane (FP-CIT), which are commercially available in Germany, are used.

Another decision option is the determination of rCBF by means of ^{18}F-FDG-PET, which can accurately separate the diseases in one examination (Hellwig, Meyer).

PET tracers are ^{18}F-DOPA and ^{18}F-Fallypride.

The tracers differ in the binding site on the receptor system.

Brain Tumors

Brain tumors (gliomas) are characterized by an increase in amino acid transporters. These can be visualized with radioactively labeled amino acids.

Three tracers are currently used, ^{11}C methionine (MET), 3-^{123}I-iodine-α-methyl-L-tyrosine (IMT) and ^{18}F-ethyltyrosine (FET). All tracers have not yet been approved in Germany.

Indications include biopsy planning, determination of the exact extent of the tumor, therapy monitoring and recurrence diagnosis (differentiation between necrosis and tumor).

A statement on the degree of malignancy is not possible. The differentiation between tumor and non-malignant changes or radionecrosis can be made by establishing quotients. Here, the uptake in the tumor tissue is significantly higher than in the other tissues (depending on the tracer cA. 1.5 to 2.2 times increased), in the context of therapy control, the quotient should fall by >10%.

■ Meningiomas

Due to the somatostatin receptors, which are detectable in many meningiomas, these changes can be detected with a somatostatin receptor scintigraphy (111-In-Oxin). Here, the differential diagnosis to an acoustic neuroma is in the foreground.

CSF Space

CSF scintigraphy allows statements to be made about the distribution, circulation, and any leaks or fistulas that may be present. In addition, a statement about the function of existing shunt systems is also possible.

CSF scintigraphy is performed after sterile puncture of the CSF space, usually the lumbar region. Only very rarely is the puncture performed suboccipitally. The patient should remain in bed after the puncture.

If leakage is suspected, tamponade of the nasal cavity is necessary. The tamponades must be weighed before insertion into the nose and after removal. After 24 h the tamponade is removed or changed, here the side indication is very important. The tamponades are measured in the borehole. In addition, a blood sample must be taken in each case, as some of the tracer enters the tamponades even without a fistula. Now the tamponade activity/blood activity quotient is calculated. If this quotient is >2, a fistula is present.

14.3.3 Valence

Christel Vockelmann

◘ Table 14.7 shows the use of the respective therapeutic options depending on the problem

◘ **Table 14.7** Value of the therapeutic procedures

	Sonography	Conventional	Fluoroscopy/ Angiography	CT	MRI	Nuk	PET
Acute stroke	N	N	W	P	W	N	N
Dementia assessment	N	N	N	P	W	W	N
Brain death diagnostics	N	N	W	N*	W	P	N

N Not indicated, *P* Primary diagnosis, *W* Further diagnosis

N* Of course, every patient who is diagnosed with brain death will receive a computer tomography of the skull. However, this cannot be used to diagnose brain death

14

14.4 Therapy

14.4.1 Interventional Radiology

Christel Vockelmann

Angiographic Interventions

In acute occlusions of the proximal middle cerebral artery with corresponding stroke symptoms, the thrombus that led to the vessel occlusion is removed with special suction catheters and stent retrievers. For this purpose, the internal carotid artery of the affected side is probed via a femoral access route. Via a long sluice, i.e. a working channel, the occluded vessel is visited and probed with a microcatheter. The thrombus is then removed by aspiration. Alternatively or complementarily, the vessel is first released by stent implantation. In this case, the thrombus is initially only pushed to the side. After a few minutes, the inserted stent, in which the thrombus has then lodged, is removed together with the thrombus.

Symptomatic stenoses of the internal carotid artery, which are typically located close to the origin, should be treated within 14 days after the initial event such as a TIA, since the risk of a further event such as a large infarction in the area supplied by the middle cerebral artery is significantly increased. The primary procedure is surgery of the stenosis, indications for interventional therapy by means of stent angioplasty are restenosis after surgery, postradiogenic stenosis or unfavorable anatomical conditions such as a very short neck or a high division of the carotid artery. For **stent angioplasty,** a transfemoral approach with insertion of a long sheath into the common carotid artery is also performed. Often, a wire-guided filter system is then first inserted into the internal carotid artery above the stenosis to prevent possible intracranial emboli caused by detached plaque materials during the course of the intervention. The filter wire is then usually used for pre-dilation before a stent is inserted. This is inserted as

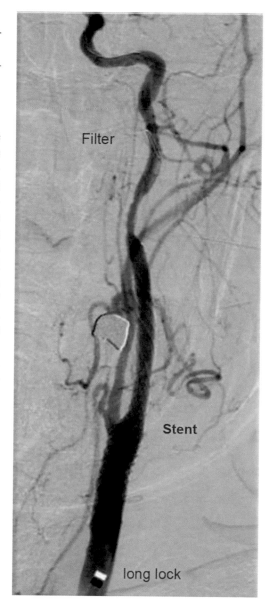

☐ **Fig. 14.13**   Carotid stent

a bifurcation-bridging stent from the ACI to the ACC, with the external carotid artery being stented over (☐ Fig. 14.13). After postdilation, the filter is then recaptured via a retrieval system and the procedure can be terminated. To avoid a vasovagal reaction due to the dilatations—comparable to an external carotid pressure—0.5 mg atropine is applied i. v. before each dilation.

14.4.2 Radiotherapy

If a tumor can be treated surgically, it is usually removed by neurosurgery and, if there are residual findings, irradiated with or without chemotherapy.

The following are used
- **Stereotaxy** (e.g. for 1–3 brain metastases) or the
- **Proton therapy** (e.g. for chordomas, chondrosarcomas)

■ Side Effects

Appetite or sleep disturbances, optic nerve in a stereotaxy >15 Gy → visual impairment in about 1/3 d. F., acoustic neuroma (vestibular schwannoma) → hearing ability↓.

■ Complications

Radionecrosis (therefore compliance with the absolute doses for the single dose of a maximum of 10 Gy per 10 mL of brain tissue).

Gliomas
Glioblastoma
■ Therapy
- Definitive radiotherapy of the tumor in case of inoperability and always postoperative radiotherapy of the tumor bed. Dose in each case 60 Gy (5×2 Gy/week) or 40.05 Gy (5×2.67 Gy/week).
- Chemotherapy, e.g. with temozolomide, especially patients with an altered DNA repair enzyme MGMT benefit from this.

Astrocytoma

Definitive radiotherapy of the tumor in case of inoperability or postoperative RT of the tumor remnant from WHO grade II. Dose 54–60 Gy each (5×1.8–2.0 Gy/week).

Oligodendroglioma

Definitive radiotherapy of the tumor in case of inoperability or postoperative RT of the tumor remnant in WHO III, dose 54–60 Gy each (5×1.8–2.0 Gy/week).

Skull Base Meningiomas
- Definitive radiotherapy of the meningioma in case of inoperability or postoperative radiotherapy of the residual finding in case of incomplete tumor removal. The 5-year progression-free survival is 40–61% after subtotal surgery and 68–95% with subsequent radiotherapy.

Acoustic Neuromas (Vestibular Schwannomas)
- Radiotherapy of the tumor: The total dose in conventional technique is around 54 Gy (1.8–2 Gy/week). In the case of a small tumor, 12–15 Gy are given stereotactically.

Pituitary Adenoma
- Definitive radiotherapy of the adenoma in case of inoperability or postoperative radiotherapy of the residual findings in case of incomplete tumor removal
- Conventional radiotherapy: 45–50 Gy (5×1.8–2.0 Gy/week)
- Particle therapy for hormone-active pituitary adenoma
- Stereotaxy with $1 \times$ or 3–5×5 Gy for prolactinoma and ACTH-producing adenomas

Chordomas, Chondrosarcomas of the Skull Base
- Conventional RT: 48–66.6 Gy
- Stereotaxy: $1 \times$ 14-16 Gy
- Protons, heavy ions (helium, carbon): 60 CGE–83 CGE

Craniopharyngeomas
- Definitive radiotherapy of the tumor in case of inoperability or in case of residual tumor postoperative RT of the residual tumor, 54 Gy (5×1.8 Gy)
- Stereotaxy and particle therapy

Childhood
Cerebrospinal Fluid Space
Investigations into medulloblastoma have shown that at the time of diagnosis, 25–40% of tumor cells are floating in the CSF, and there is also a higher risk with germ cell tumors. In these cases, the entire CSF space is therefore irradiated.

Whole Brain
In leukemias, the entire brain is irradiated due to the diffuse cell distribution.

Brain Metastases
Therapy for Multiple Brain Metastases
- Multiple brain metastases: Whole brain irradiation

Therapy for 1–3 Brain Metastases
- Surgery, whole brain radiation (increasingly with hippocampal excision and stereotactic therapy of the individual metastases are used individually either solo or in combination).
- Stereotaxy for deeper metastases up to 3 cm in size, irradiated with high single dose, e.g. 1 × 15–24 Gy.

Glioblastoma
In the case of glioblastoma, definitive radiotherapy is given to the tumor if it is inoperable, and always postoperative radiotherapy to the tumor bed. The dose in each case is 60 Gy (5 × 2 Gy/week) or 40.05 Gy (5 × 2.67 Gy/week).

Brain Metastases
- Whole Brain Irradiation.

Case Study

Volker Asmacher, 59, is woken up in the morning by the alarm clock. However, he does not manage to switch off the alarm clock with his right hand. His wife notices that the right corner of his mouth is also hanging down. She immediately calls the emergency doctor. He suspects an acute stroke. Since Mr. Asmacher woke up with the symptoms, the time window, i.e. the exact onset of the symptoms, is unclear. There is a so-called wake-up stroke. Nevertheless, the emergency physician takes the patient to the nearest stroke unit as quickly as possible and also announces the patient there as an acute stroke. Here the patient is received by the neurologist on duty, Dr. Hammer. After a quick anamnesis, Mr. Asmacher is first taken to the CT. The native cranial CT suggests a hyperdense media sign on the left as an indication of a thrombotic occlusion of the cerebral artery, otherwise it is inconspicuous. As the patient is otherwise in a very good general condition, a CT perfusion and a CT angiography are performed in addition. Perfusion imaging shows an area at risk (called tissue at risk or penumbra) in the middle mediastinal flow area, but no demarcated area yet. CT angiography confirms occlusion of the left proximal middle cerebral artery in the M1 segment. Based on the good condition and CT perfusion result, Dr. Hammer discusses with the wife and patient the option of intravenous lysis with rtPA despite the unclear time window. Additionally, Dr. Hammer advises a thrombectomy to quickly reopen the vessel. Both measures are initiated after a few minutes of consideration. In the angiography to which Mr. Asmacher is taken, the occlusion of the left cerebral artery is still present. The thrombus is removed by means of a stent retriever. The symptoms improved rapidly after the operation. Subjectively, Mr. Asmacher is symptom-free again after a few days. The MRI three days later shows only a few small punctiform diffusion disturbances in the supply area of the left cerebral artery. Bleeding due to the lysis therapy did not occur.

Practice Questions
1. How to distinguish an epidural from a subdural hemorrhage?
2. Which localizations of intracerebral hemorrhage are called typical localizations and what is the general cause of these hemorrhages?
3. How can tumor-related edema be distinguished from ischemic edema on native CT?

4. What differential diagnoses should you be aware of for space-occupying lesions in the cerebellopontine angle?

Solutions ▶ Chap. 27

14

Head/Neck

Martina Kahl-Scholz, Christel Vockelmann, Ursula Blum and Guido Heilsberg

Contents

© Springer-Verlag GmbH Germany, part of Springer Nature 2023
M. Kahl-Scholz, C. Vockelmann (eds.), *Basic Knowledge Radiology*,
https://doi.org/10.1007/978-3-662-66351-6_15

This chapter deals with the essential possibilities of radiological diagnostics, nuclear medicine and radiotherapy for diagnostics and therapy in the area of the head and neck. An introductory section provides a brief overview of anatomy and function, and a concluding section includes some practice questions on this topic.

15.1 Anatomical Structures

Martina Kahl-Scholz

Important anatomical structures from the "head/neck" area are above all the paranasal sinuses, the thyroid gland, lymph nodes and salivary glands.

The **paranasal sinuses** are the air-filled spaces in the bones close to the nasal cavity. They correspond to the lightweight principle. The sinuses include the maxillary sinus (Sinus maxillaris), frontal sinus (Sinus frontalis), ethmoidal cells (Cellulae ethmoidales) and sphenoidal sinus (Sinus sphenoidales).

The **major salivary glands** include the parotid gland (glandula parotidea), which is located in front of and behind the ear on the mandible and mastoid process. The excretory duct (ductus parotideus) opens into the oral cavity opposite the upper second molar. Other large salivary glands are the submandibular gland and sublingual gland.

The **minor salivary glands** include the lip glands (glandula labialis), palatal glands (glandula palatinae), cheek glands (glandula buccales) and tongue glands (glandula linguales).

Important components of the pharynx, which consists mainly of muscles important for the act of swallowing, are the tonsils, the thyroid gland and the larynx.

The lymphatic pharyngeal ring consists of several "defense stations", which also include the pharyngeal, palatine and **lingual** tonsils (**tonsilla palatina, pharyngea et lin-**

gualis). The most prominent of these are the palatine tonsils, which are visible in the tonsillar fossa between the two palatine arches.

■ Larynx (Larynx)

The larynx consists of cartilage, ligaments and muscles. Important forming cartilages are the thyroid cartilage (**Cartilago thyroidea**), the **cricoid cartilage (Cartilago cricoidea)** and the articular cartilage (**Cartilago arytenoidea**). The **epiglottis** closes the access to the trachea during swallowing.

The **skull** (cranium) is formed by many individual bones that have grown together in the course of development.

■ Skullcap (Calvaria)

The skullcap is formed by
- Parietal bone (Os parietale)
- Occipital bone (Os occipitale)
- Frontal bone (Os frontale)

These parts are joined together by sutures (sutturae):
- **Sutura coronalis** between frontal and parietal bones
- **Sutura sagitalis** between the two parietal bones
- **Sutura lambdoidea** between parietal bones and occipital bone
- Frontal **sutura**
- **Sutura squamosa** between parietal bone and temporal bone

■ Facial Skull

The facial skull is composed of the following bony parts:
- Frontal bone (Os frontale)
- Nasal bone (Os nasale)
- Sphenoid bone (Os spheniodale)
- Zygomatic bone (Os zygomaticum)
- Ethmoid bone (Os ethmoidale)
- Temporal bone (Os temporale)
- Parietal bone (Os parietale)
- Lacrimal bone (Os lacrimale)

- Upper jaw bone (maxilla)
- Lower jaw bone (mandible)

The **orbit** is formed by the Os sphenoidale, Os ethmoidale, Os lacrimale, Os frontale, Os zygomaticum and Maxilla.

15.2 Disease Patterns

Martina Kahl-Scholz

15.2.1 Head

Sinusitis

This is an acute, sometimes chronic inflammation of the paranasal sinuses (NNH).

■ Clinic

(Persistent) facial and headache, purulent secretion, difficult nasal breathing, tapping

and pressure pain depending on the localization of the inflammation.

■ Diagnostics

Conventional X-ray (◘ Fig. 15.1)
  CT of the NNH (in case of complications or chronic inflammation)
- **Acute** sinusitis: **mucosal wall thickening** in the NNH, mirror/shadow formation of mucous effusions within the NNH
- **Chronic** sinusitis: similar, **possibly with polypous changes of** the mucosa

Mucocele

In the case of a mucocele (◘ Fig. 15.2), cysts form within the paranasal sinuses which cannot empty because the openings in the sinuses are narrowed. If an infection occurs, this is called a pyocele.

■ Clinic

Feeling of pressure, protrosio bulbi, possibly visual disturbances

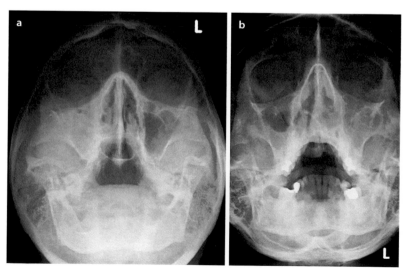

◘ **Fig. 15.1** **a** Sinusitis and **b** Pansinusitis in X-ray image

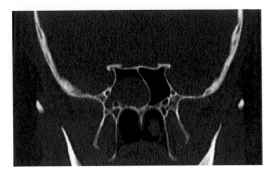

Fig. 15.2 Mucocele of the NNH

■ Diagnostics

Conventional X-ray
  The paranasal sinus is **dilated and shaded**, the **walls thinned** but **not interrupted.**

❯ DD mucocele shadowing vs. tumor shadowing of the NNH: thinning of the wall without destruction in mucocele!

CT Similarly, also extension of the NNH and thinning of the wall visible.

MRI Accumulation of mucous fluid **without enhancement**.

Tumors
Nasopharyngeal Area

These include benign (e.g. nasopharyngeal fibroma, polyp) and malignant (such as nasal pharyngeal carcinoma) space-occupying lesions of the nasopharynx.

■ Clinic
Depending on the size and location of the tumor, various symptoms may occur, such as obstruction of nasal breathing, ear pain, nasal dribbling, etc.

■ Diagnostics

CT/MRI
  For the diagnostic procedure mainly CT and MRI are used for correct differentiation. Noticeable are shadowing in the naso-pharyngeal area and destruction of the bony structures as well as a contrast image in the MRI.

❯ In case of unclear shadowing and bony destruction, think of the possibility of a nasopharyngeal tumor!

Orbit
These include benign (meningioma) or malignant (retinoblastoma) space-occupying lesions in the orbital region.

■ Clinic
Frequent symptoms are the protrusion of the eyeball (exophthalmos), mobility disorders and possibly pain.

■ Diagnostics
Both sonography (first diagnostic step) and CT and MRI are used. There are the following characteristics:
- Retinoblastoma: calcifications
- Optic glioma: dilatation of the optic canal
- Optic meningioma: calcifications around the optic nerve

Salivary Glands
The most common tumor is pleomorphic adenoma.

■ Clinic
Often the tumors remain silent for a long time and do not cause any symptoms. In some cases, only a mass is initially noticeable, sometimes with pressure pain. In the later course, pain, fascial paresis, possibly dry mouth and swelling of the lymph nodes may occur.

■ Diagnostics
Diagnostically, sonography, CT and MRI are used. Most conspicuous are inhomogeneous parenchymal patterns and an enlarged gland.

Sialography   In sialography, which can also be used to visualize salivary stones, the orifice of the respective gland is probed with a fine cannula and filled with KM to enable better visualization in conventional X-rays, CT or MRI.

Fractures
Skull Base

Fractures of the skull base are divided into frontobasal (frontal sinus posterior wall, ethmoid roof, sphenoid sinus) and petrous fractures.

▪ Clinic

The clinic varies depending on the location. Cerebrospinal fluid (CSF) hemorrhages and cranial nerve deficits may occur, while fractures of the temporal bone may lead to injuries of the middle ear with the associated clinical symptoms.

▪ Diagnostics
CT/MRI

CT and MRI are the best way to assess the extent and course of the fracture. Co-injuries to other structures and the entry of air (pneoencephalon) can also be detected in this way.

X-ray

If a skull base fracture is suspected, a CT is primarily indicated today; conventional X-rays are no longer performed in the context of these questions.

Zygomatic Bone

▪ Clinic

Decreased sensation in the supply area of the infraorbital nerve, motility disorders of the bulb and difficulties in opening the mouth may accompany a zygomatic fracture clinically.

▪ Diagnostics
Conventional X-ray

Often, images of the paranasal sinuses (NNH) or so-called bicipital images are taken in order to be able to assess the zygomatic arch. However, CT should be given generous priority, especially if more complex fractures are suspected.

Middle Face

Midface fractures are classified according to LeFort into:
- LeFort I = basal detachment of the maxilla
- LeFort II = pyramidal detachment of the maxilla including the bony nose
- LeFort III = high avulsion of the entire midfacial skeleton including the bony nose

▪ Clinic

Occlusion disorders of the dentition may occur. If the orbit is involved (LeFort II and III), eye mobility may also be restricted and bleeding may occur in the form of a monocular or spectacle hematoma.

▪ Diagnostics
Conventional Radiography

Imaging of the NNH allows assessment of the nasal skeleton, orbital walls, and shadowing/mirroring (hematosinus). A lateral image allows co-assessment of the maxilla, ethmoid cells and sphenoid sinus.

CT

In the case of a LeFort III injury, it is useful to perform a CT scan to assess any structures that may be involved.

Orbital Floor

In the case of an orbital fracture, if the force is applied directly to the eye, a so-called blow-out fracture can occur, in which the orbital floor fractures and orbital contents can enter the maxillary sinus.

▪ Clinic

The mobility of the eyeball, especially the elevation of gaze, may be impeded by entrapment of the muscles. Furthermore, enophthalmos and eyelid emphysema may occur.

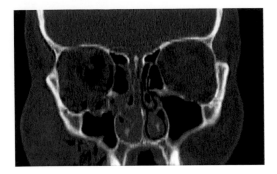

◻ Fig. 15.3   Hanging drop in blow-out fracture

■ Diagnostics
Conventional X-ray/CT/MRI

In all three imaging variants, the so-called "hanging drop" is the specific detection (◻ Fig. 15.3). This refers to the contents of the orbit, which become visible on the maxillary sinus roof.

Attention should be paid to whether a foreign body (depending on the mechanism of the accident) may also be found. In addition, mirror formation in the maxillary sinus, orbital emphysema and shadowing of the ethmoid cells may occur, depending on the localization of the fracture.

15.2.2 Neck

Laryngocele

These congenital dilations of the sacculus laryngis may be air-filled or mucus-filled.

■ Clinic
As a rule, there are no symptoms. In most cases, resistance can already be felt from the outside.

■ Diagnostics
CT/MRI

CT/MRI allows good visualization of a laryngocele as a **hypodense structure.**

Trachelastenosis

This is understood to be the narrowing of the tracheal lumen.

■ Clinic
Respiratory distress, expiratory/inspiratory stridor.

■ Diagnostics
Transillumination

This shows a **lumen variation**.
CT

A stenosis of the trachea can be detected more precisely by means of CT, especially since it is possible to assess directly what is probably causing the narrowing (enlarged thyroid gland, tumorous changes, etc.).

Cervical Cyst

A distinction is made between the lateral (at the anterior border of the sternocleidomastoid muscle) and the median cervical cyst (mainly in the region of the base of the tongue).

■ Clinic
Mostly asymptomatic.

■ Diagnostics
Sonography

This shows an anechoic **lumen**, a **smooth wall structure** and a **distal sound amplification.**
CT

This is only used if sonographic imaging is not possible.

Thyroid Gland

▶ Chapter 21, Endocrinology

Parathyroid Gland

▶ Chapter 21, Endocrinology

Tumors
Laryngeal Carcinoma

In ENT, laryngeal carcinoma is the most common malignant tumor and is most likely localized to the glottis itself.

■ Clinic
This may be silent at first and then, depending on the location, manifest as hoarseness,

foreign body sensation, difficulty swallowing and irritable cough.

■ Diagnostics

CT

A **change in density** in the tumorous tissue and, depending on the extent, **obliteration** (i.e. spreading) of the anatomical fatty tissue layers can be seen. Furthermore, the depth of infiltration and metastases can be detected.

MRI

This can also be used to assess **depth and metastasis.**

Sonography

Sonography is useful to investigate **metastatic spread to the cervical lymph nodes.**

Thyroid Carcinoma

(► Chapter 21)

Salivary Gland Carcinoma

(Section tumors)

15.3 Diagnostics

15.3.1 Diagnostic Radiology

Christel Vockelmann

Sonography

Primary imaging for the examination of the soft tissues of the neck with thyroid gland, salivary glands and lymph nodes is sonography. Color Doppler sonography is also used to assess blood flow.

Conventional X-ray Diagnostics

A typical indication for X-ray diagnostics in the head region is still the X-ray of the paranasal sinuses. As a rule, this is only performed in the occipito-mental beam path. The examination should be performed with the patient in a sitting position, since acute sinusitis leads to fluid levels that cannot be detected in the X-ray image when the patient is lying down.

Conventional radiography plays a minor role in imaging of the neck. One of the few possible indications is lateral imaging of the soft tissues of the neck to assess calcifications and spondylophytes of the cervical spine leading to narrowing of the esophagus.

Fluoroscopy/Angiography

Fluoroscopic examinations of the neck can be performed to assess the pharynx and esophagus, and in particular the swallowing act. Rare indications are visualizations of the lacrimal duct, here if necessary also with the possibility of interventional therapy of stenoses.

Computer Tomography (CT)

Conventional X-ray diagnostics often cannot reliably differentiate between reduced pneumatization and inflammatory shadowing of the paranasal sinuses. Prior to surgical treatment of sinusitis, the ENT physician would often also like to be able to assess the bony anatomy of the paranasal sinuses, as this is highly variable. For example, there are patients in whom the carotid artery runs elongated in the skull base and extends far into the sphenoid sinus with or even without bony cover. The rhinobase, i.e. the bony lamella between the frontal brain and the nose, may also be of varying depth. This is elementarily important information for the surgeon. For this reason, CT scanning of the paranasal sinuses is performed relatively frequently. Since this involves bony structures and soft tissue swelling, i.e. findings that have a high contrast, a low-dose CT of the paranasal sinuses is sufficient for the diagnosis of sinusitis or prior to surgery.

Computed tomography plays a particularly important role in staging examinations for tumor diseases or in acute diagnostics. All soft parts of the neck can be assessed, as well as the neck vessels and bony structures.

Magnetic Resonance Imaging (MRI)

MRI is particularly suitable for diagnosing the soft tissues of the neck due to its high soft tissue contrast. MRI can also be used to assess all soft tissues of the neck, as well as the neck vessels and bony structures. However, in contrast to computed tomography, it is even more necessary to adapt the sequence parameters as well as the slice direction and the examination section to the questions.

15.3.2 Nuclear Medicine

Ursula Blum

Tear duct scintigraphy and salivary gland scintigraphy have been superseded in clinical diagnostics by radiological diagnostics, especially MRI. With PET-CT, however, a newer procedure is becoming increasingly important in tumor diagnostics.

The main risk factors for the development of malignant diseases in the ENT area are smoking or regular consumption of high-proof alcohol. In the combination of smoking and drinking, the risk increases up to 30 times that of the normal population (LL Oncology 5/14/25). Other risk factors can be the HP virus, as well as poor oral hygiene.

Most cases are squamous cell carcinomas (95%). In larger tumors (T3 and 4) with lymph node involvement, secondary tumors are not uncommon.

Normally squamous cell carcinoma show good FDG storage. In primary diagnostics, PET/CT increases the diagnostic sensitivity and specificity with regard to the lymph node status. PET/CT is more important in the diagnosis of recurrence, and PET/CT can also be helpful in determining the extent of surgery or the radiation fields.

Sentinel lymph node (SLN) imaging is possible. The safety of SLN removal alone for early detected tumors has not yet been sufficiently researched in comparison to standardized elective removal of the cervical lymph nodes and is currently only permissible in the context of studies.

Skeletal scintigraphy is indicated only in individual cases.

15.3.3 Valence

Christel Vockelmann

◾ Table 15.1 shows the use of the respective therapeutic options depending on the problem.

◾ **Table 15.1**   Value of the therapeutic procedures

	Sonography	Conventional	Fluoroscopy/ Angiography	CT	MRI	Nuk	PET
Head and Neck Tumor	N	N	N	P	W	N	W
Sinusitis	W	P	N	W	W	N	N
Dysphagia	N	N	P*		N	W	N	N

N Not indicated, *P* Primary diagnosis, *W* Further diagnosis
P* High-frequency kinematography is the primary imaging method for dedicated swallowing disorders. Of course, endoscopic diagnostics should always be performed first

15.4 Therapy

15.4.1 Radiotherapy

Guido Heilsberg

Head/Neck Tumors

The irradiation of ENT tumors is nowadays almost exclusively carried out with the aid of IMRT (intensity-modulated radiotherapy). Usually both sides of the neck are irradiated.

It is important to undergo **dental rehabilitation** in advance, because the teeth and gums are affected by the radiation. The impact of the radiation on the implants/metal fillings causes additional scattered radiation, which stresses the oral mucosa. The dental splint made must be worn during the daily radiation therapy session and also serves to harden the tooth enamel with the help of fluoride-containing gels and thus make it more resistant to the radiation.

In the case of aggressive therapy concepts, a PEG system should be considered if necessary.

Acute side effects from radiotherapy include **xerostomia**, erythema, **ageusia**, and **mucositis**.

Chronic side effects include: **Xerostomia**, permanent **dark discoloration of the skin**, **fibrosis**, and **lymphedema**.

Nasopharyngeal Carcinoma (Carcinoma of the Nasopharynx)

Nasopharyngeal carcinoma occurs predominantly in the form of PLECA (squamous cell carcinoma) or lymphoepithelial carcinoma (Schmincke's tumor).

Primary radiotherapy is combined with platinum-based concurrent chemotherapy and a dose of 68–72 Gy at 5×2.0 Gy per week.

Oropharyngeal Carcinoma (Carcinoma of the Oral Cavity)

Simultaneous radiochemotherapy with cisplatin, 5-FU or MMC (mitomycin) as therapy of choice with 70–72 Gy with 5×2.0 Gy per week as IMRT with chemotherapy.

Oral Cavity Carcinoma (Carcinoma of the Floor of the Mouth, Carcinoma of the Tongue)

Adjuvant radiotherapy or platinum-based radiochemotherapy is applied to the former tumor bed 60–66 Gy and the lymphatic drainage 54–60 Gy with 5×2.0 Gy per week as IMRT.

Hypopharyngeal Carcinoma (Carcinoma of the Lower Pharynx)

Oropharyngeal carcinoma section

Laryngeal Carcinoma (Carcinoma of the Larynx)

In advanced stages, primary radiotherapy or radiochemotherapy may be considered with 56.25/63 Gy in stage T1 with 5×2.25 Gy per week, 70 Gy from stage T2.

Case Study

A 60-year-old truck driver who has been a heavy smoker since his youth has been complaining of persistent hoarseness for about two months, suffers from stridor (whistling when breathing) and has lost 8 kg. His wife sends him to an ENT specialist, who finds a clearly visible tumor on laryngoscopy and takes a biopsy. He also palpates a large swollen lymph node on the neck. The biopsy reveals a PLECA of the larynx, and the patient is referred to radiation oncology. The radiation oncologist presents the patient to an interdisciplinary tumor board to determine appropriate therapy depending on the findings and in consultation with ENT specialists. Due to the extensive findings, the patient is recommended primary combined radiochemotherapy to enable organ preservation, including the vocal cords and larynx. The patient receives a PEG device in advance in order to ensure nutrition during radiotherapy, as the side effects, such as xerostomia and mucositis, are expected to worsen the nutritional situation.

Practice Questions

1. On imaging, what is a possible distinguishing feature between mucocele shadowing vs. carcinoma shadowing?
2. What are the key features that sonographically indicate a neck cyst?
3. How are midface fractures classified?
4. In what pathology is the "hanging drop" seen?
5. For which problem is sialography used?

Solutions ▶ Chap. 27

Gynecology

*Carla M. Kremers, Guido Heilsberg, Ursula Blum,
Christel Vockelmann and Martina Kahl-Scholz*

Contents

© Springer-Verlag GmbH Germany, part of Springer Nature 2023
M. Kahl-Scholz, C. Vockelmann (eds.), *Basic Knowledge Radiology*,
https://doi.org/10.1007/978-3-662-66351-6_16

This chapter presents various options for the treatment and therapy of gynecological diseases. Diseases of the mammae are discussed as well as diseases of the pelvis. The diagnostic and therapeutic options for the treatment of benign as well as malignant masses are discussed. Diseases in young adulthood, such as extrauterine pregnancy and adnexal torsion, are also discussed in this chapter. In addition to the diagnostic and therapeutic procedures of radiology, nuclear medicine and radiation therapy procedures are also presented.

16.1   Anatomical Structures

Martina Kahl-Scholz

In addition to the mammary gland, the female reproductive organs include the ovaries, uterus, vagina and labia.

The mammary **gland** consists mainly of fatty and connective tissue, the skin with the areola mammae and the nipple (papilla mammaria). From puberty onwards, the tissue increases in size in women.

The ovary is about the size of a plum and is located in the side wall of the pelvis in the ovary fossa. From it originates the fallopian tube (tuba uterina), which is about 10–15 cm long and ends in the uterus (womb). The uterus is pear-shaped and is divided into the body (corpus uteri) and the cervix uteri. The latter passes into the vagina (vagina), which is about 10 cm long and leads to the labia majora et minora pudendi and the vaginal vestibule (vestibulum vaginae).

16.2   Disease Patterns

16.2.1   Chest

Carla M. Kremers

Breast Carcinoma

Breast carcinoma is the most common malignancy in women (a rare one, but possible in men) and continues to be a common cause of death. In order to detect these tumors as early as possible, there is (as the only preventive program working with X-rays) in Germany the mammography screening program. Women between 50–69 years of age receive invitations by mail. If a woman decides to take part in the program, she will be examined at specialized centers.

■ Clinic

Breast carcinoma hardly causes any symptoms; only in very late stages can painful retractions of the breast tissue or exulcerating masses occur.

■ Diagnostics

Sonography (◻ Fig. 16.1)

If a mass is detected in the breast, sonography is usually performed first. A breast carcinoma can then be delineated as an **echo-poor, blurred round focus**, possibly with **dorsal sound extinction** and above all with **interruption of the longitudinal connective tissue structures** (Cooper's ligaments).

Mammography

Mammograms of both breasts are taken in two planes and examined independently by two specialist radiologists. In case of any abnormality, the woman is asked to present herself again for a supplementary examination.

Mammographic signs of breast carcinoma are (◻ Fig. 16.2)
— Grouped or segmentally arranged microcalcifications
— A blurred, possibly spiculated focal finding in two planes
— Architectural abnormalities such as a tent sign (zipfel-shaped gathering of mammary gland tissue)
— A thickening of the cutis or nipple and a nipple retraction
— An asymmetry compared to the opposite side

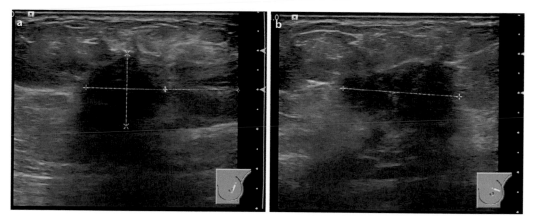

◘ Fig. 16.1 a,b Breast carcinoma on sonography. The echo-poor focus with dorsal sound extinction is not sharply delineated. The reflex-rich stripes – corresponding to Cooper's ligaments – are not displaced but interrupted. (With kind permission of Dr. Göb)

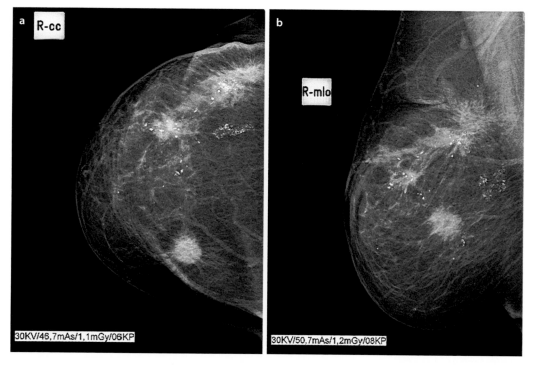

◘ Fig. 16.2 Multicentric breast carcinoma. At least three foci are visible, some of which show microcalcifications. Adjacent to the cranially located focus in mlo projection, a cutaneous retraction and can also be seen

Unfortunately, however, even in the case of a round, smoothly circumscribed round focus, a carcinoma cannot be excluded and further clarification is necessary. For further clarification of circumscribed compressions, supplementary magnification target images of the conspicuous area can equalize overlays.

In order to indicate the density and thus the assessability of the breast, a grading based on the American College of Radiology criteria is given (■ Table 16.1).

The higher the classification, the more difficult the examination is to assess and the easier it is to overlook a focal finding.

Suspected malignancy is also graded using such a scheme, the Breast Imaging Reporting And Data System (■ Table 16.2).

MRI Further unclear findings (e.g. due to dense mammary gland tissue) or malignancies, the extent of which cannot be assessed beyond doubt, require an additional MRI mammogram. To avoid motion artifacts, the patients lie prone on a coil that leaves one chamber free for each breast. The mammae are additionally compressed in these chambers.

In addition to native T1 and T2 sequences, dynamic contrast medium series are also prepared, i.e. after a native T1 sequence, contrast medium is applied i.v. and the sequence is repeated several times at different times in order to subsequently assess the contrast medium dynamics at specific locations. The contrast-enhancing focal findings can then be detected with the aid of subtraction. For this purpose, the native series is subtracted from a series with contrast medium enhancement. What remains is an almost black image in which only the structures that absorb contrast agent are illuminated. Fuzzy, spiculated foci with rapid, inhomogeneous, possibly ring-shaped contrast uptake and rapid contrast washout are suspicious. The Göttingen score has been established for assessing the dignity of contrast-absorbing lesions in MR mammography (■ Tables 16.3 and 16.4).

Biopsy Suspicious focal findings are clarified with a **histological examination.** Biopsies can be performed sonographically, mammographically or by MRI. To ensure that the location of the biopsy can be found again after the biopsy or after neoadjuvant therapy, small metal clips are often inserted during the biopsy to mark the location.

If breast-conserving therapy (BET) is planned, the malignant or suspicious lesion

■ **Table 16.1** American college of radiology criteria

ACR1	Predominantly fatty, easily assessable tissue
ACR2	Predominantly fibroglandular tissue
ACR3	Inhomogeneous dense tissue
ACR4	Extremely dense fabric

■ **Table 16.2** Breast imaging reporting and data system

BI-RADS 0	No classification possible, further imaging necessary
BI-RADS 1	No conspicuousness
BI-RADS 2	Descriptive but not malignant findings
BI-RADS 3	Unclear, probably benign findings Follow-up in six months
BI-RADS 4	Findings requiring clarification, biopsy recommended
BI-RADS 5	Highly suspicious findings, biopsy recommended
BI-RADS 6	histologically confirmed carcinoma

16

◘ Table 16.3 Göttingen score scheme

	Zero Points	One Point	Two Points
Initial contrast agent enrichment	<50%	50–100%	>100%
Postinitial contrast agent behavior	Further KM recording (>+10%)	Plateau (+/−10%)	Wash out (<−10%)
Contrast agent distribution	Homogeneous	Inhomogeneous	Annular
Form	Round, oval	Irregular, dendritic	
Limitation	Sharp	Fuzzy	

◘ Table 16.4 Score evaluation

0–1 Point	MRM BIRADS 1	Certainly benign
2 Points	MRM BIRADS 2	Probably benign
3 Points	MRM BIRADS 3	Unclear
4–5 Points	MRM BIRADS 4	Probably malignant
6–8 Points	MRM BIRADS 5	Certainly malignant

can be marked using a thin wire (◘ Fig. 16.3) to allow the surgeon to locate and safely remove it.

Galactography A possible symptom of breast carcinoma is a (bloody) secretion from the nipple. If the focus cannot be detected using the above methods, galactography is used. For this purpose, a thin button cannula is inserted into the secretory milk duct and iodine-containing contrast medium is injected above it. An intraductal mass can be detected on the basis of the contrast medium recesses within the milk duct.

Fibroadenoma

Fibroadenomas are common benign masses of the mamma and occur mainly in women of reproductive age.

▪ Clinic
Mostly asymptomatic.

▪ Diagnostics
Sonography

On sonography (which should be the method of first choice in young women), they are **smooth-bordered, low-echo**, and respect the connective tissue layers of **the breast, i.e., they displace but do not break through Cooper's ligaments.** Due to hormone sensitivity, their size may fluctuate under hormonal influence. If the findings remain unclear or the lesion shows a tendency to grow, a biopsy is indicated.

Mammography

In mammography, fibroadenomas are also round and smoothly limited in all planes. They often contain **coarse calcifications**, which facilitates their diagnosis. The **displacement of surrounding tissue** by compression during mammography can cause a **halo effect**, i.e. a ring-shaped lightening around the lesion.

Cysts

These are also possible in the breast. More often they occur in the context of fibrocystic mastopathy.

▪ Clinic
Mostly asymptomatic.

▪ Diagnostics
Sonography

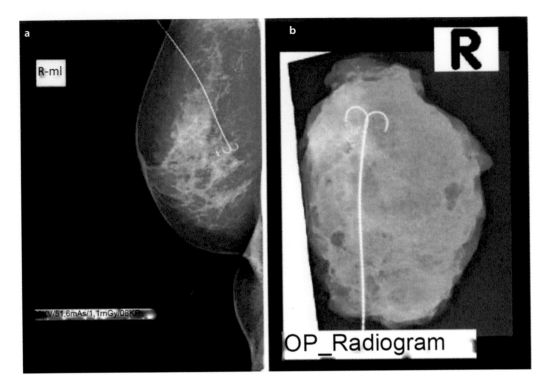

Fig. 16.3 Checking the position of a wire marker before surgery. After partial resection of the breast, the removed tissue is examined again to check whether the clip or the microcalcifications have been removed in their entirety – if parts are missing, resection is necessary

A definite sonographic diagnosis is possible if the lesion is **round, smooth bordered, anechoic** with **dorsal sound enhancement.** Also a cyst **does not break through Cooper's ligaments.** Further clarification is not necessary.

Mammography

On mammography, cysts can be delineated as **homogeneously compacted, round, smoothly circumscribed masses** that may exhibit a **halo effect** similar to a fibroadenoma due to **displacement of the surrounding tissue.**

Fibrocystic Mastopathy

Fibrocystic mastopathy makes breast diagnosis difficult. It is a remodeling of the mammary gland tissue with fibrotic alteration of the connective tissue and formation of multiple cysts, which makes the breast unclear in all imaging. Due to hormone sensitivity, size variations of the existing lesions are possible.

- **Clinic**

Depending on the cycle, feelings of tension and pain can occur.

- **Diagnostics**

Sonography

Sonographically, the cystic lesions can be easily recognized and distinguished from solid structures. Again, care must be taken that the cysts do **not** contain **any solid portions,** which may correspond to precancerous lesions.

Mammography

In mammography, a juxtaposition of **patchy shadows** is found, which makes it difficult to differentiate between individual foci. In addition, **microcalcifications** may occur, which, however, are not grouped, but are **diffusely** distributed. If grouped microcalcifications can be demarcated, they are suspicious and require clarification.

MRI

In MRI, **multiple diffusely distributed, partly planar contrast images** can be delineated, which show a rather slow enhancement.

Mastitis (Plasma Cell Mastitis)

Mastitis is a bacterial inflammation of the breast (mastitis puerpalis) that usually occurs during lactation. If such an inflammation occurs independently of the breastfeeding period, it is referred to as non-puerpal mastitis.

- Clinic

Pain, redness, swelling, possibly fever, chills, malaise.

- Diagnostics

Sonography/Mammography

Radiological imaging is not necessary for puerpal mastitis. Sonographic controls, which are mostly carried out by the colleagues of the gynecology, clarify whether an abscess is present.

Mastitis non-puerpalis must be differentiated from the special form of breast carcinoma, the inflammatory breast carcinoma. Clinically and mammographically, mastitis and inflammatory breast carcinoma look very similar: in addition to a thickened cutis, a diffusely condensed breast parenchyma can also be seen. If the clinical course and imaging are not conclusive, a biopsy may be necessary.

Typical mammographic findings of an expired so-called plasma cell mastitis (plasma cell-rich infiltrate, often asymptomatic) are linear, lancet-shaped calcifications.

16.2.2 Small Basin

Tumors of the Ovary

Ovarian tumors can take very different forms from solid to cystic due to different histological entities (different ovarian tumors as well as metastases are possible).

- Clinic

Due to the lack of early symptoms, they are often noticed late.

- Diagnostics (◻ Figs. 16.4 and 16.5)

Ovarian cysts are so named only from a diameter of 3 cm. Smaller lesions are usually functional cysts (or follicular cysts). Larger cystic findings may be benign cystadenoma. Although this is primarily benign, it can degenerate into malignancy and is then called cystdenocarcinoma. Ovarian cysts should therefore be further clarified.

In all imaging, **septations** are usually seen in cystadenomas. In addition, the content is not always **water-equivalent**, i.e. **sonographically echo-poor** but not echo-free or possibly **T1w hyperintense** or in CT around **15–25 HU**. Solid, contrast-enriched areas indicate the presence of cystadenocarcinoma.

In contrast to cystadenocarcinomas, masses of the ovary can also be solid. In principle, any solid mass of the ovary is considered suspicious. It is usually detected by (endovaginal) sonography. MRI is the method of choice for further assessment of a lesion that cannot be classified with certainty by sonography. If a carcinoma is suspected, a primary CT is indicated for staging.

Depending on the definition, an **extra-uterine pregnancy** is also a mass in the ovary – it should not normally stray into

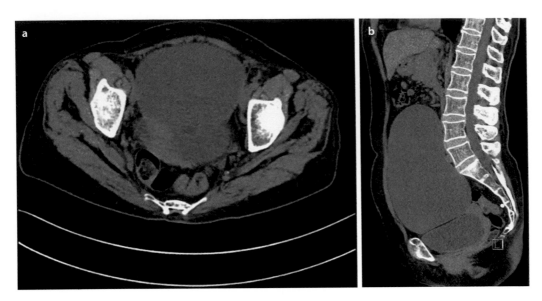

◘ Fig. 16.4 CT images of a cystadenoma originating from the right ovary. From the image alone, no distinction can be made between a cystadenocarcinoma and a cystadenoma

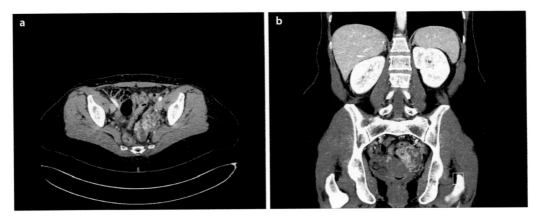

◘ Fig. 16.5 Largely solid mass of the left ovary. The finding was surgically removed. It was a dermoid

radiology. In women and girls of childbearing age with lower abdominal pain and possibly pressure pain resistance, a β-HCG test should shed light on the situation. Complementary sonography may show an empty uterine cavity or a pseudo-gestational sac (a circumscribed accumulation of fluid in the cavity) if β-HCG is positive. Depending on the size and position of the embryo, a dilated tube and possibly an amniotic sac including embryo in the area of the adnexa may also be visible.

16.2.3 **Tumors of the Uterus**

Fibroids

Myomas are extremely common and fortunately benign masses in the female genitalia – they are most frequently found in the uterus, but vaginal localization is also possible, for example. They are hormone-sensitive tumors that occur at childbearing age.

Within the uterus, they are further classified based on their location: submucosal fibroids grow into the cavum uteri. Intramural fibroids, as the name suggests, are located within the uterine wall and subserosal fibroids grow on the outside of the uterus. Myomas may be pedunculated and cause similar discomfort to tubal torsion during pedicle rotation.

- Diagnostics

Sonography

In all imaging, fibroids are round and have smooth borders. Due to frequent calcification and sometimes fat deposits the internal structure may appear inhomogeneous. Sonographically they are predominantly **hypodense** (if necessary with acoustic effacements) and usually the sonographic imaging is already sufficient.

MRI

On MRI, fibroids are primarily **hypointense to** the uterine musculature in both T1w and T2w. The pattern may become very inhomogeneous in case of calcification, fatty deposits or hemorrhage.

CT

On CT, fibroids stand out as secondary findings; they are then **smoothly circumscribed, usually calcified masses** in or on the uterus.

In contrast medium-supported examinations they show a **strong (arterial) contrast medium accumulation.** This effect can be used in the treatment of symptomatic fibroids (those that cause pain or abnormal bleeding): One possible form of therapy is embolization of fibroids. In this procedure, the artery supplying the fibroid is probed with a catheter and then sealed with the help of small particles. The myoma dies from the lack of oxygen and hopefully no longer stands in the way of the patient.

Polyps

Polyps can occur in the uterus and cervix. They are usually noticed during the gynecological examination. Sonographically, they can be delimited by an **echo** and are usually an incidental finding without relevance.

Carcinoma of the Corpus

Corpus carcinomas (= endometrial carcinomas) are conspicuous by postmenopausal bleeding and sometimes lower abdominal discomfort and are diagnosed during gynecological examination (colposcopy/abrasio).

- Diagnostics

Sonography may reveal a focal **widening of the endometrium with an echo.** If further diagnosis of the local findings is necessary for therapy planning, MRI is the method of choice in which the extension and possibly infiltration into or even into surrounding structures can be assessed (◻ Fig. 16.6). Important lymph node stations here are

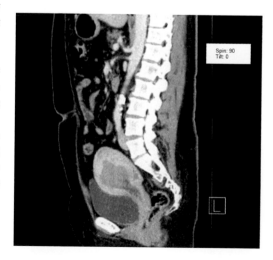

◻ Fig. 16.6 CT of an endometroid growing uterine carcinoma

above all locoregional, parailiac and sacral lymph nodes. However, direct exposure to retroperitoneal and para-aortic lymph nodes is also possible.

Cervical Carcinoma

Cervical carcinoma is ideally detected during the annual gynecological check-up.

■ Diagnostics (◘ Fig. 16.7)
Endosonography is often sufficient for imaging, in which the mass can be recognized as an **echo-poor area**. Larger findings can lead to an obstruction of the cervix and thus to **hydrometra**. If hydrometra is detected as an incidental finding on a CT scan in a postmenopausal woman, a supplementary gynecological examination should therefore be performed. If further pre-therapeutic imaging is required after sonography, MRI is indicated to assess the local finding and its spread. In T2w, a **hypointense area** is then noticed in contrast to the rest of the cervix. It is important to assess the extension: does it grow into adjacent structures? Is the surrounding fatty tissue inconspicuous (i.e. bright in T2w)? Is there a fat lamella between the rectum and the bladder? In addition,

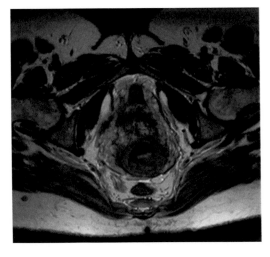

◘ **Fig. 16.7** T2-weighted image of a cervical carcinoma at the left dorsal circumference of the cervix

attention should be paid to lymph node enlargements (predominantly parametranal, sacral and inguinal, possibly para-aortic). If malignancy is detected, CT can be used to search for distant metastases.

Endometriosis

Endometriomas are to be understood as uterine mucosa scattered in unusual places, which, depending on the cycle, undergoes the same cycle of formation and degradation as the normal endometrium. They are also called chocolate cysts because of their thick old-blooded brown content.

■ Clinic
The patients often complain of menstrual pain and are accordingly examined by a gynecologist.

■ Diagnostics
Sonography
   In sonography, a very **inhomogeneous mass** can be delineated, which shows **no signal** (i.e. no blood flow) in the **Doppler flow measurement.**
   MRI
   In the case of atypical location of endometriomas (i.e. not in or on the female genitals, but for example in the abdominal wall), the search continues with MRI. In T2-weighting, a **mirror image** can be indicative in the case of larger findings: in the case of overall fluid filling, the blood degradation products (**T2w hypointense**) collect at the bottom of the mass and the upper portion is **T2w hyperintense**, as is appropriate for fluid. For smaller nodules, T1 weighting is helpful: due to the bloody content, the signal in T1 weighting is hyperintense. In order to be able to distinguish it from any surrounding fatty tissue, a fat-saturated, T1-weighted sequence should be performed (fat is then shown hypointense, i.e. dark). In addition, **endometriosis lesions also absorb contrast medium** and can thus be detected.

Cysts

Cysts exist in the female genital tract in various locations. Physiologically, follicular cysts of different sizes are found in the ovaries of childbearing women. One speaks of an ovarian cyst only when the lesion is **larger than 3 cm.** Cysts in the cervix are called ovula nabothi. They can grow up to 1 cm in size. In the vagina, there are cysts that originate from the Garnter ducts. They are called Gartner cysts.

■ Clinic

Depending on size, mostly unspecific.

■ Diagnostics (◻ Fig. 16.8)

As in all other organs, cysts in the lesser pelvis should be **fluid filled, round, smooth bordered** and delineated with a **filmy wall.** In sonography they are **anechoic.** In MRI water **T1w hypointense and T2w hyperintense.** In CT the density values should be around **0 HU.**

It is sufficient to know that they are physiologically present and have little pathological relevance.

Inflammatory Changes
Endometritis

Endometritis refers to inflammation of the inner layer of the uterus.

■ Clinic

It leads to bleeding disorders and is usually diagnosed on the basis of the gynecological examination. Pain and fever.

■ Diagnostics
Sonography

Sonographically, the endometrium is shown to be **odematous (echo-poor) thickened.** Frequently there is involvement of the myometrium.

In **myometritis**, the myometrium is correspondingly widened **oedematously.** If fluid is deposited – e.g. due to a swollen cervix— this is referred to as hydro-, hemato- or pyometra, depending on the type of fluid (◻ Fig. 16.9). While hydrometra is sonographically imaged as **anechoic fluid retention,** blood and pus collections are **anechoic.** Further imaging is rarely necessary.

MRI

In MRI, the inflamed uterine parts will show **a signal increase in T2w** and a **signal decrease in T1w** due to their edema **in** addition to a **widening.** After administration of contrast medium there is a **strong enhancement.** The content of a hydrometra **is fluid isointense in MRI,** thus **hyperintense** in T2w and **hypointense** in T1w. A hematometra is conspicuous by **high signal intensity in T1 weighting** with otherwise liquid content

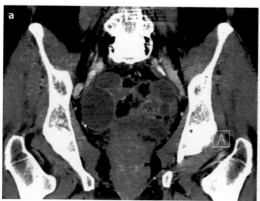
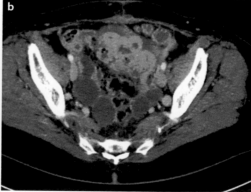

◻ **Fig. 16.8** CT of a young patient with several large ovarian cysts in coronary and axial sectioning. **a** Coronary, **b** Axial

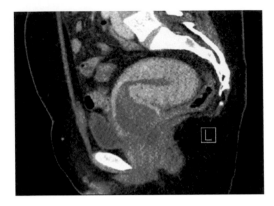

Fig. 16.9 CT in sagittal slice guidance showing a uterus filled with fluid in hematometra. The fluid has a density of approx. 50 HU

(T2w hyperintense). The signal of a pyometra varies depending on the protein content. Often air inclusions are detectable and an edge accentuated contrast uptake.

CT

CT reveals a thickened uterus with **strong contrast uptake.** The contents of the uterus can be further evaluated by its density values if sufficiently filled (water approx. 0 HU, pus >10 HU and blood >30 HU).

Adnexitis

Adnexitis is an inflammation of the ovary and the tube. If only the tube is inflamed, it is called **salpingitis**, and if the ovary is inflamed in isolation, it is called **oophoritis**.

■ Clinic

Primarily, there is an edematous swelling of the respective organ accompanied by local pain.

■ Diagnostics

Sonography

In ultrasound, the respective structure is then **inhomogeneous** due to the edema and **predominantly** echo-poor. Due to drainage obstacles, e.g. due to inflammation or in the case of scarred structures, the tube may be

filled with fluid. In this case, depending on the fluid, one speaks of a hydro-, hemato- or pyosalpinx.

The imaging of these fluids is analogous to the accumulation of fluid in the cavum uteri (see above).

MRI

In MRI, inflammatory edema leads to a **signal increase in T2w** and a **signal decrease in T1w,** just as in **the** uterus. In order to make such edematous changes particularly well visible, "fat-saturated" T2-weighted sequences can be used, in which the fat is then imaged hypointense and only fluids (i.e. also an edema) remain bright (hyperintense). The increased blood flow due to inflammation is correspondingly noticeable by a **strong accumulation of contrast medium.**

CT

Usually, cross-sectional imaging also reveals edema in the surrounding adipose tissue; on CT, this may be the only evidence of inflammation of the adnexa (■ Fig. 16.10).

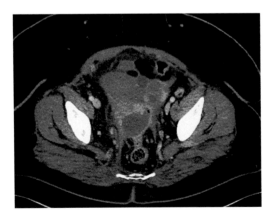

Fig. 16.10 CT of a patient with lower abdominal pain and significantly elevated inflammatory parameters. Several fluid formations can be seen, some with vigorous contrast uptake in the marginal area and some with air inclusions. Several tuboovarian abscesses were involved

Torsions

- Clinic

A **torsion of the tube or ovary** is followed by a strong, sudden (usually with a jerky movement) onset and unilateral lower abdominal pain (accompanying nausea or vomiting are also possible) with otherwise unremarkable laboratory parameters. Ideally, the history alone is sufficient to seek contact with the gynecologist – especially since this is a gynecological emergency that requires immediate surgical repair to prevent infarction of the organ. Pedunculated cysts or fibroids can also cause similar complaints.

- Diagnostics

Sonography

Sonographically, the respective organ is edematously **swollen** and in **duplex sonography the blood flow** (in contrast to inflammation) **is reduced or absent.** Accompanying ascites (fluid in the Douglas space) is often seen.

CT

In the cross-sectional image (in this case, a CT is more likely to be requested due to the acute onset of symptoms and clinical impairment), the **lack of contrast medium accumulation** can be groundbreaking due to the vessels occluded by the strangulation.

16.2.4 External Female Genitalia

The external genitals can be adequately imaged on the basis of the gynecological examination, if necessary with the aid of sonography. In the case of tumors of the vulva and vagina, radiology is rarely required for the diagnosis of spread or infiltration. Then it is important to identify the tumor spread and the involved structures as precisely as possible. MRI is then the imaging of choice.

16.3 Diagnostics

16.3.1 Diagnostic Radiology

Christel Vockelmann

Sonography

Besides the internal genitals, the female (and also male) mammary gland belongs to the field of gynecology. In the examination of the mamma, sonography is part of the basic diagnostics in addition to the clinical examination including palpation of the breast. Sonography of the breast requires a **high-resolution transducer (7.5 MHz)**. Both breasts are examined in detail, usually once completely transversally and in the second direction sagittally. As an additional plane, especially in the case of existing findings, an alignment of the transducer to the nipple is suitable. In this orientation, milk ducts in the breast can be delineated in the course.

In case of complaints, especially in younger patients (<30 years), sonography is the most important examination modality. On the basis of the findings then available, a decision is made about possible further diagnostics.

Conventional X-ray Diagnostics

Mammography is the standard in breast diagnostics with the exception of younger patients. As the only X-ray examination to date, mammography is also used as a screening method in Germany. All women between 50 and 69 years of age are invited for screening. In this population group, it has been proven that screening with mammography can save lives through early diagnosis. Mammography screening may only be performed by certified screening units. The mammograms must meet strict quality requirements. The MTRA working in a screening unit must have undergone special further training and a certification course

"Specialist for Mammography Diagnostics". A double diagnosis is carried out by two specialized and certified radiologists. Discrepant findings are discussed by a third radiologist and a consensus conference. In addition to screening, typical indications for the performance of a so-called curative mammography are suspicious palpation findings or complaints.

> Screening mammograms in asymptomatic women may only be performed by certified screening units.

Another special feature of mammography is the use of the very soft X-rays between 25–30 kV. Compression is also a special feature of mammography. This achieves, on the one hand, a reduction in scattered radiation. The second effect is a homogenization of the thickness of the breast, which of course is normally much thicker near the chest wall than in the area of the nipple.

Galactography is available as a further diagnostic option. With the advent of MR mammography, this procedure has moved into the background. However, in the case of bloody galactorrhoea and otherwise inconspicuous imaging, there are still indications for this procedure. The image itself corresponds to that of the "normal" mammogram. Beforehand, however, the radiologist probes the milk duct with a thin cannula, e.g. the plastic cannula of a blue Viggo, and injects contrast medium into it. The goal is to find contrast gaps in the milk ducts that indicate a papilloma. **Papillomas** are basically benign tumors, but they have a certain potential for degeneration and are therefore operated on in most cases.

Computed Tomography

Computer tomography plays no role in breast diagnostics. **Digital tomosynthesis** is a new procedure that is ultimately also based on images acquired with the aid of X-rays. To generate the image, images are first taken from different angles. From these images, simple back projection (remember: back projection also existed in CT image calculation) is used to calculate layered images of the breast that are free of superimposition. At present, the procedure is only used by a few, mainly large clinics. Tomosynthesis is not yet used in routine diagnostics. Advantages are offered above all in the case of breasts with very dense glandular parenchyma, where the assessability is considerably limited due to the numerous superimpositions in conventional mammograms.

Magnetic Resonance Imaging

Magnetic resonance imaging has been an established procedure in the diagnosis of certain breast changes for several years. Not every conspicuous finding is examined in conventional mammography. The indication for an MRI examination of the breast is on the one hand the young patient with very dense breasts and a high risk of disease. The confirmed lobular carcinoma is often examined in MRI in order to exclude secondary findings. A classic indication for MRI is the differentiation between a scar after breast surgery and a recurrence of a breast carcinoma.

The examination is performed in a special mammography coil. The patient lies on her chest during the examination, and there are two recesses in the coil for the two breasts. The breasts are fixed in these to minimize breathing artefacts. The administration of contrast medium is obligatory during the examination in order to achieve a dynamic examination of the breast. The background to this is that breast carcinomas show an early contrast medium enhancement 1–3 min after contrast medium administration, and in the later sequences generally show a washout or even a plateau phase of the contrast medium. Benign tumors, on the other hand, tend to accumulate contrast medium less strongly, but increasingly in the course of the examination.

16

An MRI examination of the breast always requires the administration of a contrast medium.

16.3.2 Nuclear Medicine

Ursula Blum

In gynecology, nuclear medicine examinations are mainly required after the diagnosis of a malignant disease.

Rarely, questions about renal outflow in the case of anatomical malformations or after surgical interventions (extensive operations of the lower abdomen, e.g. removal of the uterus with removal of the ovaries and lymph nodes). The determination of the side-separated kidney function can also be useful in the context of chemotherapy or a planned radiation of the abdominal cavity.

Breast Carcinoma

As part of preoperative diagnostics, **sentinel lymph node scintigraphy** (SLS, ▶ Chap. 22) is a standard examination in breast centers. A distinction is made here between a protocol on the day before surgery and a protocol on the day of surgery. In accordance with the Directive on Protection against Damage by Ionizing Radiation (StrSchV), it must be ensured that the activity in the patient at the time of surgery does not exceed the exemption limit of 10 MBq. In addition, there are different injection techniques (intradermal, subdermal, peritumoral, subaureolar, peri-areolar). So far, no injection technique seems to be superior with regard to the visualization of axillary lymph nodes. In the context of purely dermal and aureolar injections, sentinel lymph nodes outside the axilla (e.g. parasternal) may not be detected. However, these lymph nodes are usually not surgically removed. The highest correct visualization of the SLN is achieved with T1 and T2 tumors.

In the case of extensive tumor stages, preoperative chemotherapy is administered first. If necessary, the sentinel lymph node is marked and removed before chemotherapy. After chemotherapy, the sentinel lymph node may be pathologically false negative.

Skeletal scintigraphy is usually performed postoperatively as a staging examination.

If disseminated skeletal metastases are found, **palliative pain therapy**, e.g. with samarium, can be performed.

A **PET/CT examination** is currently not recommended in primary diagnostics. However, there is a benefit in the diagnosis of local recurrence and mediastinal or parasternal lymph node metastases. In the detection of distant metastases, PET/CT appears superior to other methods in some cases; exceptions are small lung metastases (<10 mm) or brain metastases. PET/CT also plays an important role in therapy monitoring.

Vulvar Carcinoma

If vulvar carcinoma is confirmed (bioptically), SLN diagnostics can be performed preoperatively if the lymph node status is clinically inconspicuous. In this case, 4 (-6) activity depots are injected intracutaneously around the primary tumor. The images were taken dynamically as well as statically up to one hour after the injection. The first presenting lymph nodes should be marked on the skin. Matching is performed during surgery with the gamma probe.

Further imaging diagnostics is only necessary for special questions from stage FIGO III.

SLN Diagnostics in Other Gynecological Tumors

Recent studies show that SLN imaging could also be helpful for other gynecological tumors (cervical carcinoma, uterine carcinoma). Further studies still have to prove the benefit.

□ Table 16.5   Value of the therapeutic procedures

	Sonography	Conventional	Fluoroscopy/ Angiography	CT	MRI	Nuk	PET
Primary diagnostics breast carcinoma	P	P	N	N	W	N	N
Vulvar cancer	P*	N	N	W	W	W	W
Ovarian cancer	P	N	N	P	N	W	W

N Not indicated, *P* Primary diagnosis, *W* Further diagnosis
P* Transvaginal endosonography

Ovarian Carcinomas

Here, too, FDG-PET/CT can be used in primary diagnostics, recurrence diagnostics and therapy monitoring.

16.3.3 Valence

Christel Vockelmann

□ Table 16.5 shows the use of the respective therapeutic options depending on the problem.

16.4 Therapy

16.4.1 Interventional Radiology

Christel Vockelmann

Stereotactic Vacuum Suction Biopsy of the Breast

Stereotaxy is a diagnostic rather than a therapeutic procedure. Today, it generally replaces the open surgical mammary biopsy in the case of focal findings that could not already be punched sonographically (usually by the gynecologist). The biopsy is mammographically guided. The patient usually lies on an examination

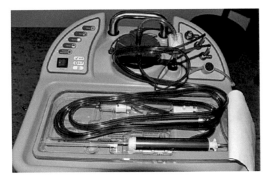

□ Fig. 16.11   Prepared device for vacuum aspiration biopsy with 11G biopsy needle

table which has a hole for the breast to be examined. The corresponding breast hangs through this hole. A mammography device is set up under the table. This is used to take two oblique images of the lesion to be biopsied, usually malignant microcalcifications, in order to localize the pathological findings. In these two images, the radiologist marks the calcification. The stored computer program can then determine the depth of the lesion in the breast and the access route from the two markings. After local anesthesia and a stab incision, the radiologist inserts the biopsy needle, most commonly an 11-G needle, with a trocar to just in front of the lesion. □ Figure 16.11 shows prepared vacuum suction device.

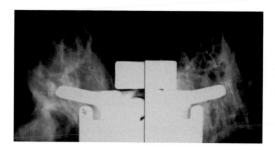

Fig. 16.12 Stereotactic control images with biopsy needle in front of the microcalcification group to be biopsied

After another X-ray to check the position, the biopsy needle is released (■ Fig. 16.12).

Then at least 12 samples are taken. The breast tissue is sucked through the vacuum into the biopsy channel and then cut out with the needle and taken. For the next sample, the needle is rotated a little so that ultimately samples are taken all around the needle.

Then the needle in the trocar is withdrawn slightly and a control image is taken. Often, no more microcalcifications can be detected at this point. In this case, a clip should be inserted through the trocar into the sampling area. If the biopsy reveals a malignancy, a follow-up operation must be performed. The clip is then used to operate on the correct area.

The samples obtained with the vacuum suction biopsy are first x-rayed using the mammography technique. This serves to send the specimens with microcalcifications (■ Fig. 16.13) to the pathologist separately, since a particularly complex processing must be carried out here.

If a stereotactically biopsied area has to be reoperated, the clip left behind is marked with a wire (■ Fig. 16.14). The localization for the wire insertion is done in the same way as for stereotaxy. The wire then serves the surgeon as a guide to the surgical area.

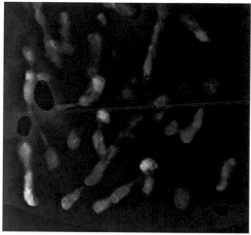

Fig. 16.13 Punch biopsies taken with microcalcifications in several samples

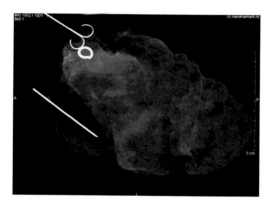

Fig. 16.14 Preparation after surgery with wire and clip in preparation

16.4.2 Radiotherapy

Guido Heilsberg

Cervical Carcinoma

Indications for radiation are: positive lymph node involvement, tumor size over 4 cm, from FIGO III primary radiochemotherapy is usually performed as combined tele- and brachytherapy, adenocarcinoma, R1/2, or narrow tumor-free resection margin.

- Percutaneous radiotherapy total dose 45–50.4 Gy, single dose 1.8–2 Gy/5× weekly.
- HDR brachytherapy with Ir-192 with GD 30–42.5 Gy/5–9 Gy per fraction

Side effects: vaginal and anal mucosal reactions, diarrhea, rectitis, frequent emptying of the bladder.

Breast Carcinoma

Breast-Conserving Therapy   50 Gy, 5 × 1.8–2.0 Gy/week, the target volume includes the entire mammary gland tissue and the adjacent thoracic wall. Boost can reduce the recurrence rate in the breast for invasive carcinomas, i.e. no boost is given for DCIS. The boost dose is (10)-16 Gy 5 × 1.8–2.0 Gy/week. The local saturation can be applied as electron standing field, photon standing field or tangent, in mixed-beam technique (electrons and photons) or as integrated boost (SIB, simultaneous integrated boost).

Mastectomy   50 Gy, 5 × 1.8–2.0 Gy/week, the target volume encloses the thoracic wall, including the surgical scar with safety margin.

Irradiation of the Regional Lymph Drainage System   Only in case of residual tumor in the axilla or >3 affected lymph nodes. Total dose approx. 50 Gy, 5 × 1.8–2.0 Gy/week.

Positioning is in the supine position, e.g. on a special "mammaboard" and with knee padding for the legs. The arms are taken above the head, comfortably and reproducibly positioned. In the planning CT the scar should be marked with a wire marker.

Side effects: Redness of the skin and swelling of the irradiated breast, moist epitheliolysis, esophagitis, pneumonitis, cardiac arrhythmias.

Vaginal Carcinoma

Primary radiotherapy depends on the size and location of the tumor and can help to preserve the vagina and its function. The primary therapy concept is percutaneous

radiotherapy in combination with brachytherapy (afterloading).

Primary percutaneous radiotherapy of the lesser pelvis 40 Gy with 5 × 1.8 Gy per week as pelvic box, or 4 × per week if as combination therapy with afterloading started after a dose of 20 Gy by percutaneous irradiation. Blocking out of the central structures during percutaneous irradiation at the start of afterloading in order to avoid exceeding the tolerance doses.

The patient is placed in the supine position, her legs are padded with a standard pad, and her arms are placed on her chest.

Vulvar Carcinoma

Primary radiotherapy of the vulva and both groins up to 50 Gy (for N0) with 5 × 2.0 Gy per week, boost of the primary up to 60 Gy. In case of lymph node involvement: in addition to the groin, irradiation of the lymph nodes in the pelvic region with 45–50 Gy, if necessary boost with 10–20 Gy to the affected lymph nodes. Postoperatively as adjuvant radiotherapy to the primaries and if necessary the inguinal lymph nodes 50–60 Gy with 5 × 1.8 Gy per week.

The patient is placed in the supine position, her legs are padded with a knee roll and spread apart in the frog position, her arms are placed on her chest.

Case Study

Mrs. Zucker had a breast carcinoma two years ago. The regular follow-ups were always fine. Now, however, the radiologist has discovered a new compression in the area of the old surgical scar. What procedures or interventions should be used to clarify the findings? MR mammography is a suitable imaging procedure for differentiating between a scar and a recurrence. If the findings are also conspicuous in MR mammography, a vacuum suction biopsy or punch biopsy is performed.

16

Practice Questions

1. What imaging signs would make you think of breast carcinoma on sonography?
2. What do you need to think about differential diagnosis of mastitis?
3. What are the treatment options for fibroids?
4. You will see a signal increase in T2w and a signal decrease in T1w in the adnexa on MRI. In the "fat-saturated" T2-weighted sequences, the fat appears hypointense and the fluids that are seen are bright (hyperintense). Furthermore, a strong contrast enhancement is seen. What does this finding indicate and what is your tentative diagnosis?
5. What are the indications for radiotherapy in breast cancer?

Solutions ▶ Chap. 2 /

Respiratory System

Martina Kahl-Scholz, Christel Vockelmann and Ursula Blum

Contents

© Springer-Verlag GmbH Germany, part of Springer Nature 2023
M. Kahl-Scholz, C. Vockelmann (eds.), *Basic Knowledge Radiology*,
https://doi.org/10.1007/978-3-662-66351-6_17

This chapter deals with the main possibilities of radiological diagnostics, nuclear medicine and radiotherapy for the diagnosis and therapy of the respiratory system. An introductory section provides a brief overview of anatomy and function, and a concluding section contains some case studies from practice.

17.1 Anatomical Structures

Martina Kahl-Scholz

17.1.1 Trachea and Lungs (Pulmo)

The trachea extends about 12 cm from the larynx to the bronchi of the lungs. It is made up of alternating cartilaginous clasps (**cartilagines tracheales**) and annular **ligaments** (**ligg. anularia**) that open backwards and can thus move along when the lung expands downwards during inhalation or when the larynx moves upwards during swallowing or when the head is tilted backwards. The posterior part of the cartilaginous braces is completed by muscles (**Mm. trachealis**).

The trachea divides into a left and right main bronchus (**bronchus principalis dexter et sinistra**). The site of division is called the **bifurcatio trachea** and the spur-like protrusion that arises there is called the **carina trachea**. The right main bronchus has a much steeper course than the left, so that when the airway is obstructed by foreign bodies (aspiration), the right main bronchus is more frequently affected. Within the lung, the bronchial tree divides further and further, see below.

The lungs are divided into the right and left lungs. The left lung, in turn, is divided into two lobes (**lobus**) and is slightly smaller than the right lung because much of the heart lies against it from the medial side and takes up space. The right lung is divided into three lobes and, in contrast to the left lung, is limited caudally by the liver pushing the diaphragm further upwards.

The **bronchus principalis dexter** and **sinister** divide into 2–3 lobe bronchi as they pass through the lung, and these in turn divide into 2–5 segmental bronchi.

> ❯ Right lung: three lobes, ten segments. Left lung: two lobes, 8–10 segments.

A special structure of both lungs is the area in which the vessels and main bronchi move in and out, the so-called lung clearing (**hilus**).

In the right lung the bronchus principalis dexter, the Vv. pulmonalis, A. pulmonalis pass through the hilus, in the left lung the bronchus principalis sinister as well as likewise the A. pulmonalis and the Vv. pulmonalis correspond.

17.2 Disease Patterns

17.2.1 Pleura

Pleural Effusion

In a pleural effusion, fluid is found in the pleural cavity (>20 mL).

- Clinic

Pleural effusion is usually a concomitant of another disease, such as pneumonia, heart failure or carcinoma. The clinical manifestations are dyspnoea and an attenuated breath sound.

- Diagnostics

Conventional X-ray
- Standing: Fluid collects on the **dorsal aspect of the phrenicocostal recess**. With small amounts <150 mL it may be difficult to detect the effusion at all. **Basal homogeneous shadowing** occurs (◘ Fig. 17.1).

17

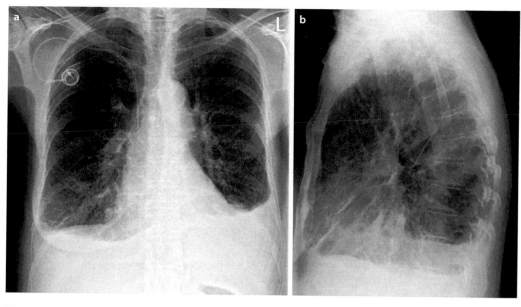

□ **Fig. 17.1**   Pleural effusion. **a** posterior-anterior. **b** lateral

— Lying down: Here the effusion is distributed and **pleural space widening** occurs. However, if the patient is lying on his back, an effusion can only be detected above 500 mL. Possible signs then are a **widening of the pleural border**, a **blurred diaphragmatic contour** and a **shadowing of the lateral sinus**.

Sonography

Transthoracic sonography can also be used to try to diagnose pleural effusion in patients (especially those who are bedridden). In this case, **anechoic parts of the pleura** are visible.

CT

CT allows detection of even **small amounts of fluid**. It is also possible to determine whether the fluid is transudate or exudate, which in turn allows conclusions to be drawn about the underlying disease.

❯ <10 U=transudate, >10 U=exudate.

Pleural Callosity

This is a scar-like change of the pleura, which can be of different genesis (traumatic, inflammatory, vascular, degenerative).

▪ Clinic

Depending on the underlying disease.

▪ Diagnostics

Conventional X-ray

Calluses can be seen as **shadowing** in two planes in the X-ray thorax. Extent, localization and degree of calcification of a pleural callus often indicate the cause: apical = probably due to expired pneumonia or tuberculosis; basal = most likely pleural effusion.

❯ A distinction callus vs. effusion is possible by taking the picture in lateral position: the effusion runs out laterally at the thoracic wall, the callus remains unchanged.

Pneumothorax

If air enters the pleural space, it is called a pneumothorax. A distinction is made between:

— closed pneumothorax (no external injuries are responsible for the pneumothorax, the air leakage is from the lungs),

— open pneumothorax (air enters due to external trauma),

- partial pneumothorax (there is a partial collapse of the lung tissue),
- total pneumothorax (complete collapse of the lungs),
- seropneumothorax (with additional fluid accumulation),
  - hematopneumothorax (there is additional bleeding),
  - pyopneumothorax (with purulent effusion),
- spontaneous pneumothorax (occurs for no apparent reason),
- bilateral pneumothorax (both lungs are affected).

The cause may be trauma, chronic lung changes such as asthma or emphysema, or an iatrogenic cause.

- Clinic

Depending on the severity of the pneumothorax, there is shortness of breath and stabbing pain as well as a dry cough.

- Diagnostics

Conventional X-ray

A pneumothorax appears on X-ray as a **transparent structure free of pulmonary vessels**. In a **mantle pneumothorax** (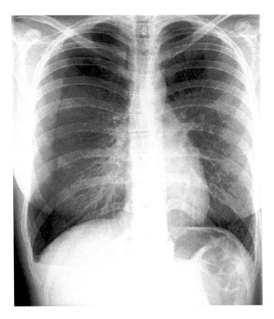 Fig. 17.2, pneumothorax in the form of a flat air mantle; is often silent percutorily and auscultatorily) only a **narrow air line** (so-called **hairline**) parallel to the thoracic wall is seen.

> The air often collects in the top of the lungs, even in small amounts, so a standing and expiratory intake is useful.

We speak of a **tip pneumothorax** when only a small amount of air enters the pleural space, which is then found mainly (see above) in the tip of the lung (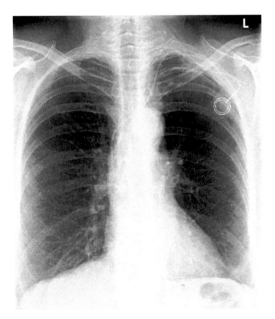 Fig. 17.3).

In seropneumothorax there is also a **fluid level.**

In tension pneumothorax, the lung is **completely collapsed** and the **mediastinum is displaced to the opposite side**. In the case

□ **Fig. 17.2**   Mantle pneumothrax

□ **Fig. 17.3**   Tip pneumothorax

of a tension pneumothorax, immediate relief by means of a drainage is necessary. In an emergency, an indwelling venous cannula in the 2nd or 3rd ICR in the medioclavicular line is also sufficient if the patient goes into shock in your radiology department.

Mesothelioma

Mesothelioma is a malignant tumor originating from the mesothelium of the pleura, which is frequently associated with exposure to asbestos. It is then a notifiable occupational disease.

- Clinic

At the beginning of the disease there are no or only nonspecific symptoms. In the further course there is increasing thoracic pain.

- Diagnostics

Conventional X-ray

There may be an accompanying pleural effusion (section pleural effusion). Furthermore, in the further course of the disease, **elongated or garland-like pleural thickening** and **extensive growth** may be seen on the X-ray.

CT

CT can be used primarily to examine the **extent** and **course of the disease**. Here, a **pleural thickening** encompassing the entire inner thoracic wall, **nodular contours** and possibly the **involvement of the** septa can also be seen. Furthermore, pleural calcifications and effusions may be manifested.

17.2.2 Emphysema

Lung emphysema is the irreversible over-expansion of the smallest air-filled structures. It represents the endpoint of a number of chronic lung diseases (COPD, bronchial asthma). A distinction is made between the following forms:

1. Centrilobular emphysema = most common type, COPD-associated, localized in the upper part of the lung with the formation of larger emphysema bubbles and dilatation of the bronchiolii respiratorii.

2. Panlobular emphysema = mostly genetic (congenital deficiency of alpha-1-antitrypsin), localized in the lower part of the lung

3. Old-age emphysema = lungs lose elasticity with increasing age

- Clinic

Cough, dyspnoea (especially on exertion) and fassthorax.

- Diagnostics

Conventional X-ray (▢ Fig. 17.4)

In order to be able to detect emphysema on a normal X-ray, it must already be in an advanced stage, otherwise it is difficult to distinguish between emphysema and "normal lung".

Important signs of emphysema are:
- increased lung transparency or rarified vascular bed
- flattened diaphragmatic domes
- enlarged retrosternal space and sterno-vertebral diameter (also called deep diameter)

CT

CT may be able to detect bullous changes earlier than conventional X-ray.

17.2.3 Bronchiectasis

This leads to irreversible dilatation of the bronchial tubes.

- Clinic

Cough, sputum ("mouthful expectoration" with three-layer sputum: foamy, mucous, purulent), recurrent infections, possibly drumstick finger.

- Diagnostics

Conventional X-ray

There are **streaky condensations** following the course of the bronchovascular structures, so-called **tram lines (rail track**

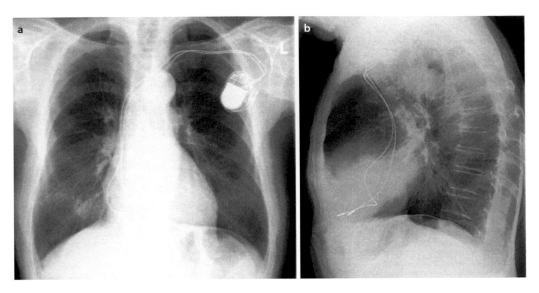

□ Fig. 17.4   Lung emphysema. **a** pa. **b** Lateral

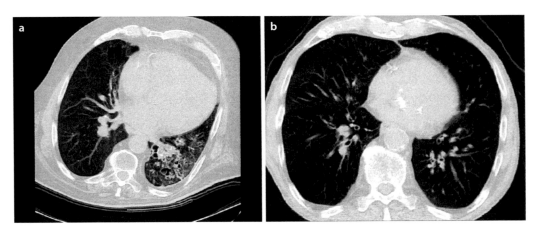

□ Fig. 17.5   a,b Bronchiectasis on CT

phenomenon) due to thickened bronchial walls, ring shadows due to saccularly dilated bronchi.

CT (□ Fig. 17.5)

Dilated bronchi, possibly **punctate/finger-shaped/micronodular condensations** (due to mucus-filled dilated bronchi) can be detected.

Bronchiography

KM is applied via the bronchoscope to visualize the bronchial tree. However, this method is almost completely replaced by CT.

17.2.4 **Pulmonary Oedema**

There is an accumulation of fluid in the lungs, which can be interstitial or interalveolar. Often an underlying cardiac disease is the cause, but also drugs, infections or carcinomas can cause pulmonary edema.

■ Clinic

Dyspnoea, cough (cardiac asthma), rales, possibly tachycardia, cyanosis, pallor.

■ Diagnostics

Conventional X-ray

The x-ray shows the following character-istics:

- Kerley B/C line = interstitial edema in the interlobular septa in the form of a reticular pattern.
- "Frosted glass phenomenon" due to intralobular edema.
- Peribronchial cuffing = edema formation in the peribronchial interstitium.
- "washed-out" hilus.
- Subpleural edema.

17.2.5 Pulmonary Fibrosis

Pulmonary fibrosis, which can be caused by various pathologies (e.g. ARDS, sarcoid-osis), leads to irreversible fibrotic remodel-ing of the lung.

■ Clinic

Initially, exertional dyspnea, tachypnea, and a dry, irritable cough may be present. Later, cyanosis, drumstick fingers, clock glass nails and cor pulmonale as well as terminal respi-ratory insufficiency may develop.

■ Diagnostics

Conventional X-ray/CT (■ Fig. 17.6)

The x-ray usually shows a proliferation of drawings in the lung structure. Due to connective tissue remodeling of the paren-chyma, the lung borders shift cranially. This can also be seen in the X-ray thorax in the form of fixed and raised diaphragmatic legs. In late stages a honeycomb lung is present. The structure of the lung can be determined even more precisely than with an X-ray examination by means of a high-resolution computer tomography. In spe-cial cases, this is performed in the prone

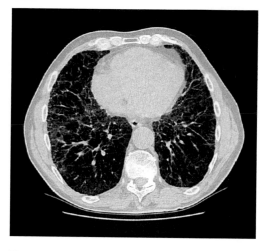

■ **Fig. 17.6** Pulmonary fibrosis with bronchiectasis

position in order to avoid reduced ventila-tion due to positioning.

17.2.6 Infectious Diseases

Pneumonia

Pneumonia describes an inflammation of the lung tissue. Pneumonias are divided into the following forms:

1. Alveolar pneumonia: the inflammation is located within the alveoli of the lungs
   - Bronchopneumonia = multifocal focal pneumonia, usually in several lobes of the lung
   - Lobar pneumonia = affection of an entire lobe of the lung (further subdi-vision into lower lobe, middle lobe and upper lobe pneumonia)
2. Interstitial pneumonia: the inflammation is localized in the interstitium, often called atypical pneumonia
   - Acute interstitial
   - Chronic interstitial
3. Community-acquired pneumonia
4. Nosocomial acquired pneumonia
5. Primary pneumonia
6. Secondary pneumonia (due to an exist-ing underlying disease)

■ Clinic

Increased respiratory rate, possibly dyspnea, fever, cough (dry or productive depending on etiology).

■ Diagnostics (◻ Fig. 17.7)

Conventional X-ray

The radiographic signs of pneumonia depend on the type of pneumonia (◻ Table 17.1).

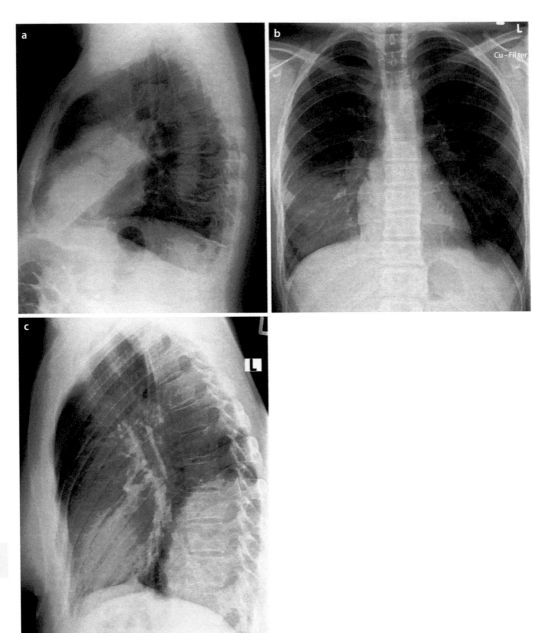

◻ **Fig. 17.7**   Types of pneumonia. **a** Lobar pneumonia. **b, c** Lower lobe pneumonia

◘ Table 17.1 Types of pneumonia

Interstitial Pneumonia	Alveolar Pneumonia		Fungal Pneumonia
	Broncho Pneumonia	Lobar Pneumonia	
– Interstitial shadowing pattern due to thickening of the interlobular septa – Predominantly strip-shaped condensations – Finely-spotted foci – Diffuse milky glassy haze	Confluent shading	Segmental shading	– Aspergilloma: homogeneous round shadow with ring-/sickle-shaped air accumulation – Candidiasis: infiltrates in the bronchiopulmonary region – Hematogenous seeding: even distribution throughout the lungs – *Pneumocystis carinii*: interstitial drawing proliferation, initially mainly perihilar, then rapid spread to mid/lower field
	– Extensive shadowing in the area of the lung lobes – Shading sharply defined by the lobe borders, blurred to the rest of the parenchyma		

CT

Similar to conventional X-ray.

Tuberculosis

Tuberculosis (short: Tbc or Tb) is an infectious disease that is most often caused by *Mycobacterium tuberculosis*. The bacteria are mainly transmitted by air, so that the lungs are often affected first. However, organ manifestation and involvement of the nervous system can also occur in the further course of the disease. The following stages of the disease can be distinguished (◘ Table 17.2).

▪ Clinic

B-symptomatics, in case of formation of a pulmonary primary complex: cough, hemoptysis, local lymph node swelling, dyspnoea.

▪ Diagnostics

Conventional X-ray (◘ Fig. 17.8)

The X-ray shows the so-called **primary complex** (usually intrapulmonary), which is also called **Ghon's focus.** Possibly a **primary cavern** develops, which can spread bronchogenically or hematogenically, with **"minimal lesions"** in the lung, which often appear as spotted shadows in the lung apex (=**Simon apex**) and possibly other organs. **Assmann's early infiltrates** (=flat, infraclavicular Felck's shadows) are, in addition to the reactivation of Simon's lace foci, a sign of post-primary TB.

An expired TB is often indicated by a **calcified primary complex** on x-ray.

CT

If primary tuberculosis is suspected, a chest CT may be performed for a more specific diagnosis.

Ascaridosis

Roundworm infestation with *Ascaris lumbricoides* is widespread worldwide (it is estimated that about ¼ of the population is infected). Transmission is oral (and then via the small intestine and bloodstream, including to the lungs).

◻ **Table 17.2**   Stages of tuberculosis

Stage	Designation	Clinic	Radiological Signs
I	Latent tuberculous infection	Positive tuberculin reaction without evidence of organ findings	Primary complex (=Ghon hearth)
II	Primary tuberculosis	Symptomatology due to a first organ manifestation	When spreading, it can come to the scattering in the bronchial system possibly also in other organs. In the lungs: shadowing and ring shadows (caverns), possibly atelectasis, pleurisy, Simon foci
III	Postprimary TB	Organ tuberculosis due to endogenous reactivation	Most often, first reactivation of Simon spikes foci, which melt down and break into the bronchial system. Then there is expansion to the lungs and other organs

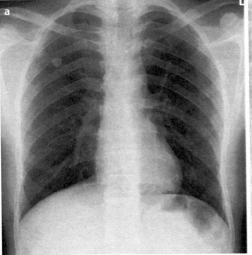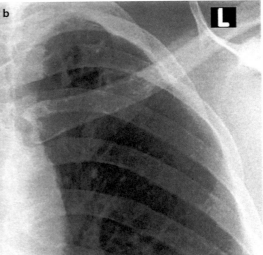

◻ **Fig. 17.8**   a,b Tbc in the posttuberculous state with (b) scar

■ Clinic

Bronchitis, shortness of breath, intestinal colic and diarrhoea, loss of appetite, possibly allergic skin reactions.

■ Diagnostics (◻ Fig. 17.9)

Conventional X-ray

Confluent spot shadows that "migrate across the lung" are seen on the X-ray. This migration is also called **Löffler infiltrate** (◻ Fig. 17.9) (which can also occur with some drugs such as penicillin). It is present when the infiltrate is no longer detectable after a maximum of ten days, eosinophilia is present, and relatively mild (pulmonary) symptoms are present.

Echinococcal Infection

Echinococcosis can be caused by different echinococci, but *Echinococcus cysticus* (dog tapeworm) and *Echinococcus multilocularis* (fox tapeworm) are the most likely.

17

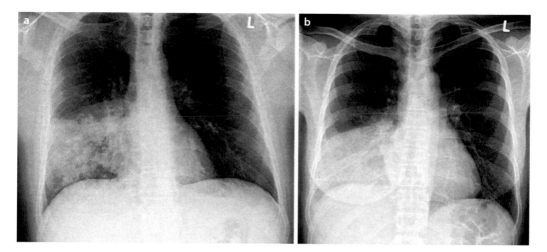

Fig. 17.9 Löffler infiltrate in ascaridosis. **(a)** Middle lobe, **(b)** Lower lobe

■ Clinic

Especially the liver and lungs are affected. There can be years of symptomlessness. The larvae (hyatids) can form a cyst, which can cause pain when ruptured. Furthermore, coughing and dyspnoea may occur and, depending on the size of the hyatids, tissue may be displaced.

■ Diagnostics

Conventional X-ray

Individual, smooth-edged round foci appear, which are **homogeneous.** After cyst rupture, a water level may also be visible on which the echinococcus wall floats (so-called **water lily sign**). Sometimes there is also the formation of a so-called **meniscus sign**, if the membrane does not lie tightly against the capsule wall, but some air exists in between.

17.2.7 Interstitial Lung Disease

Interstitial lung disease (ILD) affects the interstitial tissue of the lungs and the alveoli. Pneumoconiosis (also known as "pneumoconiosis") is the term used to describe lung diseases caused by the inhalation of dust and its deposition in the lungs.

Silicosis

Silicosis refers to pathological changes in the lungs caused by long-term inhalation of quartz dust particles (silica crystals). Silicosis is an occupational disease for which compensation is payable.

■ Clinic

The disease can be asymptomatic for years/decades. Acute symptoms are dyspnoea, cyanosis, chest pain and cough. Signs of a chronic course are lung rigidity (due to scarring), shortness of breath, dry cough, possibly dark sputum.

■ Diagnostics

Conventional X-ray

Initially, **the lung pattern** is **enhanced.** Later, especially in the middle and upper lung field, **dense** spotted **shadows** develop, the so-called **silicosis nodules.**

The following breakdown by size is made (□ Table 17.3):

As the disease progresses, the spotted shadows may become more pronounced and **calcifications** may be added (so-called shot lung).

Scarring leads to emphysema areas and larger calluses. A so-called **eggshell silicosis** develops due to shell-like calcifications

Table 17.3 Size classification of stain shadows in silicosis

Abbreviation	Meaning	Size in mm
P	Pinhead	1.5
Q	Micronodular	1.5–3
R	Nodular	3–10

under the capsule of the lymph nodes, especially at the pulmonary hilus.

CT

CT allows earlier and more accurate detection of the changes caused by silicosis (see above).

Asbestosis

Asbestosis is caused by inhalation of dust containing asbestos (fiber length >5 μm, fiber thickness <3 μm), which may also have carcinogenic effects.

- Clinic

In most cases, dyspnoea, dyspnoea, sputum and cyanosis may occur years to decades after exposure. Later, a general lung insufficiency with disability may result.

- Diagnostics

Conventional X-ray

The X-ray shows **fibrosis** of the middle and lower fields with a **reticulated, striated spread**. In contrast, **emphysema** (▶ Sect. 17.2.2) is often seen in the upper lung field. **Pleural plaques** and calcifications may also be seen.

CT

CT allows earlier and more accurate detection of the changes caused by silicosis (see above).

Organic Dusts

Exogenous allergic alveolitis is an allergic inflammation of the alveoli triggered by inhalation of fine dust (e.g. organic dusts such as molds, chemical substances).

- Clinic

A few hours after exposure there is fever, cough, dyspnea.

- Diagnostics

Conventional X-ray

An X-ray is rather unspecific, especially in the early stages, and can be difficult to distinguish from pneumonia of a different origin. There may be **streaky or nodular confluent** changes in the lower and middle fields of the lung.

CT

For a precise diagnosis (which should always be made in the context of the other anamnestic parameters such as lung function test, laboratory values, etc.), a high-resolution CT (HR-CT) should be performed. This also makes it possible to differentiate between inflammatory and already scarred areas.

17.2.8 Pneumonitis Radiation

Irradiation of tumors in the thoracic region can lead to co-irradiation of the lungs and, as a result, to reactive-toxic inflammation.

- Clinic

The symptoms are divided into an early and a late phase. The early phase may be asymptomatic, possibly accompanied by irritable cough, dyspnoea and pain. Either healing or, with repeated exposure, remodeling of the lung tissue and permanent pulmonary fibrosis then occur.

17

■ Diagnostics
Conventional X-ray

In the early phase, a **homogeneous shadowing of** the affected area is seen. In the later, fibrotic state, **striated scars with shrinkage of** the lung tissue are formed. The extent of the change corresponds very exactly to the (mostly angular) radiation field.

17.2.9 Lymphangiosis Carcinomatosa

Lymphangiosis carcinomatosa manifests itself in the lungs as malignant interstitial lung disease, but can also affect other areas such as the skin (e.g. the mamma). The cancer cells spread along the lymphatic vessels.

■ Clinic
B-symptomatics, possibly dyspnea.

■ Diagnostics
Conventional X-ray/CT (■ Fig. 17.10)

A **reticular pattern** with fine **nodular condensations** is seen, possibly accompanied by a pleural effusion (section Pleural effusion).

17.2.10 ARDS

Acute respiratory distress syndrome (ARDS) is an acute and life-threatening lung dysfunction that can be caused by shock, aspiration, sepsis, etc. The ARDS is classified into four stages (■ Table 17.4). ARDS is divided into four stages (■ Table 17.4).

■ Clinic
Depending on the underlying cause, dyspnea, cyanosis…

■ Diagnostics
Conventional X-ray (■ Fig. 17.11)

■ Table 17.4, there is initially **patchy indistinct compression** (without cardiac enlargement or pleural effusion) in the sense of edema, which then changes to a **reticular pattern in** the final stage.

17.2.11 Sarcoidosis

Sarcoidosis (also known as Boeck's disease) is an inflammation, the cause of which is not

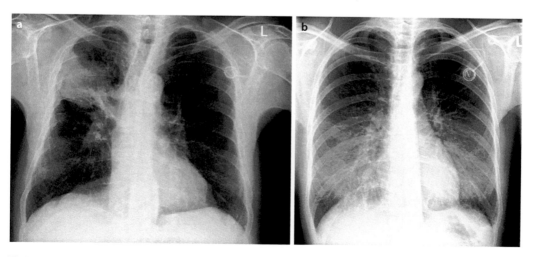

■ **Fig. 17.10** **a** Lymphangiosis carcinomatosa on the right in BC; **b** Basally accentuated lymphangiosis carcinomatosa on both sides

◻ **Table 17.4**   Stages of ARDS

Phase	Time Course	Description	Radiological Signs
Initial Phase	Until 1 h	Formation of interstitial pulmonary edema	Blotchy fuzzy condensations
Early Stage	1–24 h	Alveolar pulmonary edema, microthrombi…	Rapid fusion to homogeneous compactions
Intermediate Phase	1–7 days	Microatelectasis, fibroblast proliferation	Regression to spotty shading
Late Stage	>7 days	Pulmonary fibrosis	Regression of the spotted shadows, reticular pattern (=irreversible fibrosis)

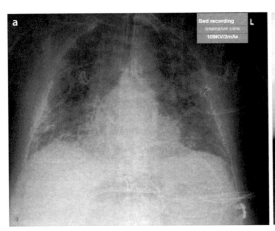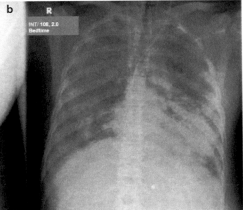

◻ **Fig. 17.11**   ARDS. **a** Stage II, **b** Stage III

yet fully understood, in which epithelioid cell granulomas are formed.

▪ **Clinic**

Acute (=Löfgren's syndrome): erythema nodosum, arthritis, adenopathy, possibly infection, fever.

Chronic: Irritable cough, dyspnea, iridocyclitis, uveitis, and many others.

▪ **Diagnostics**

Conventional Radiology/CT (◻ Fig. 17.12)

Depending on the stage, the following characteristics may be seen in the radiograph or cross-sectional diagnosis (◻ Table 17.5).

17.2.12 Tumors

Benign tumors of the lung (which are quite rare) include hamartoma, carcinoid, and benign mesothelioma. Malignant tumors, which are discussed in the following sec-

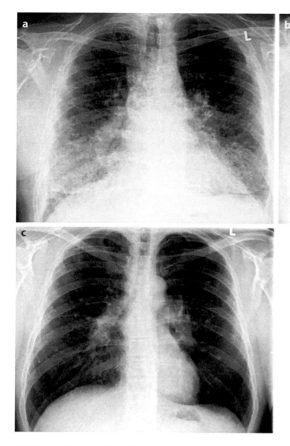

□ **Fig. 17.12** **a–c** Sarcoidosis with **b** bihilary lymphadenopathy and **c** bipulmonary round foci

□ **Table 17.5** Stages of sarcoidosis

Stage	Radiological Features
I	Symmetrical bihilar adenopathy (□ Fig. 17.12b)
II	Involvement of the parenchyma with interstitial reticular drawing proliferation
III	Pulmonary fibrosis (▶ Sect. 17.2.5)

tions, are primarily bronchial carcinoma, malignant lymphoma, and metastases to the lung from other tumors.

Bronchial Carcinoma

A bronchial carcinoma is a malignant neoplasm of cells in the lower airways (bronchi). With 25% of all carcinomas, bonchial carcinoma is a relatively frequent diagnosis, and men are more frequently affected than women.

A distinction is made between different forms of bronchial carcinoma (□ Table 17.6).

Most bronchial carcinomas are found centrally (75%), but peripheral or diffuse localization is also possible.

Metastasis often occurs to the **liver**, **brain**, **adrenal glands** and **skeletal system**, especially the spine.

◻ **Table 17.6**   Bronchial carcinoma variants

Form		Frequency in %	Localization	Metastasis
Small cell lung carcinoma		15	Mostly central	Early
Non-small cell lung cancer		85		
Of this:	Squamous cell carcinoma	40	Mostly central	Late
	Adenocarcinoma	35	Mostly peripheral	Relatively fast
	Large cell carcinoma	10	Central and peripheral	Early

■ Clinic

In the early stages usually initially asymptomatic, then possibly cough, chest pain, whistling breathing, shortness of breath (shortness of breath), hemoptysis (bloody tinted sputum), hoarseness and swelling of the face/throat.

Pancoast tumor is a special variant of bronchial carcinoma. It is initially located at the apex of the lung, but rapidly affects the thoracic wall, border cord and brachial plexus, which may lead to Horner's syndrome with miosis, ptosis and enophthalmos.

The term bronchioalveolar carcinoma, which belongs to the adenocarcinomas, is no longer found in the current classifications. Radiologically, this form, which is currently pathologically designated with a lepidic growth pattern, impresses as a **pneumonia-typical infiltrate,** which, however, shows no response to appropriate antibiotic therapy.

■ Diagnostics

Conventional X-ray

There are initially non-specific clues that may raise suspicion of carcinoma on x-ray. These include:

- **Atelectasis due to bronchial stenosis**
- **Persistent infiltrate**
- **Lung tip shadowing**
- **Mediastinal widening**
- **Unilateral hilar enlargement**
- **Upper congestion**
- **Diaphragmatic herniation (phrenic nerve paresis)**
- **Pleural effusion of unknown origin (possibly pleuritis carcinomatosa)**

Other chest x-ray findings suspicious for carcinoma may include:

- **Central tumor with hilifugal endobronchial spread**
- **Tumor with melting (tumor cavern)**
- **Hilar tumor shadow**
- **Chest wall infiltration**
- **Segmental bronchus closure**
- **General tissue displacements**

❯ Since adenocarcinoma is usually found in the periphery (◻ Table 17.6), it may also initially appear like a pneumonic infiltrate.

CT   For precise diagnosis and tumor staging, a CT should be performed if there is a justified suspicion. The administration of CT can also improve the assessment of possible vascular occlusions. If histological confirmation is not possible by bronchoscopy, a CT-guided puncture can be performed. The risk of pneumothorax can be reduced by positioning the patient on the side to be punctured.

17

> A puncture is contraindicated if it is a potentially primary operable finding!

Malignant Lymphoma

Malignant lymphoma is a neoplastic disease of the lymphatic system, which usually manifests itself in the lymph nodes, but can also affect other organs, such as the spleen, liver, lungs.

- Clinic

General B-symptomatology and swelling of the lymph nodes, cough, dyspnoea and pain if the lungs are affected.

- Diagnostics

Conventional X-ray

Mediastinal and **hilar lymph node enlargement** may present. Both hilus and mediastinum may appear widened. If the involvement is pronounced, the mediastinum appears widened like a chimney.

CT

CT is used for the precise assessment of the lymph node involvement and a possible pulmonary manifestation with mostly somewhat blurred circumscribed condensations. However, pulmonary lymphoma involvement can cause very different patterns and should therefore always be considered if the underlying disease is present.

Metastases

Lung metastases occur in about 75% of cases of renal carcinoma, in about 60% of cases of thyroid carcinoma, breast carcinoma and malignant melanoma and in about 40% of cases of prostate carcinoma.

- Clinic

In most cases, it is the primary tumor that first causes symptoms.

- Diagnostics

Conventional X-ray

Foci with a size of >10 mm can be detected. Characteristics are **multiple nod-**

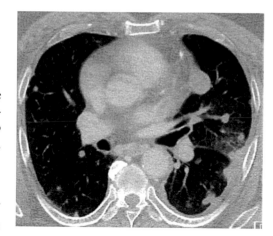

◘ **Fig. 17.13** Lung metastases (in the lung window CT) in NCC as primarius

ules (of different sizes) with **sharp margins** and **symmetrical involvement** (often the subfields are affected). If necessary, there may be fusion or calcification.

CT (◘ Fig. 17.13**)**
See above.

17.2.13 **Pulmonary Embolism**

Pulmonary embolism is the occlusion of a pulmonary artery branch by a displaced thrombus (usually from the venous pelvic/leg circulation).

- Clinic

Symptoms may be absent or nonspecific. Depending on the size of the affected area, there may be shortness of breath and/or accelerated breathing, palpitations, chest pain, anxiety, coughing and/or hemoptysis. Laboratory chemistry shows elevated D-dimers, a breakdown product of fibrin. In addition, ECG and cardiac echo show right heart strain.

- Diagnostics (◘ Fig. 17.14)

Conventional X-ray

Conventional X-rays show a regional reduction in blood flow, which **reduces the**

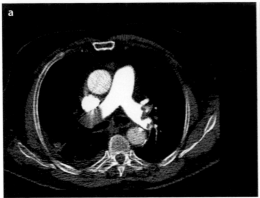 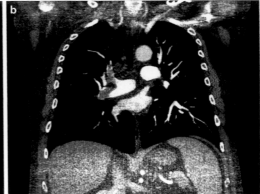

◻ Fig. 17.14 Pulmonary embolism. **a** Axial, **b** Coronary

diameter of the **vessel** and results in a **secondary increase in transparency** (so-called **Westermark sign**). Furthermore, there is the so-called **knuckle sign**, an enlargement with a jump in caliber, which results from the **ballooning of the central artery** and a **resulting clear difference in size** to the continuing vessels. Another characteristic is the shadowing district (**Hampton's hump**), in which a hemispherical shadowing (=alveolar hemorrhage) sitting on the pleura can be seen (but only after about 1–4 days post embolism). Further findings may be a diaphragmatic herniation and squamous atelectasis.

CT

Since in most cases an X-ray can be unremarkable, CT angiography (CTA) in pulmonary arterial phase is the means of choice. Among other things, it allows direct detection of the embolus via a **filling defect** or **termination of the CM column**.

Scintigraphy

▶ Section 17.3.2.

17.2.14 Childhood

See also ▶ Chap. 24.

Surfactant Deficiency Syndrome

▶ Section 24.1.1.

Hemorrhage

Pulmonary hemorrhage in infancy describes pulmonary hemorrhage due to a coagulation disorder and left heart failure, which can occur especially in premature infants or as a complication of respiratory distress syndrome.

■ Clinic

Acute dyspnea, possibly bloody secretion.

■ Diagnostics

Conventional X-ray

Depending on the location, a **patchy confluent lung shadowing** is seen, but it is usually difficult to differentiate from pneumonia or respiratory distress syndrome.

Pulmonary Emphysema

Congenital lobar emphysema describes hyperinflation of one or more lobes of the lung in the newborn/infant.

■ Clinic

Dyspnea, tachypnea.

■ Diagnostics

Conventional X-ray

As in adult emphysema there is a mostly unilateral **increase of transparency**, possibly with **displacement of the mediastinum** to the opposite side.

Lung Cyst

This is a congenital cystic malformation of the lung.

- Clinic

Dyspnea.

- Diagnostics

Conventional X-ray

A **sharply bordered, round lightening area** is visible, depending on the size of the cyst with mediastinal displacement.

Transient Neonatal Tachypnea

(See also ▶ Chap. 24). This is an intraalveolar fluid retention (synonym also "wet lung disease") and a respiratory distress syndrome caused by it, which can affect premature infants in particular.

- Clinic

Retractions at sternum and intercostal spaces, tachypnea >60/min, attenuation of breath sounds, pale gray skin coloration, cyanosis.

- Diagnostics

Conventional X-ray

The characteristics depend on the stage (◘ Table 17.7):

A bronchopneumogram results from inflammatory or other infiltrations in the

◘ **Table 17.7** Stages of respiratory distress syndrome

Stage	Radiological Signs
I	Fine granular transparency reduction
II	Additional positive aerobronchogram extending beyond the cardiac contour
III	Additionally further reduction of transparency with blurring of the diaphragm and heart contours
IV	White lung, the heart contours cannot be differentiated from the lung parenchyma

lung parenchyma, which cause an edematous peribronchial density increase. Due to the peribronchial compressions, the lumen of the bronchi becomes radiologically more transparent to the surrounding tissue, which is called a positive bronchopneumogram.

Meconium Aspiration

▶ Section 24.1.2.

17.3 Diagnostics

17.3.1 Diagnostic Radiology

Christel Vockelmann

Sonography

Sonography is very well suited for detecting pleural effusions, i.e. fluid in the pleural cavity. In the case of larger amounts of effusion, sonographically guided puncture of the effusion is also an excellent option. As a rule, this is performed by internists, since they often primarily treat patients with relevant pleural effusions.

Conventional X-ray Diagnostics

The basic diagnosis of the lungs and bronchi is the chest X-ray. In individual cases, a tracheal image is taken to detect tracheomalacia caused by an enlargement of the thyroid gland.

> Often the radiographic thorax is x-rayed with the question of a pneumothorax in expiration. However, recent studies show that there is no significant difference in the detection of pneumothorax between images taken in inspiration and expiration.

Fluoroscopy/Angiography

Fluoroscopic examinations of the thorax have become relatively rare. Fluoroscopy can be used, for example, to assess the mobility of the diaphragm or to further clarify a questionable compression in the X-ray thorax. Often, however, a computer tomography of the thorax is performed as a much more sensitive procedure.

Computed Tomography

In the meantime, computed tomography is not only a complementary diagnostic method to X-ray thorax for the clarification of diseases of the thorax. In many cases, CT of the lung is performed as the primary diagnostic method. In the case of certain diseases, e.g. rectal carcinoma, many oncological centers primarily perform a CT of the lung to exclude metastasis. The advantage of CT compared to conventional radiography is the possibility of detecting even small round foci corresponding to metastases.

Magnetic Resonance Imaging

Magnetic resonance imaging has not yet proved its worth in the assessment of the lung parenchyma. On the one hand, this is due to the detection of minute changes in an organ that is dependent on breathing and thus difficult to immobilize. Then, small calcifications are very important for the assessment of changes. Like air, these are signal-free in MRI, so these findings escape MRI. For these reasons, MRI of the lung is not a common diagnostic technique today. Nevertheless, in many examinations, such as a cardio-MRI or an examination of the upper abdomen, the lungs are at least partially included in the examination area and should always be examined as well in order not to miss any relevant findings.

17.3.2 Nuclear Medicine

Ursula Blum

Pulmonary Ventilation Scintigraphy

Ventilation scintigraphy is acquired after inhalation of gases, aerosols or vaporized carbon particles. The patient should be well informed about the examination procedure. Practice with the still inactive system with the mouth tightly closed and the nose closed is useful. This procedure ensures that the inhaled radioactive air remains trapped in the filter system provided for this purpose and does not contaminate the staff or the immediate environment. If necessary, the bronchial system can be dilated with a metered-dose aerosol (e.g. Berodual) before inhalation. The patient should be instructed to cough and take deep breaths in and out to loosen mucus plugs, the lungs expand. The target activity usually does not exceed 10–20 MBq, so that the ventilation study must precede the perfusion study.

In order to prevent the release of thrombi, the patient is carefully positioned. He lies on his back. The arms are positioned comfortably and stably above the head using appropriate positioning aids. Planar scintigrams are obtained from eight views: ventral (RVL); dorsal (LDR); left lateral; right lateral; and right anterior oblique and left anterior oblique (RAO/LAO) and right posterior oblique and left posterior oblique (RPO/LPO). For the evaluation of complex findings, the acquisition of SPECT images (64 views à 24 s/matrix 128×128) has proven to be useful. A SPECT/CT offers the possibility to combine functional and morphological imaging in a low-dose technique.

Ventilation can also be carried out with other gases, but this is associated with extensive logistical requirements. ^{133}Xenon requires special structural radiation protection measures, while ^{81m}krypton, daughter nuclide of ^{81}rubidium, requires the daily procurement of a new generator system due to its extremely short HWZ.

Lung Perfusion Scintigraphy

Immediately following and in the same position, 150–200 MBq ^{99m}Tc labeled human albumin aggregates (MAA) are injected, which are larger than the lung capillaries and block approximately every 10,000th capillary. The regional distribution of the particles corresponds to the relative perfusion of the lung. If there is constriction or occlusion of a pulmonary artery, the subsequent flow area is only partially or not at all reached, and there is an under-occupation of the corresponding section of the lung in a typical wedge shape. A commercially supplied kit containing the inactive particles is connected to the generator eluate according to the manufacturer's instructions and under exclusion of air. Before taking the required amount of activity of approx. 200 MBq ^{99m}Tc MAA, the kit vial must be shaken, as the particles settle in the bottom of the glass and cannot otherwise be taken out in the correct dosage (approx. 100,000 to 200,000 particles).

The activity is shaken again before application and then injected i. v. slowly and lying down over several deep breaths. The venous access must not contain a filter. Aspiration of blood to control the position of the access must also be avoided, as otherwise thrombi will form which carry relatively high activities and lead to an inhomogeneous distribution of the nuclide with focal hot spots. Regional perfusion is position-dependent. If the patient is sitting, the caudal lung sections are more perfused, which may be useful for examination in other indications. The MAA particles are degraded intrapulmonary via proteolysis with a HWZ of 2–3 h. The count rate of perfusion uptake must be a factor of five higher than that of ventilation in order to achieve a reliable superposition of the ventilation study. The study protocol is the same as that of ventilation for comparability of both studies.

Evaluation

Normal findings show a homogeneous activity distribution in ventilation and perfusion in all lung segments.

In the so-called **match findings, there** is a reduction in activity or a loss of activity at the same site in both ventilation and perfusion. Such a scintigraphic distribution pattern indicates pulmonary space occupying lesions, infections, pleural effusions, consequences of obstructive or restrictive lung diseases or old pulmonary embolisms and is caused by the Euler-Liljestrand reflex.

Mismatch findings are characterized by markedly reduced or abolished perfusion with intact ventilation. A mismatch finding manifests the pathology of recent pulmonary embolism. In rare cases, other pathologies of the lung also show mismatch findings. To increase the specificity of the result, a recent radiograph should be available at baseline. Alternatively, SPECT in combination with low dose CT can be used in the diagnosis of acute pulmonary embolism.

Determination of Postoperative Pulmonary Function

To predict postoperative lung function, perfusion scintigraphy is obtained before a planned pneumectomy or lobectomy. The radiopharmaceutical is injected in a sitting position to account for gravity-induced perfusion changes. First, static images are acquired ventrally and dorsally using a planar technique. Then, regional distribution in upper, middle, and lower lobes of both sides is quantified via the placement of ROIs. The percentage uptake of the lung area to be removed is subtracted from the total function and the result is multiplied by the preoperative forced expiratory volume (FEV). If this results in a postoperative FEV of less than 0.8 L, the upcoming operation must be critically questioned.

Right-Left-Shunt

Even in healthy individuals, about 2% of the blood circulating in the pulmonary circulation is removed from the oxygenation process. Various pathological changes or malformations can increase the proportion of blood flowing past the pulmonary circulation, resulting in a global oxygen deficiency. After application of ^{99m}Tc MAA particles, in case of pathologically increased right-left shunt, accumulation occurs in organs where the particle size exceeds the capillary diameter (e.g. brain, liver and kidneys). After planar imaging of the lungs and kidneys in anterior and posterior views, the percentage shunt can be calculated. A renal cardiac output of 25% is assumed.

$$\text{Shunt}\,(\%) = \frac{\text{Nierenzählrate} \times 4}{\text{Nierenzählrate} \times 4 + \text{Lungenzählrate}}$$

Pulmonary Hypertension

In patients with chronic recurrent pulmonary embolisms, the pathological pressure increase in the pulmonary circulation can be detected via pulmonary ventilation perfusion scintigraphy. If ^{99m}Tc MAA is applied in a sitting position, the lung base of the healthy person must show a higher activity accumulation than the upper lung sections due to gravitation.

In pulmonary hypertension there is no difference in the distribution, sometimes even the upper lung sections are more perfused.

Lung PET

In the diagnosis of unclear solitary lung findings, the ^{18}F-FDG PET/(CT) provides a diagnostically valuable gain, especially if the patient's general condition does not permit a biopsy. Round tumors smaller than 1 cm may escape imaging due to the inadequate spatial resolution of the device and the patient's respiratory motion during acquisi-

tion. Tumors of different histology show different memory behavior. While squamous cell carcinoma of the lung shows a high ^{18}F-FDG uptake, the tracer of adenocarcinomas of the lung is acquired very inconstantly. In small cell bronchial carcinoma, the procedure is used when the location of the primarius and lung function permit surgical intervention and distant metastases have not been detected on any imaging modality. If PET and CT findings are negative, mediastinoscopy can be omitted. If a mediastinal lymph node is found in one of the two diagnostic procedures, it requires histological clarification.

17.3.3 Valence

Christel Vockelmann

◘ Table 17.8 shows the use of the respective therapeutic options depending on the problem.

◘ **Table 17.8** Value of the therapeutic procedures

	Sonography	Conventional	Fluoroscopy/ Angiography	CT	MRI	Nuk	PET
Pneumonia	W	P	N	W	N	N	N
Bronchial carcinoma	N	P	N	P	N	N	W
Pulmonary embolism	N	N	N	P	N	W	N
Pulmonary fibrosis	N	P	N	P	N	N	N

N Not indicated, *P* Primary diagnosis, *W* Further diagnosis

17.4 Therapy

17.4.1 Interventional Radiology

Angiography

Angiography is used as a therapeutic procedure, e.g. for removing a torn port catheter or a CVC. For this purpose, a venous puncture is made in the femoral vein. The pulmonary artery is then probed with a catheter, in which the catheter is advanced to the right heart via the inferior vena cava. From the right ventricle, the pulmonary artery is probed. Then a snare loop, a lasso-like loop, is used to capture the lost catheter and remove it via the sheath in the femoral vein.

Another field of application of angiography is the treatment of hemoptysis. This term describes a coughing up of blood caused, for example, by pulmonary bleeding from the bronchial arteries. If such a condition cannot otherwise be treated by bronchoscopy, the bronchial artery of the corresponding side is probed. A microcatheter is then advanced into the bronchial artery and the artery is occluded with small particles. The procedure is feasible without leading to necrosis of the lung, since the lung tissue is not only supplied via the bronchial arteries, but also still via the pulmonary arteries.

Computed Tomography

For the treatment of primary bronchial carcinoma or pulmonary metastasis, thermoablation can be considered in certain cases. This is performed in particular in the lungs under computer tomography control. Thermoablation ultimately means the coking of tissue. For this purpose, a probe is inserted into the tumor and heat is then applied. In order to hit the tumor exactly and also to achieve a sufficient safety distance, the puncture is CT-guided. As the coking is very painful—the tissue is heated to at least 75 °C, so imagine you are touching a hot hotplate—the procedure is often performed under intubation anesthesia, or at least under analgesia. Indications for such a procedure include patients who are inoperable for general reasons or single metastases of certain tumors such as colorectal carcinoma. Local recurrence of bronchial carcinoma, e.g. after radiotherapy, can often be treated by thermoablation.

The coking of the tumor tissue leads to the death of the cells. In the course of the thermoablation, a scarring shrinkage of the area occurs.

17.4.2 Radiotherapy

Bronchial Carcinoma

Positioning is supine with the arms above the head.

- Therapy of Non-Small Cell Lung Cancer (NSCLC)

The total dose for definitive radiochemotherapy is 60–70 Gy, and that for adjuvant therapy is 50–60 Gy.

- Therapy of Small Cell Lung Cancer (SCLC)

Four to six cycles of chemotherapy followed by radio-chemotherapy of the primary tumor and adjacent lymphatic drainage area.

After completion of chemotherapy and exclusion of metastases, prophylactic whole-brain irradiation (PCI: Prophylactic Cranial Irradiation) with a total dose of 30 Gy is performed.

Side effects: Skin irritation, esophagitis, pneumonitis, pericarditis.

Case Study

Mr. Tuschka, a 76-year-old man, has noticed hemoptysis lately. His wife has been telling him to quit smoking for 30 years. However, he never got off it. Now, he has also lost weight in the last month. Due to the many years of nicotine abuse and weight loss, bronchial carcinoma is suspected. After a chest X-ray, which revealed a round focus in the right lower lobe of the lung, a computer tomography was performed. The suspicion of bronchial carcinoma is confirmed. CT-morphologically no mediastinal lymph node metastases are found. The left adrenal gland is slightly thickened. The radiologist gives the tumor stage as cT1bN0Mx. Incidental findings include marked bullous emphysema. The radiologist recommends a completion of the staging. He is especially concerned about the left adrenal gland. First, a bronchoscopy is performed, but the tumor is too far peripherally in the lung to be punctured bronchoscopically. In addition, an FDG-PET-CT scan and an MRI of the neurocranium are performed. The MRI is necessary because cerebral metastases can only be inadequately detected in the FDG-PET due to the high sugar metabolism of the brain. For the definite exclusion of cerebral metastases, the MRI examination is performed with contrast medium, although the native images show no abnormalities. Mr. Tuschka was lucky. Apart from the tumor in the lung, no other malignant findings are found. Actually, due to the favorable tumor stage without metastasis, surgery would now be the primary option. However, the lung function test showed that an operation is not possible due to the pronounced emphysema. To confirm the diagnosis and histologically determine the exact tumor entity, a CT-guided puncture is performed. In this case, there is a significantly higher risk of pneumothorax due to the pronounced emphysema, but this can be treated well with a drainage. After the diagnosis has been confirmed, the patient is presented to the tumor conference of the clinic. The conference, which is attended by the oncologist, the radiotherapist, the radiologist, the pulmonologist, the thoracic surgeon and the pathologist, decides that the patient should undergo radio-chemotherapy. Mr. Tuschka agrees to the procedure. He comes through the therapy well. A few side effects occur (such as tingling in the extremities and also hair loss). The blood values were also changed in the meantime due to anemia. However, he did not develop any complications of the radiation such as dermatitis. However, he feels quite weak during the treatment and the first time afterwards. After two years the CT thorax shows an increase of the scar in the area of the tumor. The radiologist suspects a recurrence. To confirm the diagnosis, Mr. Tuschka is again sent for a PET-CT. Here the radiologist's suspicion is confirmed. In the tumor area there is an increased glucose utilization as a sign of a vital tumor. The PET-CT is examined jointly by the nuclear medicine specialist Dr. Blümchen and the radiologist Dr. Vau. Based on the size of the recurrence of 2.5 cm, the radiologist recommends discussing a thermoablation in the tumor conference. Another irradiation of the area is out of the question. Chemotherapy alone has only very limited chances of success in Mr. Tuschka. Therefore, the conference agrees to thermoablation, which is performed in the clinic under CT guidance. Mr. Tuschka survives the procedure well, even though he has a pleural drainage for a few days due to a pneumothorax. The further CT checks and follow-up examinations with the oncologist show no recurrence in the next months and years.

Practice Questions

1. In a pleural effusion on CT, what characterizes a transudate and what characterizes an exudate?
2. What are signs of pulmonary edema on x-ray?
3. What do the abbreviations "p", "q", and "r" stand for in the size classification of spot shadows in silicosis?
4. What are the stages of ARDS and what are the radiological findings depending on the stage?
5. When do Westermark signs and Knuckle signs show up?

Solutions ▶ Chap. 27

Gastrointestinal Tract

Christel Vockelmann, Ursula Blum, and Guido Heilsberg

Contents

© Springer-Verlag GmbH Germany, part of Springer Nature 2023
M. Kahl-Scholz, C. Vockelmann (eds.), *Basic Knowledge Radiology*,
https://doi.org/10.1007/978-3-662-66351-6_18

The gastrointestinal tract includes all organs that serve to absorb and process food, i.e. the esophagus, gaster, duodenum, jejunum, ileum, colon and rectum, as well as the liver, pancreas and biliary system. In addition to inflammatory changes, tumorous changes play a major role in medicine and thus also in imaging techniques, which are indispensable in the diagnosis and therapy of these diseases.

18.1 Anatomical Structures

Christel Vockelmann

The digestive tract begins with the mouth and pharynx (▶ Chap. 15) and then continues through the thorax with the approx. 25 cm long **oesophagus** into the abdomen. Here the **stomach** lies subdiaphragmally on the left. The duodenum lies retroperitoneally in the middle section up to the flexura duodenojejunalis   (Treitz's   ligament). **Jejunum** and **ileum** lie intraperitoneally, via Bauhin's valve the digested food pulp reaches the **colon**, which is fixed retroperitoneally in the ascending and descending part.

The arterial supply of the small and large intestine up to the right flexure is via the superior mesenteric vein, the descending colon and rectosigmoid are supplied via the inferior mesenteric artery. Venous outflow is via the mesenteric vein to the portal vein (V. porta).

The **liver** lies intraperitoneally in the right upper abdomen and is protected in large parts by the thorax. The liver is fused to the diaphragm only via the pars affixa, in the remaining area there is a covering with the peritoneum. This runs out into the ligaments falciforme, hepatograstricum and hepatoduodenale as well as teres hepatis. The surgical anatomy and segmentation, which is therefore also relevant in clinical practice, is based, among other things, on the falciform ligament, which divides the liver into the right and left hepatic lobes. The individual segments are formed by the branches of the portal vein with the accompanying bile ducts and the venous drainage areas.

The **gallbladder is** located at the lower border of the liver at the surgical border between the right and left liver lobes. It is the reservoir for bile. The outflow of bile takes place via the dexter and sinister hepatic ducts into the common hepatic duct. After union with the ductus cysticus, bile flows via the ductus choledochus (clinically DHC) into the duodenum via the papilla vateri.

The pancreas lies secondarily retroperitoneal. It fulfils exocrine and endocrine functions. Sonographically, the lienal vein (V. splenica) serves as a guide structure, which runs along the upper edge of the pancreas. The arterial supply of the liver, gallbladder and pancreas is via the truncus coeliacus.

18.2 Disease Patterns

Christel Vockelmann

18.2.1 Pharynx, Oesophagus

Oesophagitis

These are inflammatory changes of the mucosa. Nowadays, the diagnosis is made endoscopically. The reason for this, in addition to reflux, which leads to irritation especially in the distal esophagus, is a restricted immune system with then infection of the esophagus by mainly fungi (Candida). Thermal or chemical damage can also lead to esophagitis.

The complications of rupture of the esophagus due to vomiting is called **Boerhaave syndrome.** Other reasons for rupture are iatrogenic perforation in about 55–60% of cases.

■ Clinic

Burning thoracic, pain on ingestion of fluids and food.

■ Diagnostics

Radiological diagnostics are mainly used in the evaluation of complications. Sometimes the esophageal swallow is still used as a diagnostic procedure to assess the extent of reflux and the contractility of the esophagus.

Conventional X-ray (□ Fig. 18.1)

Air in the mediastinum can be detected by demonstrating **lines of lightening along the mediastinal pleura** or even the pericardium. If **pneumomediastinum** is suspected, a CT scan should always be followed up to better assess the extent of the injury and the possible cause.

Transillumination

Fluoroscopy allows assessment of contrast passage and contractile waves of the esophagus as well as the location of the cardia below the diaphragm, observation of possible reflux of contrast.

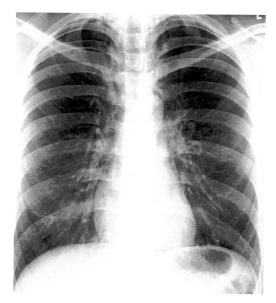

□ Fig. 18.1 Pneumomediastinum

CT

Computed tomography is used to assess the complications of inflammatory diseases of the esophagus. Possible abscesses in longstanding changes can be reliably detected. The extent of pneumomediastinum can also be reliably assessed.

Diverticula of the Oesophagus

Diverticula are divided into the following variants:

- **Zenker's diverticulum**: 70% of all diverticula, cervical pulsatile diverticulum. Preferred in men of older age. Large pseudodiverticulum localized dorsally at the upper esophageal jugular predominantly on the left side.
- **Bifurcation diverticulum**: True diverticulum due to scarring, e.g. after TBC.
- **Epiphrenic pulsatile diverticulum**: Pseudodiverticulum above the hiatus, often combined with a hiatal hernia or achalasia (sec. Achalasia)

■ Clinic

Mostly only Zenker diverticula become symptomatic by food retention with regurgitation or bad breath. Complication can be aspiration pneumonia.

■ Diagnostics

Fluoroscopy (□ Fig. 18.2)

The esophageal swallow is used to assess the location and size in addition to endoscopy.

❯ A Zenker diverticulum may sonographically mimic a left retrothyroidal mass.

Swallowing Disorders

Swallowing disorders are distinguished between:

- **Dysphagia**: A feeling of tightness or pain when swallowing. This can be caused by a wide variety of diseases, e.g. diverticula, tumors, inflammations or even cere-

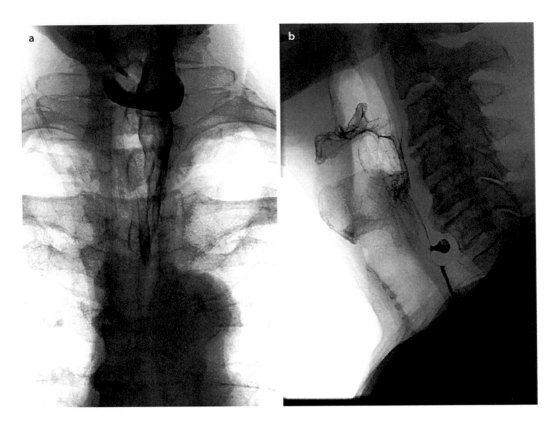

◘ Fig. 18.2   a, b Zenker diverticulum

bral ventricle diseases such as infarctions resulting in cranial nerve failures.

- **Aspiration**: transfer of food, liquids or saliva into the trachea with the risk of pneumonia.
- **Tertiary contractions**: Non-propulsive contractions especially of the distal esophagus as a disturbance of the swallowing act. Frequent incidental finding in older patients, may be combined e.g. with a hiatal hernia or reflux. Possible cause is also a diabetic neuropathy of the gastointestinal tract.

■ Clinic

Irritable cough on aspiration, pain on swallowing, globus sensation (often localized higher than the actual pathology, e.g. in the mid-thorax in case of bolus occlusion of the distal esophagus).

■ Diagnostics

In addition to the unspecific diagnosis of esophageal swallowing, kinematography can be performed in cases of dysphagia, especially with aspiration.

Fluoroscopy (◘ Fig. 18.3)

It allows the observation of the onward transport of contrast medium or contrast medium-soaked food pulp from the mouth into the upper esophagus and makes it possible to exclude a transfer into the trachea (aspiration).

Achalasia

Achalasia is a narrowing of the lower esophageal sphincter with sectular dilatation of the esophagus. It is a rare condition with an incidence of 1:100,000 population/year. Peak incidence 3rd–5th decade of life.

18

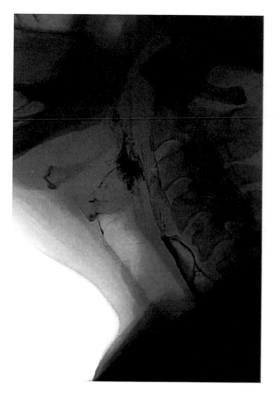

◘ Fig. 18.3 Aspiration

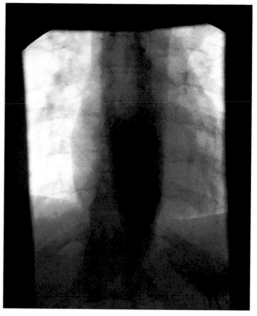

◘ Fig. 18.4 Achalasia

■ Clinic

Dysphagia with frequent after-drinking, bad breath, retrosternal feeling of fullness.

■ Diagnostics

Fluoroscopy (◘ Fig. 18.4)

The oesophageal swallow with water-soluble contrast medium shows a pathogno-monic chalice-like dilatation of the distal oesophagus. In contrast to carcinoma this has a smooth border of the esophagus.

Oesophageal Carcinoma

This is a malignant epithelial tumor of the esophagus – frequently squamous cell carcinoma (approx. 40% age peak 55 years), adenocarcinoma (approx. 60%, age peak 65 years) (=Barrett's carcinoma) in the distal esophagus, rarely undifferentiated. The tumor is frequently localized at the three physiological strictures at the esophageal constriction, at the level of the aortic arch and in the diaphragmatic fossa. Risk factors include concentrated alcohol, hot drinks, smoking, nitrosamines, reflux disease, achalasia, papillomavirus.

Metastasis occurs to the upper esophagus with early infiltration to adjacent organs due to lack of serosal coating and early lymphogenic metastasis. Hematogenous metastasis to liver, lung and bone is rather late.

■ Clinic

Dysphagia, possibly weight loss. Often late symptoms with characteristic complaints.

■ Diagnostics

CT (◘ Fig. 18.5)

CT is used for the diagnosis of spread. PET-CT, as the most sensitive method, enables the detection of distant metastases, but is currently not primarily used. Usual staging: endoscopy and CT, if operability is given → diagnostic laparoscopy to exclude peritoneal carcinomatosis (also not reliably detectable on PET-CT).

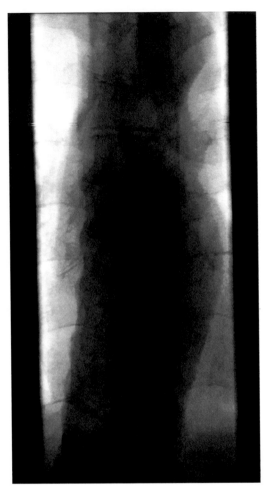

Fig. 18.5 Esophageal carcinoma

Postoperative/Posttherapeutic Changes

Significantly relevant changes in radiology here include:

- **Gastric elevation**: stomach displaced into the thorax after resection of the distal esophagus.
- **Colonic interposition**: Replacement of the esophagus by the colon, then usually with cervical and abdominal anastomosis, elevation mostly retrosternal or intrathoracic, occasionally subcutaneous.

■ Clinic

With insufficiency fever, septic picture.

■ Diagnostics (☐ Fig. 18.6)

In the case of complications, a CT should be performed for clarification, and in the case of suspected insufficiencies, positive oral contrast medium (as a diluted, approximately 3% solution) should be used if necessary.

18.2.2 Stomach and Duodenum

Gastritis, Ulcers and Complications

These are inflammatory changes of the gastric mucosa. The cause is often exogenous noxae such as alcohol excess or drugs (corti-

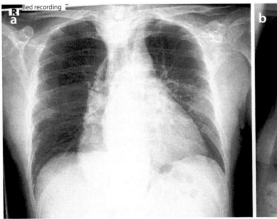
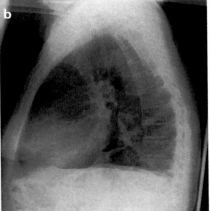

Fig. 18.6 **a, b** Stomach elevation

costeroids, ASA, non-steroidal anti-inflammatory drugs, chemotherapeutic drugs).

Complication: Ventricular or duodenal ulcer (ratio about 1:3) with bleeding or perforation. After healing, scarring with stenosis occurs.

Atypically localized ulcers must be suggestive of malignancy.

■ Clinic

Nausea, loss of appetite, upper abdominal pain, feeling of pressure. With complications "acute abdomen", upper GI bleeding.

■ Diagnostics

The primary diagnosis is usually made endoscopically.

Conventional X-ray

Furthermore, an X-ray abdomen, usually in a lying position and on the left side, is taken to detect free air.

CT

Frequently, CT is also primarily used as a much more sensitive method for detecting free air and hollow organ perforations.

❯ To detect free air, patients should lie on their left side for at least 5 min before the radiograph is taken in the left lateral position.

Free air is recognizable in the left lateral position as a **lightening** between the abdominal wall and the liver under the diaphragm. If the patient cannot be positioned in the **left lateral position for a** sufficiently long time, a standing X-ray of the thorax and abdomen may be helpful, where the free air can be detected as a lightening in the form of a **black crescent between the liver and diaphragm.** In the **supine x-ray,** the air usually collects centrally in the upper abdomen and may then be demarcated as a **roundish increase in transparency ("football sign").**

Duodenal ulcers may also perforate retroperitoneally. Here one has to look for a lightening fringe along the **psoas shadow** as a sign of retroperitoneal perforation.

In acute upper GI bleeding, diagnosis and treatment are usually performed endoscopically. If a bleed in a duodenal ulcer cannot be stopped endoscopically, endovascular therapy can be attempted (▶ Sect. 18.4.1).

18.2.3 Duodenal Diverticulum

This is an outpouching of the duodenal wall, mostly para- or juxtapapillary, frequency increasing with age (about 3% of the population).

■ Clinic

Mostly symtpomeless, may possibly cause outflow obstruction of DHC or D. wirsungianus.

■ Diagnostics

It is a frequent incidental finding with an air- or contrast-filled cavity directly related to the duodenum on CT or fluoroscopy examinations (◻ Fig. 18.7), usually without pathological significance.

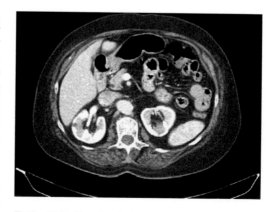

◻ **Fig. 18.7**   Duodenal diverticulum

Benign Tumors

These include polyps or mesenchymal tumors (lipomas or neurofibromas). They are rare overall.

- Clinic

Mostly asymptomatic.

- Diagnostics

Primarily an endoscopic diagnosis is performed.

CT

A CT is used in the clarification of mesenchymal tumors. Here, a **smoothly bounded mass** is seen in **the stomach wall**. In the case of lipoma, there is evidence of **fat isodense density values**.

Gastric Carcinoma, Duodenal Carcinoma

This is a malignant mass of the stomach, mostly adenocarcinoma. Duodenal carcinomas are very rare.

The Siewert classification of adenocarcinomas of the esophagogastric junction (AEG) is important for treatment.
- AEG I (actually Barrett's carcinoma): 1–5 cm orally down the cardia.
- AEG II (actually cardiac carcinoma): Oral <1 cm and aboral <2 cm from the cardia.
- AEG III (subcardiac gastric carcinoma): >2 to 5 cm from the cardia.

Metastasis occurs relatively early lymphogenically; hematogenically first to the liver, then also to the lungs, bones and brain. Per contingent breath, peritoneal carcinomatosis with ascites may occur (this must usually be excluded laparoscopically in the case of surgically apparent carcinomas from the preliminary diagnosis).

Krukenberg tumor is a drip metastasis in the ovaries or in the Douglas space.

- Clinic

Upper abdominal discomfort, B symptoms, aversion to meat, acute bleeding.

- Diagnostics

The primary diagnosis is made endoscopically.

CT

The staging is determined by means of CT diagnostics. The primary tumor is often not assessable. Lymph node metastases are detectable by lymph node enlargement. Liver metastases appear as flat hypodense lesions in the portal venous phase. Ascites may be interpreted as a sign of peritoneal carcinomatosis.

> ❯ In the hepatoduodenal ligament, lymph nodes up to 2 cm in size may be normal.

Gastrointestinal Stromal Tumors (GIST)

Gastrointestinal stromal tumors, GIST for short, are rare sarcomas of the gastrointestinal tract. The most frequent localization is the stomach. Characteristic is a submucosal location of the tumors in contrast to gastric carcinoma. Risk factors for the development of GIST are not known. Affected are mainly older patients in the 6th and 7th decade of life. Staging is performed according to the TNM classification, whereby the tumor size is decisive for the T-stage and not, as is usually the case, the infiltration into the surrounding area and neighboring organs.

- Clinic

No specific symptomatology, with progressive disease B-symptomatology.

- Diagnostics (◨ Fig. 18.8)

CT/MRI

Primary diagnosis by endoscopy and CT-diagnostics. Because of the good vascularization in the arterial phase **enhanced contrast enhancement in** CT and MRI. The tumor **is T1w isointense** and **T2w hypo- to isointense**, so that contrast medium administration significantly improves the detection of the tumor.

18

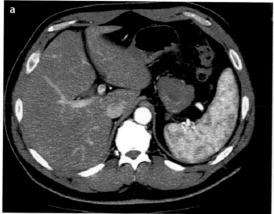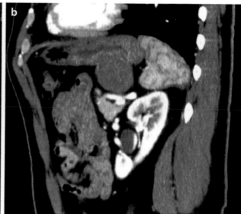

⬛ Fig. 18.8   a, b GIST

In particular, **PET-CT** with 18F-FDG is increasingly used for follow-up examinations and for the primary diagnosis of spread, since GIST tumors show a strong enhancement.

Postoperative Changes

These include:

- **Gastrectomy**: Complete gastric resection, oesophagojejunostomy with jejunal pouch
- **Gastric resection**:
  - Formerly **Billroth I**: Resection of the distal 2/3 of the stomach, gastroduodenostomy.
  - **Billroth II**: Resection of the distal 2/3 of the stomach. Blind closure of the duodenal stump, gastrojejunostomy by means of Braun footpoint anastomosis or Y-Roux anastomosis.

- ▪ Clinic
- ▬ Early dumping: abdominal pain, vomiting within the first 30 min after eating.
- ▬ Late dumping: symptoms of hypoglycemia about 2–3 h after eating.

- ▪ Diagnostics
The altered anatomy is problematic postoperatively. End-to-side anastomoses may become bulging. It is therefore important to know the previous operations and anastomoses. It is helpful, if possible, to talk to the surgeon or to have a look at the surgical report. An anastomosis insufficiency is indicated by a **contrast medium leakage** with **oral positive contrast** in CT (diluted CM!) and fluoroscopy. Often more sensitive are **air pockets** and **fluid collections** at the anastomosis. Dumping syndromes are characterized by **accelerated passage time of contrast** or **radiopaque tracers**, with the diagnosis made primarily clinically and imaging obtained to rule out other causes.

18.2.4   Jejunum and Ileum

Inflammatory Diseases

These include:

- **Diverticulitis** of the jejunum or ileum: inflammation of one or more small intestinal diverticula. Very rare overall.
- **Morbus Whipple**: Systemic infection with *Tropheryma whipplei.*

- ▪ Clinic
Nonspecific, abdominal pain up to acute abdomen.

- ▪ Diagnostics
Sonography/CT

Sonography, supplemented by CT diagnostics in the case of pronounced symptoms. Whipple's disease may be associated with enlarged mesenteric lymph nodes. Diverticulitis of the small intestine shows a comparable picture to diverticulitis of the large intestine with **surrounding reaction of the small intestine** when a diverticulum is detected.

Coeliac Disease

This is an intolerance to gliadin, a component of gluten. The prevalence in Germany is 1:500.

- Clinic

Including diarrhea, malabsorption syndrome, iron deficiency anemia, chronic hepatitis.

- Diagnostics

In a gastrointestinal passage shows accelerated passage time and mucosal swelling.

Meckel's Diverticulum

Meckel's diverticulum is a remnant of the omphaloenteric duct and is present in about 2% of the population. The localization in adults is about 100 cm proximal to the ileocecal valve, the length is up to 8 cm.

- Clinic

Mostly asymptomatic, due to ectopic gastric mucosa possibly ulceration with clinical picture similar to appendicitis or occult bleeding. Possible cause also of a volvulus (section hernias).

- Diagnostics

In case of complication with clinical picture of hemorrhage or acute abdomen CT is recommended.

Small Intestinal Tumors

Spatial lesions of the small intestine are very rare overall. Benign variants are e.g. leiomyomas, lipomas, angiomas, familial polyposis syndromes, small bowel endometriosis.

Malignant tumors are malignant lymphomas or neuroendrocrine tumors (NET). These are localized mainly in the ileum and appendix.

- Clinic

Often incidental finding. Depending on the size, passage problems. Carcinoid syndrome with flushing symptoms in hepatic metastasis of a NET.

- Diagnostics

MR Sellink

Oral contrast with sorbitol leads to distension of the small intestinal loops. Butylscopolamine is administered to decrease intestinal peristalsis. Detection of **contrast-enhancing space-occupying lesions** may occur.

Postoperative Imaging/ Complications

Short bowel syndrome: malabsorption and bile acidosis syndrome. It can occur from a resection length of 40 cm of the ileum.

- Clinic

Diarrhoea, megaloblastic anemia due to vitamin B deficiency$_{12}$.

- Diagnostics

Imaging is only performed as a supplementary procedure, e.g. MR-Sellink or gastrointestinal passage.

18.2.5 Colon and Rectum

Acute Inflammatory Diseases

Inflammatory diseases include:
- **Colitis**: Inflammation of the colon, e.g. due to ischemia, toxins (pseudomembranous).
- **Diverticulitis**: Inflammation of one or more diverticula with an inflammatory environmental reaction. In the sigmoid colon (90% of cases) pseudodiverticula

due to constipation, increasing with age. In the coecum true diverticula. A classification is shown in ◘ Table 18.1.

◘ Table 18.1	Classification of diverticulitis	
	Designation	**Clinic/Imaging**
Type 0	Asymptomatic diverticulosis	Diverticula detection
Type 1	Acute uncomplicated diverticulitis	
Type 1a	Without ambient response	Clinical symptoms, at most wall thickening visible on imaging
Type 1b	With phlegmonous environmental reaction	Streaky compaction of the surrounding area with thickening of the wall with evidence of diverticula
Type 2	Uncomplicated diverticulitis as 1b, plus:	
Type 2a	Microabscess or minimal perforation	Fluid content ≤1 cm, tiny paracolic air pockets
Type 2b	Macroabscess >1 cm, also paracolic or mesocolic, covered perforation	Liquid content >1 cm with rim enhancement, air pockets locally
Type 2c	Free perforation, free fluid, generalized peritonitis...	Air under the abdominal wall at a distance from the local findings, ascites
Type 3	Chronic diverticular disease	
Type 4	Diverticular bleeding	Detection of the source of bleeding

- **Appendicitis**: Acute inflammatory change of the appendix vermiformis.
- **Appendicitis epiploicae**: Spontaneous necrosis of an appendix epiploicae.

According to S2K guideline on diverticular disease (AWMF, May 2014)

- Clinic

Diarrhea, pain, fever, blood in the stool.

Appendicitis: Periumbilical pain moving to the right lower abdomen. Release pain, fever.

Appendicitis epiploicae: Picture of diverticulitis.

- Diagnostics

Sonography

In acute symptomatology, sonography is performed with evidence of a **cocard** in circumscribed wall thickening.

CT

In the case of diverticulitis: CT of the abdomen with rectal application of contrast medium (H_2O) to assess the **extent of inflammation** and **clarify complications** (perforation, bleeding, abscess).

Pseudomembranous colitis shows a **long-distance (pancreatic) hypodense wall thickening of** the colon. **Ischemic colitis is** often a consequence of microangiopathic vascular changes. Indication of an ischemic genesis is a correlation to the arterial flow areas.

To look for bleeding, an **arterial and a venous phase of** the abdomen should be obtained on CT to find a contrast leak. If these two phases are not clear, a late phase after 2–3 h may be helpful.

Appendicitis presents as a **cocard** >7 mm. The wall is **thickened** to **>3 mm**. Often a calcified appendicolith is detectable. The surrounding area is infiltrated with inflammation. Air in the appendix or a retrograde CM filling speaks against appendicitis. The **mucocele of the appendix** must be differentiated, which can be distinguished as a **fluid-filled, distended appendix**. Intraoperative rupture of this benign change

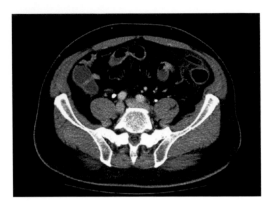

□ Fig. 18.9   Appendicitis epiploicae

□ **Table 18.2**   Differential diagnosis of IBD according to Herold: Internal Medicine 2015

	Ulcerative Colitis	Crohn's Disease
Localiza-tion	Colon	Entire digestive tract
Rectal Involve-ment	Always	20%
Ileum Involve-ment	Rarely	Up to 80%
Spreading	Continuous	Discontinuous
Typical Complica-tions	Toxic mega-colon, bleeding	Fistulas, fissures, abscesses, stenoses
Typical X-ray Signs	Petren loss → Bicycle inner tube	Cobblestone relief, short segmental stenoses, fissures

is followed by **pseudomyxoma peritonei** (▶ Sect. 18.2.5).

❯ A mucocele of the appendix must not rupture intraoperatively to avoid a pseudomyxoma peritonei.

Appendicitis epiploicae presents pathognomonic as an **oval fatty isodense lesion on the colon** with **central hypodensity** and **annular adipose tissue inhibition** (□ Fig. 18.9).

Chronic Inflammatory Bowel Disease (IBD)

These include Crohn's disease (MC) and ulcerative colitis (CU). The incidence in Germany is about 6/100,000/year. The peak incidence for CU is 25–35 years of age, for MC 15–35 years of age.

■ Clinic

Pain, diarrhoea, bloody-mucous in CU.

Complications of IBD: Extraintestinal symptoms (erythema nodosum, eyes, joints, liver with primary sclerosing cholangitis – 5% in MC, more common in CU).

In MC: fistulas (40%), anorectal abscesses (25%).

In CU: colorectal carcinomas (correlating with extent of colonic involvement and duration of disease).

■ Diagnostics

The diagnosis is based on clinical findings, endoscopy, sonography with thickening of the intestinal wall if necessary. A differential diagnosis is shown in □ Table 18.2.

MR-sellink after oral contrasting with mannitol or sorbitol. **Axial and coronary T2w sequences** as well as **T1w sequences** are obtained **natively and after contrast medium.** The inflammatory altered bowel sections are detectable **wall thickened** with **enhanced enhancement.** In particular, fistulas and abscesses can be detected in the contrast-enhanced sequences. MR-Sellink has completely replaced conventional Sellink fluoroscopy.

Voiding Disorders/Dysfunction of the Pelvic Floor

These include constipation or incontinence.

■ Clinic

Constipation, incontinence. Most often in women with childbirth, obesity.

■ Diagnostics

Defecography

In the case of a functional disorder, conventional defecography or MR defecography can provide information. The advantage of conventional defecography is the natural sitting posture during defecation, compared to MR defecography. The disadvantage is the inability to assess the soft tissues such as the vagina and bladder and the radiation exposure, which should not be underestimated.

Pathological findings:

- **Enterocele**: Displacement of the small intestine, omentum, or sigmoid into the Douglas space.
- **Rectocele**: The most frequent finding is an anterior rectocele with a ventral protrusion of the anterior rectal wall.
- **Intussusception**: folding of the rectal mucosa during defecation. This is often the cause of defecation-obstruction syndrome.
- **Cystocele**: Descensus of the urinary bladder with subsidence of the anterior compartment of the pelvic floor.
- **Uterovaginal prolapse:** descensus of the vagina and uterus or often of the vaginal stump after hysterectomy.
- **Anismus**: absent or paradoxical contraction of the puborectal loop. In the imaging impression of the posterior wall of the rectum, narrow anal canal, reduction of the anorectal angle during pressing.

Polyps of the Colon

This is a mucosal protrusion, by definition no statement about the dignity of the mass is possible. Polyps can be detected in about 10% of adults, increasing with age.

■ Clinic

None, possibly blood in the stool.

Degeneration possible, endoscopy with polyp removal is "real" cancer screening.

■ Diagnostics

Endoscopy, only in case of incomplete and not possible colonoscopy a virtual colonoscopy by CT is performed.

Colorectal Carcinoma

These are malignant tumors of the colon or rectum. The borderline between colon and rectum is a distance of 16 cm between the aboral edge of the tumor and the anocutaneous line, measured in rigid rectoscopy. Colorectal carcinoma is the second leading cause of death in men (after bronchial carcinoma) and women (after breast carcinoma).

Localization: Rectum (50%) > Sigma (30%) > Ascending colon (10%) > Remaining colon.

Metastasis: lymphogenic, hematogenic liver (in distal rectal carcinoma also primary lung), lung.

■ Clinic

Peranal bleeding, constipation, changing bowel habits, B-symptomatics.

■ Diagnostics

CT

First endoscopy, a virtual CT colonoscopy is performed if colonoscopy is incomplete. Furthermore, also a CT abdomen, CT thoracic abdomen for staging in rectal cancer.

MR (◻ Fig. 18.10)

An MR rectum is used to assess local findings and distance from the mesorectal fascia in lower and middle third rectal cancer.

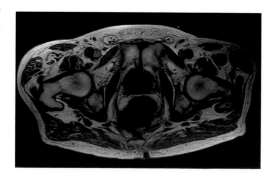

◻ **Fig. 18.10**   Mesorectal fascia (red arrow) with carcinoma

Postoperative/Posttherapeutic Changes and Complications

These include:

- **Anastomosis insufficiency**, knowledge of the anastomosis technique (e.g. end-to-side or end-to-end) is helpful here,
- **Anastomosis Stenosis,**
- **Postradiogenic changes after irradiation,** e.g. of a rectal carcinoma, are the almost regularly detectable transformation of the covered bone marrow into fatty marrow. In case of irradiation of bladder and intestine, inflammatory changes of the mucous membranes with cystitis or colitis develop.

▪ Clinic

Anastomosis insufficiency with postoperatively increased infection parameters up to sepsis.

Anastomotic stenosis leads to constipation.

▪ Diagnostics

CT/Fluoroscopy

In this case, **contrast medium leakage** occurs in case of insufficiency.

Inflammatory changes of involved organs in the irradiation field lead to **wall thickening with hypodense imaging** on CT.

MR

MR shows a **postradiogrenous fat marrow** with corresponding **hyperintense imaging in T1w sequences** as well as a very sharp border to the non-irradiated bone marrow.

18.2.6 Mesentery, Peritoneum and Abdominal Wall

Hernias

Hernias are caused by the contents of the abdominal cavity passing through fascia of the abdominal wall or mesentery.

A distinction is made between the following **diaphragmatic hernias**:

- **Hiatal hernia** with passage through the esophageal hiatus; axial hiatal sliding hernia (>90%): Cardia intrathoracic; paresophageal hiatal hernia: cardia abdominal; mixed hernia; special form: thoracic stomach (upside-down stomach) with herniation of more than 2/3 of the stomach to intrathoracic, risk of gastric volvulus
- **Bochdale hernia** in the dorsal part of the diaphragm bds. with prolapsing fat
- **Morgagni hernia** in the ventral part near the sternum

Furthermore, there are different **abdominal wall hernias**:

- **Paraumbilical hernia** at the level of the navel
- **Epigastric (above the umbilicus) or hypogastric (below the umbilicus) hernia:** passing through the midline
- **Spieghel hernia** between internal and external transverse abdominal muscles paramedian infraumbilical

Scar hernias are classified according to the previous operations:

- **Internal hernias**: Passage through the mesenteric root
- **Inguinal hernias**: directly through the Hesselbach triangle or indirectly along the inguinal canal
- **Femoral hernias**: medial along the femoral vessels; predominantly in women
- **Obturator hernias**: Passage between obturator muscle and ridge muscle

▪ Clinic

Protrusion, passage problems up to ileus with a picture of acute abdomen, in case of entrapment also danger of vascular strangulation; in case of hiatus hernia thoracic tightness, reflux.

▪ Diagnostics

Sonography

The first diagnostic test is sonography.

CT

A CT is used to evaluate the hernial orifices and contents.

Conventional X-ray (⬛ Fig. 18.11)

A hiatal hernia is a frequent incidental finding on chest x-ray with retrocardiac space with mirror formation.

Positional Changes of Organs of the Abdominal Cavity

These include:

— **Situs inversus totalis**: thoracic and abdominal mirror-image arrangement of organs

— **Malrotation**: arises in the 5th–6th embryonic week
  – Nonrotation: large intestine on the left, small intestine on the right in the abdomen
  – Malrotation I: Coecum and ascending colon lie in front of the small intestinal loops

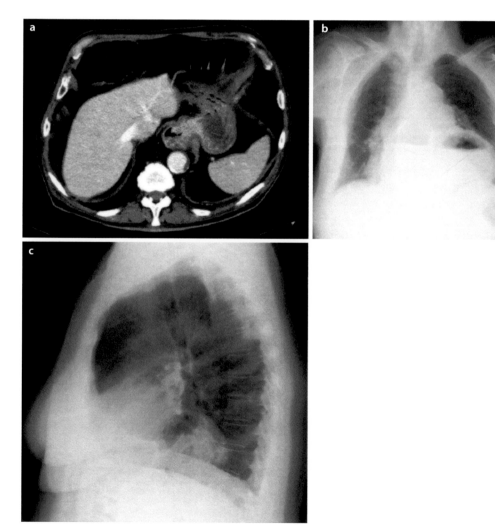

⬛ **Fig. 18.11**   Hiatal hernia. **a** In CT, **b** In X-ray p. a. and **c** Laterally

– Malrotation II: the colon lies behind, the distal duodenum in front of the mesenteric root
▬ **Sigmavolvulus**: rotation of the sigmoid colon around its mesenteric axis

▪ Clinic

Sigmavolvulus: acute abdomen with ileus, common in patients >70 years of age.

▪ Diagnostics

Situs inversus and malrotations are often incidental findings on radiographs, sonography, and CT imaging of the abdomen.

In sigmoid volvulus (◨ Fig. 18.12) the **coffee bean sign** is pathognomonic, in CT rotation of the mesenteric root as whirlpool-sign (◨ Fig. 18.13).

Benign Changes of the Mesentery and Abdomen

Benign changes include:
▬ **Panniculitis mesenterialis**: Chronic fibrosing change of the mesenteric root. Often incidental finding, may be associated with retroperitoneal fibrosis and Whipple's disease and lead to wall thickening of small bowel loops
▬ **Lipoma**: Fatty tissue tumor
▬ **Endometriosis**: Functional endometrial tissue outside the cavum uteri

▪ Clinic

Endometriosis: typical triad with dysmenorrhea, dyspareunia and infertility.

▪ Diagnostics

Endometriosis cysts are up to 15 cm in size; if they are hemorrhagic, they appear as chocolate cysts. Endometriosis lesions are often only a few mm in size and are hardly visible on imaging. Laparoscopy remains the gold standard; transvaginal ultrasound and MRI can be used to attempt detection.

MRI

MRI shows **T2w hypointense lesions with single hyperintense spots.** Hemorrhages can be **hyperintensely** delineated in a **fat-saturated T1w sequence.**

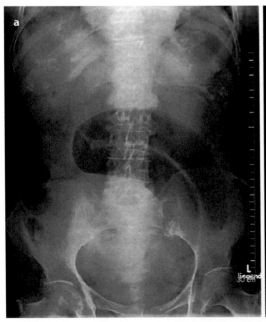
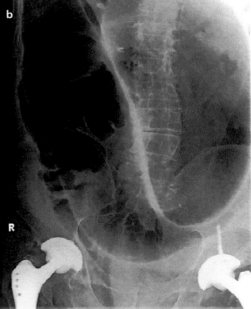

◨ **Fig. 18.12   a, b** Volvulus

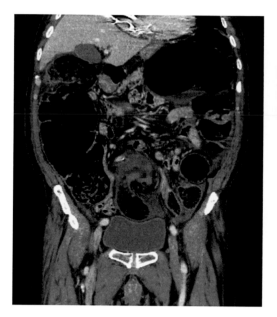

Fig. 18.13 Whirl-pool-sign

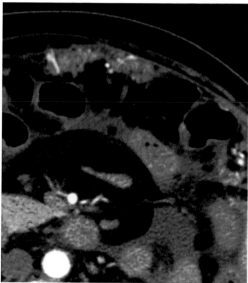

Fig. 18.14 Omental cake

Malignant Changes of the Peritoneum and Abdomen

Peritoneal carcinomatosis is the most common malignant disease of the peritoneum and occurs mainly in tumors of the ovary, stomach, colon, mamma, pancreas and lung.

A rare special form is **pseudomyxoma peritonei** with gelatinous implants in primary tumors of appendix and ovary.

Sarcomas, liposarcomas, or primary peritoneal carcinomas are rare forms of primary malignancy of the peritoneum or abdomen.

- Clinic

B-symptomatics due to tumor disease, ascites with abdominal circumferential proliferation.

- Diagnostics

Sonography/CT

Sonographically and CT-morphologically ascites can be easily detected. However, the exclusion of ascites does not mean a definite exclusion of peritoneal carcinomatosis. Peritoneal tumor nodules as **CM enhancement** can rarely be detected.

A typical manifestation of peritoneal carcinomatosis in ovarian carcinoma is the so-called **"omental cake"**, which can be delineated on CT as a **pronounced nodular-surfaced compression of the omentum majus. Calcifications** in the peritoneum are also indicative of ovarian carcinoma as the primary tumor (**Fig. 18.14**).

18.2.7 Liver and Biliary System

Fatty Liver (Steatosis Hepatis)

35–40% of the adult population in industrialized nations show increased fat storage in the hepatocytes. The fatty liver shows different degrees of severity up to micronodular cirrhosis. Non-alcoholic fatty liver disease is mainly caused by the metabolic syndrome. Approximately 5–10% of the population in Western Europe has alcoholic fatty liver.

■ Clinic

Early stages asymptomatic, in late stages clinic of liver cirrhosis.

■ Diagnostics

Sonography

In the ultrasound image the liver is rich in echoes, well demarcated in comparison to the kidney.

CT

On CT the liver is more hypodense (normal value 55–65 HU), the hepatic vessels can be demarcated hyperdense to the liver tissue in the native image.

Storage Disorders

This includes:
- Iron: Primary **hemochromatosis, hemosiderosis** (transfusion- or nutrition-related); deposition also in myocardium
- Copper: **Wilson's disease** with pathognomonic Kayser-Fleischer corneal ring, deposits also in the basal ganglia

■ Clinic

Hepatomegaly, liver enzyme elevation.

■ Diagnostics

CT/MRI

Storage diseases usually lead to **increased density of** the liver on CT (>70 HU) or to a **signal drop of the liver** on MRI in **T2w sequences.**

Liver Cirrhosis

This leads to the destruction of the liver parenchyma and the formation of fibrosis and regenerative nodules. The incidence in Europe is approx. 250/100,000/year. The etiological cause is alcohol abuse in up to 40% of cases and viral hepatitis in about 55%.

■ Clinic

Hepatic insufficiency, portal hypertension.

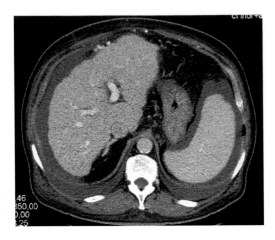

■ **Fig. 18.15** Liver cirrhosis with collaterals and splenomegaly

■ Diagnostics

CT (■ Fig. 18.15)

Imaging shows a **small- or coarse-nodular remodeling of** the liver with an undulating surface of the liver. The **parenchyma** is **inhomogeneous**, the **liver margin rounded**. In portal hypertension, portal venous bypasses via the splenic vein, esophageal varices, or recanalization of the umbilical vein can be demonstrated.

Regenerative nodules can often not be distinguished from hepatocellular carcinoma (section liver cirrhosis) with ultrasound and CT. Here, MRI of the liver with liver-specific contrast agent helps. In contrast to HCC, regenerated nodules retain the contrast medium and are isointense to the liver tissue in late T1w images.

Benign Tumors of the Liver and Biliary Tract

These include:
- **Hemangioma**: The most common benign liver tumor with about 10% in autopsy specimens.
- **Hepatocellular adenoma**: Relatively rare, frequent in women of childbearing age, hamartoma of the hepatocytes, sometimes very large (>10 cm); surgical indi-

cation especially for large and superficially located adenomas; risk of degeneration in adenomatosis with >10 adenomas.

- **Focal nodular hyperplasia (FNH)**: Predominantly women, frequent with oral contraceptives, hamartoma of normal liver tissue.

■ Clinic

Asymptomatic, incidental finding, rarely bleeding complication in hemangioma or large adenomas.

■ Diagnostics

Step-by-Step Diagnostics

A stepwise imaging diagnosis with color duplex sonography, CE-ultrasound, multiphase CT, MRI; PET-CT for differentiation from malignant tumors is recommended:

- Hemangioma: Sonographically echorich, typical garland-shaped arterial enhancement, "closing" in portal venous and later phase with hyperdense imaging in CT compared to surrounding liver parenchyma.
- Hepatocellular adenoma: Small tumors isoechogenic, arterial enhancement, venous iso- to hypodense.
- FNH: Arterial enhancement, rapidly parenchymisodens; central scar with late enhancement in MR (■ Fig. 18.16).

Cystic Lesions of the Hepatic Cavity

Cystic hepatic space claims are subdivided into:

- Dysontogenetic multiple or solitary liver cysts: Frequent incidental finding
- Echinococcosis: Caused by larvae of the fox tapeworm, incubation period 10–20 years, usually asymptomatic
- Abscess: Consequence of bacteremia through the portal vein, e.g. in diverticulitis or appendicitis; multiple small peripheral abscesses in cholangitis
- Liver hematoma: Hemorrhage into the liver; caveat: free perforation with bloody ascites, concomitant splenic injury

■ Clinic

Abscess with typical clinic (fever, laboratory constellation); liver hematoma after trauma with upper abdominal pain.

■ Diagnostics

CT

A **fluid isoechogenic or -isodensic picture is** seen centrally. The cysts are **sharply delineated without rim enhancement and with sonographic dorsal sound enhancement.** An abscess is seen with **thickened capsule and rim enhancement**, bleeding is **hyperdense** to the liver on CT depending on the stage (■ Fig. 18.17).

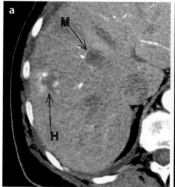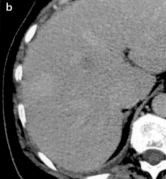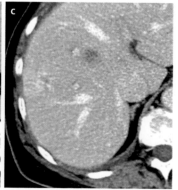

■ **Fig. 18.16**   Liver hemangioma H and metastasis M, **a** arterial, **b** late, **c** venous

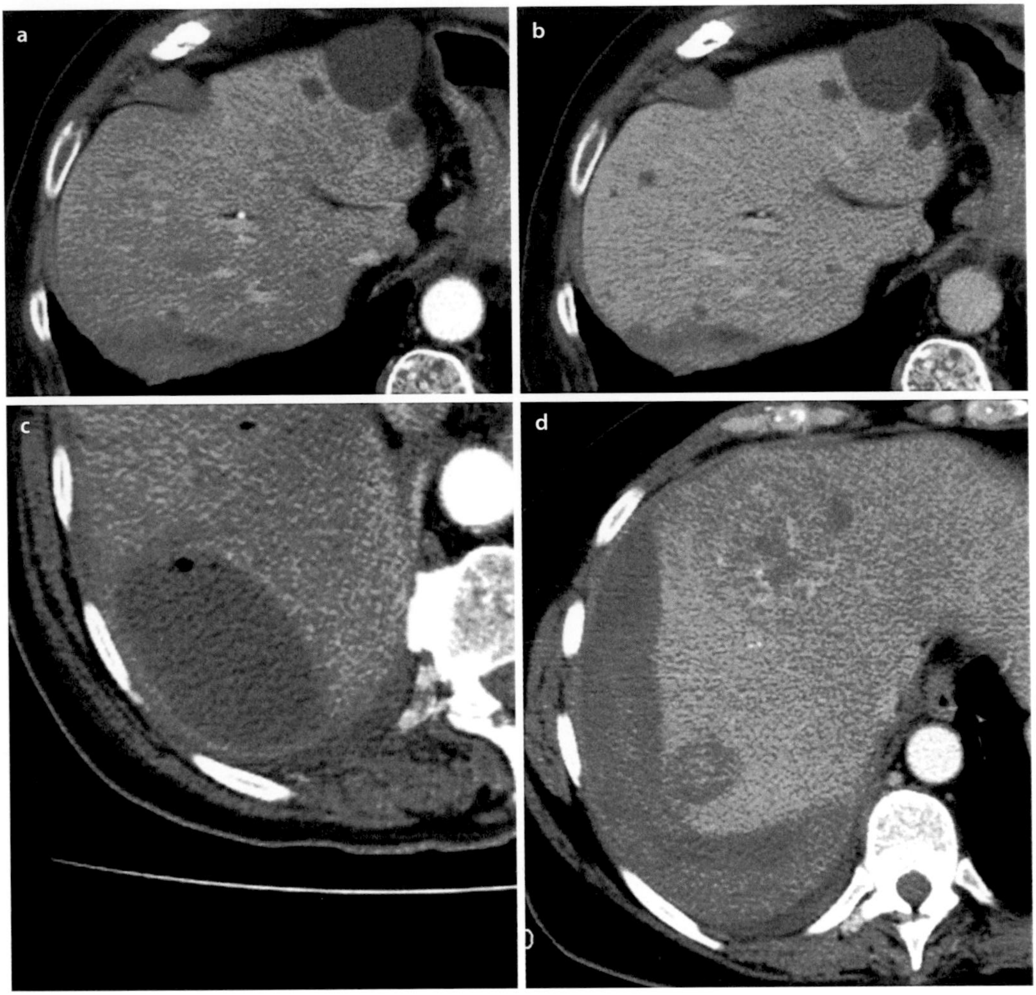

◘ Fig. 18.17 Liver cysts **a** arterial and **b** venous. **c** Liver abscess. **d Liver** hematoma with sarcoma metastases

Pseudotumours

This is a focal textural disturbance of the liver that may mimic a mass. Especially often it is a focal excess or deficiency of fat.

▪ Clinic

Asymptomatic.

▪ Diagnostics

A focal multiple fatty lesion is seen on sonography to be **anechoic, sharply** demarcated, more **map-like** than round; CT and MRI show evidence of fat, **hypodense to the surrounding parenchyma. The** most frequent localization is at the falciform ligament; a lesser degree of fatty degeneration is more echoic on sonography.

Budd-Chiari-Syndrome

It is the occlusion of the venous outflow from the liver, in the typical picture with occlusion of the large hepatic veins and the hepatic venous sternum.

▪ Clinic

Hepatomegaly due to the outflow obstruction, lack of flow signal in the hepatic veins.

■ Diagnostics

MRI

There is hepatomegaly with detectable **increased T2 signal** and occlusion of the hepatic veins.

Malignant Tumors of the Liver and Biliary Tract

These include:

- **Hepatocellular carcinoma**, usually as a result of liver cirrhosis (>90%), at the time of diagnosis in 50% of patients multilocular growth, metastasis mainly in lymph nodes and also bones
- **Liver metastases**: Most common form of malignant liver disease, often multiple; primary tumors often gastrointestinal or mammary

■ Clinic

In HCC usually associated with liver cirrhosis; liver metastases with B-symptomatics; with large tumor burden capsular pain.

■ Diagnostics

- HCC: Arterial early **enhancement with wash-out**. A typical finding on two imaging modalities is considered conclusive in the presence of liver cirrhosis (■ Fig. 18.18).
- Liver metastases: Different appearance depending on the primary tumor, **often**

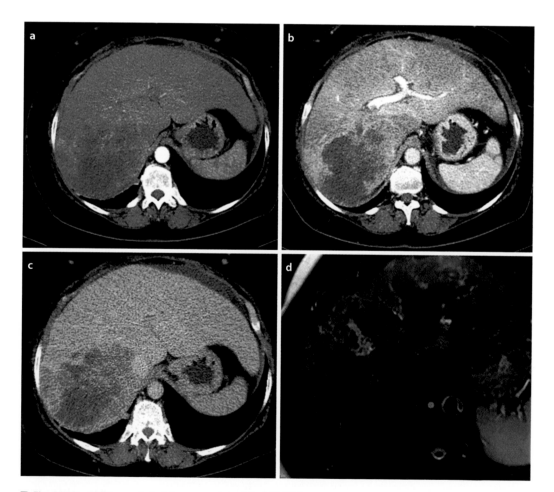

■ **Fig. 18.18** HCC. **a–c** Arterial, venous, late, **d** In MR T2fs

echo-poor halo, **rim enhancement** on CT, predominantly **hypodense** but not liquid isodense (◘ Fig. 18.19).

> Tumor puncture of HCC should be avoided at potentially curative stage to avoid implantation metastases (about in 2%).

◘ Table 18.3 once again provides an overview of differential diagnostic factors.

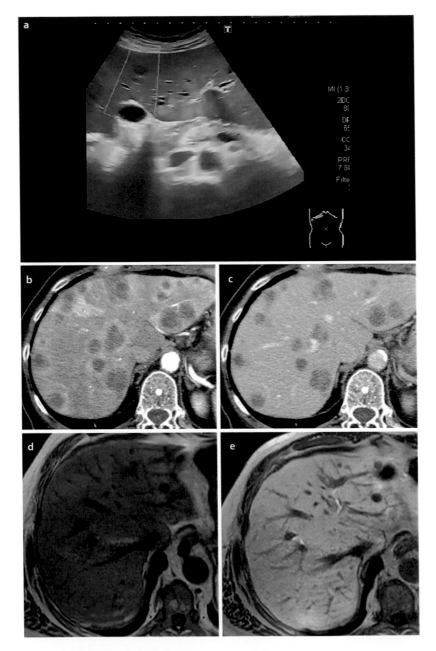

◘ **Fig. 18.19**   Liver metastases. **a** Sono, **b** Arterial, **c** Venous, **d** T1, **e** T2

18

■ Table 18.3 Differential diagnosis of liver diseases

Tumor Entity	Ultrasound	CT Density	MRI Signal	Morphology	CM Behavior
Cyst	Echo-free, dorsal sound amplification	Liquid isodens	T2w strongly hyperintense, T1w hypointense	Sharply defined, round	No enhancement
Hemangioma	Echo rich, variable with increasing size	Blood isodens	T2w hyperintense, "light bulb phenomenon" with increasing signal intensity with increasing T2 weighting	Sharp, larger hemangiomas often lobulated and somewhat inhomogeneous	Garland-like early enhancement in the marginal area, "closing" in portal venous and especially in the helpful late phase
Adenoma	Isoechogenic, variable with hemorrhages	Iso/hypoden	Non-specific; T1w iso/hypointense, T2w iso/hyperintense	Often in larger findings inhomogeneous with hemorrhages and necroses	Short-term enhancement, late approximation to the parenchyma or washout
FNH	Iso-, slightly hyperechogenic	Iso/hypoden	T1w isointense, T2w iso-, possibly hyperintense	Central scar, wheel spoke pattern	Rapid enhancement, then alignment with liver, late enhancement of scar
Abscess	Echo-free to echo-poor with fringe	Hypo to liquid isodens	T2w hyperintense, T1w hypointense	Especially at the beginning rather blurred delimitable with hypodense rim	Marginal CM enhancement
HCC	Echo rich, cirrhosis of the liver	Slightly hypodense	Variable, T1w hypointense, T2w hyperintense	Complex imaging for hemorrhages and necroses, rarely also fat detection possible	Irregular arterial enhancement not only in the tumor margin, portal venous wash-out
Liver metastasis	Often echo-poor with fuzzy echo-poor rim (target sign)	Iso/hypoden	T1w hypointense, T2w hyperintense	Blurred boundaries, often multiple	Rim enhancement depending on the degree of vascularization

18.2.8   Gall Bladder and Bile Ducts

Cholecystolithiasis

These are concretions formed mostly in the gallbladder, of which 80% are cholesterol stones, 20% bilirubin stones. Pigment stones sediment at the bottom of the gallbladder, cholesterol stones float in the gallbladder. The prevalence in women is about 15%, in men about 7.5%. Choledocholithiasis occurs simultaneously in 10–15%.

■ Clinic

75% asymptomatic; 25% with colicky complaints in the right upper abdomen, unspecific with a feeling of pressure/fullness, intolerance e.g. of fatty foods.

Complications: acute cholecystitis, cholangitis; recurrent cholecystitis can lead to shrinking gallbladder and porcelain gallbladder, late complication gallbladder carcinoma; choledocholithiasis with colicky pain and possible cholangitis.

■ Diagnostics

Sonography (◘ Fig. 18.20)

An ultrasound is very sensitive with **echo-rich lesions in the gallbladder** showing dorsal acoustic extinction.

CT

Gallstones are often not visible on CT. In cholecystitis there is an **increased enhancement of the gallbladder bed in** the arterial CM phase with sonographically and CT-morphologically **thickened, three-layered gallbladder wall.**

MRI

In MRI, **signal extinction** occurs **in MRCP** due to stones; in this case, a very sensitive detection of choledocholithiasis is possible (◘ Fig. 18.20).

Gall Bladder Polyp

The gallbladder polyp is a primarily benign polyp-like growth of the gallbladder wall. In 95% it is not a true polyp, but cholesterol deposits in the mucosa. A cholecystectomy is recommended from ≥1 cm with an increased risk of carcinoma.

■ Clinic

Incidental finding.

■ Diagnostics

Polypoid thickening of the wall, a DD to gallstones is possible sonographically by repositioning the patient.

Primary Sclerosing Cholangitis (PSC)

PSC is a sclerosing chronic inflammation and destruction of the intra- and extrahepatic bile ducts. It frequently occurs between the 30th and 50th year of life, the incidence is approx. 1/100,000/year.

■ Clinic

In the early stage incidental finding, in the further course jaundice with itching; biliary cirrhosis as complication.

■ Diagnostics

ERCP (gold standard) or MRCP show a **pearl cord-like duct irregularity**. In case of doubt, histological confirmation is required.

Gallbladder Carcinoma

This is a maglinoma of the gallbladder, mainly >70th year, risk factors: cholelithiasis and chronic cholecystitis as well as porcelain gallbladder.

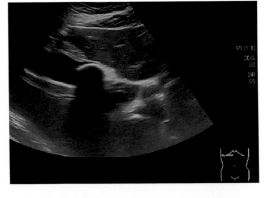

◘ Fig. 18.20   Cholecystolithiasis on sonography

18

- Clinic

Incidental finding, in case of symptoms late finding with icterus or palpable tumor in the gall bladder bed.

- Diagnostics

Wall thickening and **infiltrative growth** into the liver are seen; in the early stages, the carcinoma is often not recognizable on imaging.

Cholangiocellular Carcinoma (CCA), Klatskin-Tumor

This malignant tumor originates from the bile duct epithelium, and the majority of cases are adenocarcinomas.

Classification: Intrahepatic CCA; perihilar CCA (Klatskin tumor), here further classification according to the Bismuth classification to assess also a potential operability; distal CCA below the outlet of the D. cysticus.

- Clinic

No early signs. Clinically classic painless jaundice and palpably enlarged gallbladder (=Courvoisier sign); laboratory chemically cholestasis parameter.

- Diagnostics

Sonography, endosonography, MRI with MRCP; CT abdomen, ERCP. In all procedures, evidence of the **biliary obstruction** can be obtained, the tumor itself may be detectable by endosonography, in CT and MRI usually only in relatively large tumors.

18.2.9 Pancreas

Pancreas Divisum and Pancreas Anulare

Pancreas divisum is the most frequent malformation of the pancreas (prevalence approx. 6%), caused by a lack of fusion of the ventral and dorsal pancreatic anlagen. This results in a complete or incomplete separation with the opening of two ducts in the papilla major and papilla minor.

Pancreas anulare is a very rarely occurring malformation with a constriction of the duodenum. The infantile form is manifested in the first days of life, the adult form between the 20–50th year.

- Clinic
- Pancreas divisum: Mostly asymptomatic
- Pancreatic anulare: Stenosis symptoms, ulcers, chronic pancreatitis.

- Diagnostics

MRCP

The MRCP shows a morphological gait representation.

MRI

In anulare pancreas, MRI shows **constriction of the duodenum** by pancreatic tissue.

Acute and Chronic Pancreatitis

This is an acute or chronic inflammation of the pancreas. Men are more frequently affected than women. Etiology: biliary tract diseases, e.g. choledocholithiasis, alcohol abuse, hereditary, drugs.

Special form: autoimmune pancreatitis, which leads to chronic pancreatitis due to fibrosis.

- Clinic

Belt-shaped upper abdominal pain, elevated pancreatic enzymes (especially lipase), ascites, fever. Clinic up to hypotension and signs of shock, also ECG changes possible.

- Diagnostics

Sonography/CT

In the acute situation, sonography and later a CT scan are performed for further clarification. The degrees of severity range from oedematous pancreatitis, which is often barely detectable in terms of image morphology, to exudative pancreatitis with peripancreatic fluid accumulation (often misleadingly referred to as "necrotic pancreatitis"), to necrotising pancreatitis with cell death of the pancreatic tissue. This can be demonstrated on CT by **absent or reduced contrast of** pancreatic portions.

In chronic pancreatitis, **pancreatic calcifications** are evidential. **Pancreatic duct stones** and pearl cord-like changes in the ductus wirsungianus are also signs of chronic pancreatitis.

MRI

Autoimmune pancreatitis shows a **segmental distention of the pancreas** with a **narrowed ductus wirsungianus**. Late **enhancement** with late **CM accumulation** is characteristic in **late MRI** images. An important DD in all forms of (chronic) pancreatitis is pancreatic carcinoma, which can often only be excluded surgically.

Pancreatic Laceration

This is a contusion or rupture of the pancreatic parenchyma, especially in the corpus section due to pressure on the upper abdomen, so that the pancreas is compressed in front of the spine, e.g. in a bicycle accident by the bicycle handlebars.

- Clinic

History, signs of pancreatitis, possibly active bleeding.

- Diagnostics

CT

CM-CT is the method of choice for abdominal trauma. In the area of injury, there is **reduced CM enhancement**, possibly also **CM leakage in the case of active bleeding as** well as exudates peripancreatitically.

Pancreatic Carcinoma

This is a malignant mass of the pancreas, usually originating in the ductal system. It is most frequently localized in the pancreatic head. The incidence is 15/100,000/year, the mean age of onset is 70–75 years. Histologically, most are adenocarcinomas. Papillary carcinomas show a significantly better prognosis.

- Clinic

Symptoms usually only at an advanced stage. Icterus especially with localization pancreatic head and papilla.

- Diagnostics

Endosonography

Endosonography is the most sensitive method and is clearly superior to CT and MRI. An important sign is a **dilatation of the ductus wirsungianus**.

CT

In CT, an additional CM spiral should be run over the pancreas late arterially (delay 25–30 s), here the tumor can be delineated **hypodense to** the remaining, rapidly accumulating pancreatic tissue. The question of **vascular infiltration** as well as signs of **lymphogenic** or **peritoneal metastasis** is important for the clarification of operability. Preoperatively, the vascular anatomy of the liver should always be assessed, since variant vascular supply requires a corresponding adaptation of the surgical procedure.

Cystic Pancreatic Neoplasms

These include primarily cystic tumors that originate from the ductal epithelium. Cysts arise due to the formation of mucus.

Classification: IPMN from the main duct (60%), side duct IPMN (mainly proc. uncinatus), solid pseudopapillary pancreatic neoplasia (SPN), mucinous cystic pancreatic neoplasia (MCN), serous cystic pancreatic neoplasia. Overall, about 25–40% are malignant tumors.

- Clinic

Usually asymptomatic, possibly clinic as in chronic pancreatitis.

- Diagnostics

Incidental finding in sonography or CT. Clarifying diagnosis with endosonography and, if necessary, endosonographic cyst puncture (elevated CA19-9 in the cyst indicates malignancy), MRCP, ERCP to show communication with the ductal system. DD e.g. pseudocysts in chronic pancreatitis (calcifications?) or serous/mucinous cystadenoma (both show no connection to the ductal system).

In cases of suspected malignancy as well as IPMN, surgical resection is usually performed.

Pancreatic Endocrine Tumors

The group of neuroendocrine tumors of the pancreas are divided into insulinomas, gastrinomas, VIPomas, glucagonomas, etc. depending on the leading hormone secretion. Insulinomas are mostly benign, all other endocrine pancreatic tumors are often malignant.

▪ Clinic

Depending on the hormone secretion.

▪ Diagnostics

Sonography/Endosonography

Sonography and endosonography show an **echo-poor, well-defined mass** in the pancreas. Thereby the masses can show an enormous size of up to 40 cm in the glucagonoma.

CT

However, they are often small findings (<3 cm) with **hypervascularization in the arterial, venous or late phase** (multiphase CT of the pancreas). Usually there is no obstruction of the ductus wirsungianus.

18.3 Diagnostics

18.3.1 Diagnostic Radiology

Sonography

Sonography represents the primary imaging modality for all abdominal diagnostics. A systematic approach with adherence to standard planes is important. In addition, image documentation of pathological findings must be performed. B-mode sonography is supplemented and expanded by power or color duplex procedures and, especially in the clarification of pancreatic processes, an endosonographic procedure.

Conventional Diagnostics

Conventional imaging is increasingly regressive in the diagnosis of abdominal diseases, as CT provides disproportionately more information at increasingly lower doses. For the detection of free air, the abdominal overview must be performed either in the standing position or, more frequently, in the left lateral position (LSL). In this case, the image should not be taken before 5 min have elapsed in appropriate positioning, as the air needs time to collect. Air in the GI tract should be low detectable in all bowel segments. Air-fluid levels in the LSL are indicative of ileus in the affected intestinal segment. However, ileus can also be associated with fluid-filled loops of bowel only, which then escape conventional diagnosis and are readily detectable sonographically. Oral contrast medium administration as gastrointestinal passage (MDP) is often performed in subileus conditions, e.g. postoperatively, in order to delineate possible passage obstructions. Often the contrast medium also has a therapeutic effect and has a prokinetic effect.

Swallowing Study

For the diagnosis of swallowing disorders of the pharynx, **fluoroscopy** is performed in the lateral beam path. It is important to record the entire pharynx up to the upper esophagus (image borders: anterior row of teeth, hard palate, cervical vertebral bodies, at least 3 cm below the epiglottis). For the evaluation of the physiological movements of the swallowing act with elevation of the hyoid and closure of the epiglottis, higher image frequencies of 15–30 images/sec are necessary. If necessary, an examination of the swallowing act with different consistencies (solid, mushy, liquid) is necessary. For this purpose, bread or biscuits and yoghurt mixed with contrast medium can be swallowed by the patient during the exposure.

Esophageal Swallow

As a rule, the **esophageal swallow** is nowadays performed with water-soluble contrast medium. This has the disadvantage of significantly poorer assessability of the mucous membranes, but this is the domain of endoscopy anyway. The pure function with assessment of contractility and reflux are usually sufficiently detectable with water-soluble contrast medium. If there is a tendency to aspiration, imaging of the neck with detection of the upper esophageal orifice is crucial. In principle, all sections of the esophagus should be imaged in two planes; the thoracic section is better imaged in an oblique image than in the lateral beam path. For reflux testing, the patient must be placed in a head-down position during the examination. Reflux can sometimes also be provoked in the prone position and under Valsalva maneuver. An esophageal examination usually includes an image of the stomach with documentation of the outflow of the contrast medium into the duodenum and the downstream loops of the small intestine.

CT Abdomen

CT examinations for clarification of the abdomen are performed after intravenous and oral (negative) contrasting whenever possible. If malignancy is suspected, a multiphase CT with arterial coil should be performed over the upper abdomen. A multiphase CT with a late spiral, if necessary, is also helpful in the search for bleeding in order to be able to detect a contrast medium leak. Liver and pancreas diagnostics are also performed as multiphase CT in the case of suspected tumors. Rectal contrast fillings are helpful in the evaluation of inflammatory or tumorous colonic processes. In cases of suspected ileus, oral or rectal contrast is disturbing because it can obscure the caliber jump as a sign of mechanical ileus.

A special form of colon diagnostics is **virtual colonoscopy**, which should be performed in particular in the case of incomplete colonoscopy. For this purpose, rectal air or, because it is better tolerated, CO_2 is insufflated. Butylscopolamine suppresses peristalsis and leads to dilatation of the intestine. The evaluation is done with special computer programs, where a virtual colonoscopy and other special reconstruction are calculated. The examination is usually performed in the supine and prone position. A low dose is sufficient for the evaluation of the colon, but at least in the absence of contraindications and previous images, it is advisable to perform the supine series as a diagnostic CT with also intravenous contrast.

Colonic Contrast Enema, Conventional and MR Defecography

Nowadays, **colon contrast enema** has been replaced by endoscopy and, if necessary, CT diagnostics. One of the few remaining indications is the examination of an anastomosis in case of suspected insufficiency or prior to re-displacement, whereby CT is increasingly used here as well.

Defecography is again gaining in importance with increasingly differentiated treatment of pelvic floor disorders. For this purpose, rectal contrasting and, in the case of conventional imaging, also oral and, if necessary, vaginal contrasting is performed. The advantage of conventional imaging is the natural sitting position, the advantage of MR defecography is the lack of radiation exposure and excellent soft tissue assessment. The images are taken in the lateral beam path or in sagittal slice guidance. Single images at maximum tension of the pelvic floor and during the Valsalva maneuver are helpful. Subsequently, a series of images is taken during defecation.

MRI Liver

Liver lesions can be very well differentiated using an **MRI scan of** the liver. The use of fat-sensitive sequences is important, for example, in the assessment of focal multiple fatty lesions, usually with an in- and opposed-phase sequence. Liver-specific contrast agent can very accurately differentiate healthy liver tissue that stores the contrast agent in the hepatocytes and, for example, metastases.

MR-Sellink and MR-Rectum

Small bowel examination is nowadays the domain of MRI. A good distension and fluid filling of the small intestine is necessary. This is achieved by an oral administration of 1–2 L of mannitol or sorbitol, which the patient should drink in the last two hours before the examination. Butylscopolamine is administered to decrease motility of the bowel for the examination. Typical sequences include fast axial and coronary T2w sequences (e.g., HASTE) and axial and coronary fat-saturated T1w images before and after contrast administration. Increasingly, additional diffusion weighting is obtained, which can sensitively detect pathologic processes as signal enhancement despite the low spatial resolution. T2w images provide a good overview of the intestine, inflammatory small bowel processes show wall thickening with **increased enhancement**. Fistulas can also be detected well in an MR-sellink.

For local staging of rectal carcinoma, an MRI of the rectum is nowadays usually performed in addition to endoscopic and endosonographic diagnostics. Rectal contrasting is helpful; sonogel, which the patient can hold relatively well and which provides a high T2 signal, is usually used for this. In addition to sagittal and, if necessary, coronal sequences, paraaxial sequences T1w and T2w tilted towards the tumor are mainly prepared. It is important to avoid fat saturation, as the tumor extensions can then be detected **hypoin-tense in the perirectal fat tissue.** Contrast medium is usually not necessary and tends to overestimate the extent of the tumor. Important in the evaluation of a rectal MR for therapy and prognosis is, in addition to the local lymph node status, the assessment of the depth of infiltration into the perirectal fat tissue and the distance of the tumor extensions from the mesorectal fascia.

18.3.2 Nuclear Medicine

Ursula Blum

Oesophagus

Nuclear medical functional examinations of the esophagus have become very rare in clinical routine and have been replaced by endoscopy, ph-metry and esophageal manometry.

Stomach
Gastric Function Examination

Most diseases of the stomach are detected by endoscopic examination. Scintigraphy is requested in patients with altered gastric passage (e.g. delayed in the context of diabetes mellitus or too rapid passage).

The examination is performed with either radiolabelled liquid, semi-solid or solid meal (◻ Table 18.4). The various techniques and meals have not been standardized to date. Therefore, both test meals and the standard values of gastric emptying vary greatly.

Normal half-life is about 30 min for liquids and about 90–120 min for solid meals.

Gastric Carcinoma, Gastrointestinal Stromal Tumors (GIST)

The ^{18}F-FDG-PET/CT shows only limited sensitivity in the staging of gastric carcinoma. In particular, lymph node metastases can only be assessed to a limited extent.

In the case of GIST tumors, a strong enhancement is found, here PET/CT is used

◻ Table 18.4 Procedure for gastric scintigraphy

Patient Preparation	Sober, nicotine abstinence, suspend tablets if necessary
Activity	Depending on the investigation Liquid: 20–40 MBq ^{99m}Tc-DTPA, -MAA or nanocolloid Semi-solid: 70 MBq ^{99m}Tc-tin colloid in 400 mL gruel Solid: 40–100 MBq ^{99m}Tc-DTPA, -MAA or nanocolloid in test meal (boiled egg, scrambled egg)
Application	Oral
Acquisition	Dynamic sequence over 60–90 min, 20 s/frame; 64 * 64 matrix
Special Features	If both liquid and solid phases are to be assessed in one test, the solid phase can be labelled with ^{111}In-DTPA
Evaluation	ROI technique

especially with regard to a tumor response to therapy.

Liver

Liver perfusion scintigraphy to estimate the arterioportal blood flow ratio as well as hepatobiliary function scintigraphy or cholescintigraphy to assess bile production and the biliary excretory system are very rarely performed today. Liver blood pool scintigraphy for the differentiation of various liver tumors has also been superseded by methods such as multiphase CT, CM sonography and MRI with liver-specific contrast medium.

Liver Perfusion with MAA, Calculation of A Liver-Lung Shunt (◻ Table 18.5)

For malignant diseases of the liver (HCC, HCA, metastases), various non-surgical therapy options are available today. These include chemotherapy (possibly also intrahepatic as TACE), thermal ablation and SIRT.

In particular, before SIRT, a MAA examination of the liver must be performed, including calculation of a liver-lung shunt.

The evaluation is performed visually, and special attention should be paid to extrahepatic nuclide accumulations. In case of detectable intra-abdominal accumulations, a repetition of the angiography with occlusion of further collateral vessels (if necessary, surgical intervention) is indicated, and a repetition of the MAA liver examination is mandatory.

The lung shunt is calculated quantitatively using the following formula:

$$\frac{Counts_{Lunge}}{Counts_{Lunge} + Counts_{Leber}} \times 100 = Lungenshunt \quad (\%)$$

with indication of the mean value from both projections.

Liver Tumors and PET/CT

— **Hepatocellular carcinoma (HCC):** Hepatocellular carcinomas show different behavior with regard to FDG storage. So far, there is no general recommendation for PET/CT.

— **Cholangiocellular carcinoma (CCC):** Cholangiocellular carcinoma shows more marked enhancement than HCC in most cases. Distant metastases can be visualized relatively reliably, whereas regional lymph node metastases can only be visualized to a limited extent.

— **Metastases:** Many primary tumors metastasize to the liver. Only for metas-

◘ Table 18.5 Procedure for SIRT

Patient Preparation	30 min before angiography thyroid blockade with 400 mg perchlorate First angiography of the liver with occlusion of existing collateral vessels, catheter left in place
Activity	150 MBq ^{99m}Tc-MAA (<1,000,000 particles)
Application	Intra-arterial via the horizontal catheter in the liver If necessary, division of the activity according to the vascular supply of the tumor
Acquisition	Static images ap, pa of the abdomen or whole-body scintigraphy Static images ap, pa of the thorax including the liver SPECT(/CT) of the abdomen LEHR
Evaluation	Visual, quantitative

◘ Table 18.6 Procedure for scintigraphy with ^{99m}Tc-labelled erythrocytes

Patient Preparation	30 min before the examination thyroid blockade with 400 mg perchlorate
Activity	In vitro labeling of erythrocytes: Draw sufficient patient blood (heparinized tube) Marking with tin pyrophosphate according to manufacturer's instructions Incubation for 30 min or according to manufacturer's instructions Add 700 MBq ^{99m}Tc-pertechnetate Test for mark yield (>85%), then Reinjection In vivo labelling or in vivo/in vitro labelling is possible in emergency cases, but the labelling yield is significantly worse than in vitro labelling
Application:	i. v.
Acquisition	Dynamic 1 min/image over 60 min from ventral (Kuwert) Thereafter, ventral static images every 15–30 min up to a maximum of 24 h p. i. From bleeding detection dynamic recording over 30–60 min 128 * 128 matrix
Evaluation	Visual

tases of colorectal cancer there are sufficient studies. Here, PET/CT is of great importance, especially for therapy planning. A single liver metastasis can in principle be cured by surgical resection. In these studies, PET/CT usually showed a higher sensitivity than CT or MRI. In addition, previously unknown extrahepatic metastases can be detected. In the case of recurrence, PET/CT also allows a more precise diagnosis due to the altered anatomy of the liver; in addition, therapy monitoring with chemotherapy is possible at an early stage.

Intestine
Bleeding Source Search

Intra-abdominal sources of bleeding are easily detectable in endoscopically accessible sections and may also be directly treatable. However, a large proportion of the small intestine cannot be reached endoscopically.

Here, scintigraphy with ^{99m}Tc-labelled erythrocytes can detect bleeding from 0.05–1.0 mL/min (◘ Table 18.6).

Intestinal Carcinomas
- Carcinomas of the Small Intestine

Carcinomas of the small intestine are rare tumors; they are frequently neuroendocrine tumors. These tumors generally have an increased number of somatostatin receptors, which are accessible to nuclear medicine diagnostics and therapy. Here, either ^{111}In-

◘ Table 18.7 Scintigraphy with ^{111}In-Ctreotide	
Patient Preparation	Discontinuation of somatostatin analogues
Activity	111 MBq ^{111}In-octreotide
Application	Slow i. v.
Acquisition	Whole body scintigraphy and SPECT 4 h and 24 h p. i. If necessary, static recordings, late recordings up to 48 h p. i. Medium-energy collimator
Evaluation	Visual, ROI technique if necessary
Special Features	Laxative measures between examinations High radiation exposure with 12 mSv

◘ Table 18.8 Scintigraphy with ^{68}Ga-somatostatin analogues	
Patient Preparation	Discontinuation of somatostatin analogues, not fasting
Activity	100–150 MBq ^{68}Ga-somatostatin analogue
Application	i. v.
Acquisition	20–60 min p. i. 3–4 min/bed position
Evaluation	SUV determination
Special Features	Only in the context of a therapeutic trial, as the radiopharmaceutical is not approved for diagnostic use High physiological activity in liver, spleen and kidneys Radiation exposure approx. 2–3 mSv

octreotide can be used (◘ Table 18.7), or in PET/CT (PET/MRI) radioactively labelled ^{68}Ga-somatostatin analogues (◘ Table 18.8), mostly DOTA-TOC; more rarely DOTA-NOC, or DOTA-TATE. A ^{18}F-FDG-PET/CT is only suitable for poorly differentiated, fast-growing tumors.

Depending on the findings, a nuclear medical therapy with radioactively labelled (^{90}Yttrium or ^{177}Lutetium) somatostatin analogues can follow.

■ Colorectal Carcinomas

PET/CT has a 1a-indication in recurrence diagnostics and a 1b-indication in therapy monitoring.

Limitations exist with changes whose diameter is smaller than twice the maximum resolution of the PET scanner (partial volume effect). As a rule, these are lesions with a diameter of less than 10 mm.

Pancreas

Pancreas diagnostics is the domain of endoscopic sonography. In unclear cases, nuclear medicine can be used as further diagnostics.

Especially small pancreatic carcinomas can be detected by FDG-PET/CT with a relatively high specificity and sensitivity. PET/CT is also useful for the diagnosis of distant metastases and therapy monitoring.

In the case of neuroendocrine pancreatic tumors, tumors larger than 2 cm can be detected with a high degree of certainty using ^{111}In-octreotide. In PET/CT, Ga-labelled somatostatin analogues are available here with[68], showing an even higher sensitivity of the diagnosis. If the neuroendocrine tumors show a higher accumula-

Table 18.9 Value of the imaging procedures in the gatrointestinal region

	Sonography	Conventional	CT	MRI	Nuk	PET
Clarification ileus	P	(P)	W	N	N	N
Acute abdomen	P	N	P	N	N	N
Staging of GI tract tumors	P	N	P	W	W	W
Bleeding search	P	N	P	W	W	N
Clarification of liver focus	P	N	W	W (liver-specific CM, if applicable)	N	W

N Not indicated, *P* Primary diagnosis, *W* Further diagnosis, * CT in contraindications for MRI

tion, a therapy with radioactively labeled (^{90}Yttrium or ^{177}Lutetium) somatostatin analogues can be performed.

18.3.3 Valence

Christel Vockelmann

◻ Table 18.9 once again summarizes the areas of application of the respective imaging techniques.

18.4 Therapy

18.4.1 Interventional Radiology

Christel Vockelmann

Puncture and Drainage

For clarification or histological confirmation of **liver lesions**, these can often be **punctured** sonographically or also CT-guided. For this purpose, the lesion is localized with the appropriate procedure and the puncture route is planned. In the case of CT-guided puncture, it must be borne in mind that the puncture is usually performed in a breathing position with the patient awake and the puncture route is in the slice plane. It is

therefore necessary to plan the puncture route sufficiently, in particular to avoid injuring the lung with a pneumothorax. Sufficient coverage of the findings by healthy liver tissue must also be aimed for in order to avoid intraperitoneal bleeding. The puncture itself is usually performed using the **coaxial technique.** For this purpose, a guide needle is brought forward to the finding, through which several punching cylinders can then be obtained.

A **liver abscess** is usually treated by means of a drainage, a surgical procedure is not necessary. The **trocar technique** should be used for liver abscesses. Here, the drainage catheter is advanced directly with the puncture needle. The advantage is that no germs or at least fewer germs are carried along the puncture path than with the **seldinger technique**. In this technique, the abscess is first punctured with a needle, followed by dilatation of the puncture path via an exchanged wire, and then the drainage is advanced to the abscess via the wire. This technique is mainly used for difficult puncture routes, e.g. retroperitoneal for superinfected pancreatic pseudocysts, if these cannot be relieved endoscopically via the stomach.

Thermal Ablation of Liver Metastasis

Thermoablation is usually performed in the liver as radiofrequency ablation or microwave ablation. In both procedures, the metastasis is punctured with the ablation probe and the area around the probe is then heated to 60–80 °C. The metastasis is then ablated with the ablation probe. Because the metastasis is painful and easier to puncture, this procedure is usually performed under intubation anesthesia. The smaller the metastasis, the better the possibility of curative treatment. From a size of 3 cm, the risk of local recurrence increases, even though metastases of up to 5 cm can be approached. Ultimately, the procedure can be used almost as often as desired. A combination with a surgical procedure (e.g. left hemihepatectomy and RFA of a metastasis in the right liver lobe) is also very possible.

Transjugular Intrahepatic Portosystemic Shunt (TIPSS)

The TIPSS is an artificially created short-circuit connection between the portal vein and the hepatic veins to reduce portal hypertension in liver cirrhosis. Indications for this are complications of portal hypertension such as hepatorenal syndrome or massively bleeding esophageal varices. To create the TIPSS, a curved puncture needle is inserted into the right hepatic vein via the jugular vein. From here, the puncture is made ventrally in the direction of the right portal vein branch. Sonographic control of the puncture is helpful here. After the correct reaching of the portal vein is ensured by an angiographic series, dilatation of the parenchymal tract through the liver and subsequent stent insertion is performed. TIPSS insertion is complex and often unsuccessful despite multiple puncture attempts. A complication of TIPSS is hepatic encephalopathy due to insufficient detoxification of the blood. In this case, the flow through the TIPSS can be reduced with a reducing stent.

Acute GI Bleeding

Duodenal ulcers can usually be controlled endoscopically. However, if this is exceptionally unsuccessful, closure of the gastroduodenal artery with coils can be performed in addition to a surgical procedure. In this case, access is via the coeliac trunk. It is important that the distal parts of the gastroduodenal artery are closed first to prevent bleeding by retrograde feeding of the gastroduodenal artery from the superior mesenteric artery. After reaching the desired position, anchoring coils, small metal coils chosen large enough to anchor to the site, are first released. Additional coils are then inserted until the desired section of the vessel is occluded. Prior to completion of the procedure, imaging should be performed via the superior mesenteric artery to ensure that the bleeding has been adequately managed.

Vascular Occlusions and Stenoses

In the case of occlusion or stenosis of the visceral arteries leading to acute or chronic ischemia, the affected vessels are reopened via catheter intervention, especially in the case of changes close to the origin. In the case of chronic changes, a stent is usually inserted. In acute thromboembolic occlusions, interventional thrombectomy with aspiration catheters and also intra-arterial lysis can be performed in consultation with surgery. In addition, an exploration of the abdominal cavity is necessary afterwards in order to resect necrotic parts of the intestine.

Portal Vein Embolization

In the case of a planned extended right hemihepatectomy, the remaining left liver lobe is often too small. Embolization of the right-sided portal vein branches leads to growth of the left liver lobe. Embolization is performed by percutaneous puncture of a right-sided portal vein branch. Then the desired portal vein branches are occluded via various catheters. For this purpose, so-called occluders are often used, a kind of double metal umbrella that effectively serves to occlude even larger vessels.

18.4.2 Radiotherapy

Guido Heilsberg

Oesophageal Carcinoma

- Depending on the tumor stage, therapy is definitive or neoadjuvant radiochemotherapy, if necessary with endoscopic clip marking of the tumor for radiation planning.
- Recommended radiation dose: Between 50 and 60 Gy with a fractionation of 5 × 2 Gy/week or 5 × 1.8 Gy/week. In neoadjuvant therapy, dose values of 40 Gy are applied.
- Side effects: Esophagitis, pharyngitis.

Rectal Cancer

- Tumor stage cT3 and cT4 neoadjuvant pretreatment with radiochemotherapy.
- Treatment of tumors in the small pelvis: Filling of the organs to be aimed at, especially urinary bladder and rectum.
- Combination with the administration of 5-FU as a chemotherapeutic agent.
- For preoperative irradiation, the dosage is 45 Gy with 5 × 1.8 Gy/week.
- Postoperatively, 50.4 Gy are given with additional small-volume dose increase (boost) to the former tumor region by another 5.4–9 Gy in the same fractionation.

Case Study

An engineer in a responsible position has worked in a company for many years. Therefore, he was also assigned special tasks, such as personnel support. He found this activity very nerve-racking, especially when it came to taking into account the holiday wishes of all colleagues equally. To relax, he would often have resorted to cigarettes or chocolate, knowing full well that this would exacerbate the acid regurgitation and stomach pains that had long plagued him. Since he retired, he has been doing light endurance sports regularly and has given up sweets in order to get rid of his excess weight. He has not yet succeeded in giving up smoking. The only thing that worries him is his still existing upper abdominal pain, which he attributed to trouble at work when he was working, and which he cannot explain now, because he feels absolutely relaxed. Your suspicion goes in the following direction: the pain could stem from a chronic stomach ulcer or even from a deep-seated oesophageal carcinoma. A clarification should definitely be made. In the esophagogastroscopy, the mucous membrane is assessed and, if there is a suspicious change, a tissue biopsy is taken for examination by a pathologist.

Practice Questions

1. What does a pearl cord-like gait irregularity in ERCP/MRCP suggest?
2. What are the diverticula of the esophagus and how they differ?
3. What is a Krukenberg tumor?
4. What is typical on imaging for appendicitis?
5. When does the coffee bean sign show up?

Solutions ▶ Chap. 27

Urogenital

Carla M. Kremers, Guido Heilsberg, Ursula Blum,
Christel Vockelmann and Martina Kahl-Scholz

Contents

© Springer-Verlag GmbH Germany, part of Springer Nature 2023
M. Kahl-Scholz, C. Vockelmann (eds.), *Basic Knowledge Radiology*,
https://doi.org/10.1007/978-3-662-66351-6_19

This chapter deals mainly with the diagnostic but also therapeutic possibilities in diseases of the urogenital tract and the retroperitoneal space. Both the harmless cyst and renal cell carcinoma are discussed. Diseases of the urinary tract such as tumors and urinary stones as well as diseases of the male reproductive organs such as prostate carcinoma are also covered in this chapter.

19.1 Anatomical Structures

Martina Kahl-Scholz

The urogenital system includes the kidneys, ureters, bladder and urethra.

The **kidneys** lie in the retroperitoneal space ventral to the 12th rib, the right kidney being displaced more caudally than the left kidney by the overlying liver. The kidneys are about 4 cm thick, 7 cm wide, and 11 cm long (like the spleen). They show a lateral and medial margin (margo medialis et lateralis), an anterior and posterior surface (facies anterior et superior) and an upper and lower pole (extremitas superior et inferior).

The kidney is divided into medulla, cortex and renal pelvis. From the renal pelvis, the ureter carries urine through an abdominal and a pelvic part (pars abdominalis et pelvica) 30–50 cm to the urinary **bladder** (vesica urinaria). The urinary bladder is the most anterior organ in the lesser pelvis. It lies adjacent to the symphysis pubica. The urinary bladder is divided into a tip (apex vesicae), a body (corpus vesicae), a base of the bladder (fundus vesicae) and a neck of the bladder (collum vesicae), which merges into the urethra. The urethra is about 3–5 cm long in women, but 25–30 cm long in men.

The prostate gland is about the size of a chestnut, surrounds the urethra and lies in front of the bladder. It is divided into a base and a conical end (base et apex prostatae). A further distinction is made between the isthmus prostatae and a lobus dexter, sinister et medius.

19.2 Disease Patterns

19.2.1 Urinary Tract

Carla M. Kremers

Urinary Retention
The most common pathology of the ureter is urinary retention, in other words, obstructed outflow into the bladder, which can have a variety of causes.

- ▪ Clinic

Kidney/flank pain, urinary retention.

- ▪ Diagnostics

Sonography
Initial imaging should be sonography, with which **dilatation of the renal pelvis** and also of the **ureter** (which can be seen sonographically only if dilated) can be well assessed.

Congestion is divided into 4° of severity (▫ Table 19.1).

19.2.2 Urolithiasis

Urolithiasis is the most common cause of painful urinary retention. The exit of the kidney stone occludes the ureter at one of its physiological constrictions (exit from the renal pelvis, crossing of the psoas musculature and iliac vessels and confluence with the bladder ostium), so that the urine flowing in painfully dilates the proximal part of the ureter. Injuries of the ureter by the concrement often result in hematuria.

- ▪ Diagnostics

CT (▫ Fig. 19.1)
The diagnostic instrument of choice is a low-dose CT of the abdomen, which, depending on the device, is hardly higher in radiation dose than an X-ray of the abdomen—which is a diagnostic alternative for estimating stone size and localization if a

19

Grade I	**Grade II**	**Grade III**	**Grade IV**
Renal pelvis dilated Renal calices normal Parenchyma width regular	Renal pelvis and calices dilated Preserve papillae tips Parenchyma width regular	Renal pelvis and calices strongly dilated Papilla tip flattened Incipient parenchymal narrowing	Differentiation between dilated renal pelvis and renal calices no longer possible Parenchyma trophy

Table 19.1 Severity of the backlog

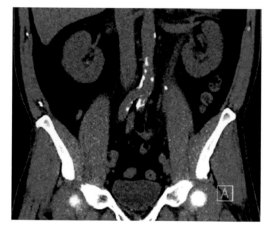

Fig. 19.1 CT ureteral concretion on the left, dilated ureter proximal to it and edematous surrounding reaction (fatty tissue inhibition)

corresponding computer tomograph is not available. The information obtained is relevant for further therapy planning: small calculi can be eliminated naturally under analgesia. In the case of large calculi, urological intervention may be necessary.

❯ If urolithiasis is suspected, a native low-dose CT is the diagnostic method of choice, if available. The radiation exposure corresponds to an X-ray examination of the abdomen in two planes.

Compression: Urinary retention can also be caused by an external pressure effect. Reasons for this are manifold and range from malignant tumors in retroperitoneum

and pelvis to severe diseases like retroperitoneal fibrosis (Ormond's disease), post-inflammatory scarred strictures to curious benign things not relevant for examination like a pronounced coprostasis (extremely rare).

19.2.3 Urothelial Carcinoma

Urothelial carcinomas are usually localized in the urinary bladder and can be detected there both sonographically and in cross-sectional imaging—if they are large enough and the bladder is well filled so that its wall texture can be assessed and the tumor (usually low-echo and polyp-like) growing into the bladder lumen can be detected. More rarely, urothelial tumors are localized in the renal pelvis or ureter.

▪ Clinic
Painless hematuria, usually late pain and urinary retention.

▪ Diagnostics
Sonography
Sonographically a **focal widening of the urinary bladder wall protruding into the bladder lumen** may be noticeable in a well-filled **bladder.**
MRI/CT

❯ A mass of the urothelium can only be evaluated well if the cavity is well filled.

Accordingly, in the clarification of a suspected urothelial carcinoma (e.g., due to an unclear hematuria), a urographic phase with well-filled ureters and renal pelvis in a CT is very helpful to detect **contrast medium voids** caused by space-occupying structures. In order to assess contrast medium accumulation of such a structure (and thus distinguish it from a blood coagulum, for example), preceding (native/arterial/venous or nephrographic) contrast medium phases are helpful.

Urography Due to the almost universal availability of computer tomography and the often significantly greater information gain, i. v. urography, which was previously used to assess the urinary tract, has declined significantly. This involves conventional X-ray images of the abdomen before and after intravenous administration of contrast medium, which can be used to assess ureters or their outflow obstructions (◻ Fig. 19.2).

Bladder Fistulas and Leaks

These are occasionally undesirable consequences after surgical interventions or, rarely, side effects of an underlying disease with fistula formation (e.g. in Crohn's disease).

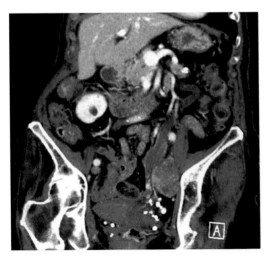

◻ **Fig. 19.2** Urothelial carcinoma in the distal ureter. The dilated and tortuous ureter proximal to the ureter is clearly visible

■ Clinic
Urine is not discharged via the urethra, but via the respective fistula route via the intestine, vagina or skin.

■ Diagnostics
Transillumination
   To check the tightness of the bladder after intraoperative injury, a **fluoroscopic examination** with a few individual images is sufficient (retrograde cystography). For this purpose, the bladder is sterilely filled with contrast medium via a bladder catheter to the extent tolerated by the patient. The individual images should show the filled bladder in different planes **in order** to detect, for example, **a dorsal leakage of contrast medium.**
   CT (◻ Fig. 19.3)
   If a fistula is suspected, the question of the exact **course of the fistula** and also the end must often be answered, then a CT is recommended. For this purpose, too, the bladder is retrogradely filled as well as possible with sterile, diluted contrast medium via a permanent catheter and the lower abdomen is then imaged on the CT. In this way, it may be possible to determine the exact location of the fistula opening and whether there is a connection to the intestine or other adjacent structures.

Bladder Emptying and Micturition Disorders

■ Clinic
Sometimes, e.g. in case of recurrent urinary tract infections, micturition disorders are asked for.

■ Diagnostics
Fluoroscopy (◻ Fig. 19.4)
   In order to see the bladder and urinary tract, the bladder is also filled with contrast medium via a bladder catheter. After removing the bladder catheter, the patient is then X-rayed during micturition. Important landmarks of the examination are the orifices of the ureters into the bladder: is there **reflux of contrast medium** here (**vesicoure-**

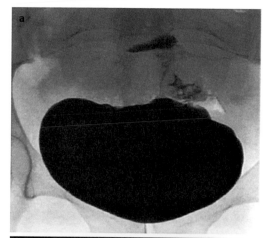

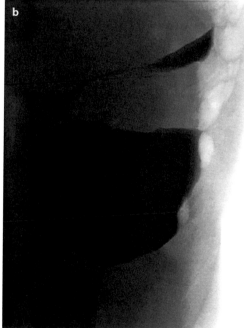

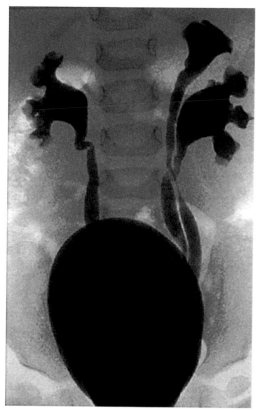

■ Fig. 19.4 MCU

■ Fig. 19.3 **a** Cystography with postoperative fistula. **b** Cystography with postoperative leakage laterally

thral reflux)? The bladder itself: Is it round? Is it compressed anywhere? Does it empty quickly and completely? And the urethra: Can the urine flow freely? Are there any constrictions in the urethra?

   Sonography

   If, for example, in neurological diseases with bladder emptying disorders, the amount of residual urine is required, the procedure is reversed: the patient is asked to empty the bladder as well as possible and the amount of fluid remaining in the bladder is assessed. An ultrasound with imaging of the bladder in two planes is sufficient for this. The amount of residual urine can be estimated from the diameters measured in this way (■ Fig. 19.5).

19.2.4 Kidney Diseases

Inflammatory Renal Changes

In most cases, the diagnosis of **acute pyelonephritis** can be made solely on the basis of the patient's history, clinical examination and the corresponding changes in laboratory parameters.

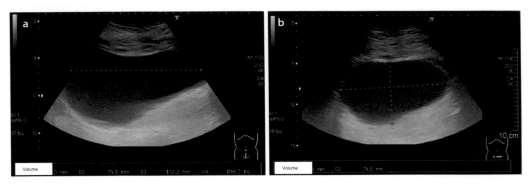

Fig. 19.5 Bladder with residual urine. **a** 1st level. **b** 2nd level. Formula: $a * b * c * 0.5$ = bladder volume

■ Clinic

Fever, chills, dysuria, flank pain, possibly belt-like pain as in pancreatitis, possibly back pain.

■ Diagnostics

Sonography (Fig. 19.6)

Ideally, the diagnosis is made by means of targeted sonography. Here, the inflamed kidney is conspicuous by a **parenchymal swelling**, i.e. it is enlarged in a lateral comparison and due to the edema it shows a lower echogenicity than the healthy counterpart. The parenchymal swelling can also cause the **calyces to** appear **constricted**. If you are already holding the transducer in your hand, it makes sense to look for complications right away: are the ureters dilated? Is there a higher degree of urinary retention? If there are accompanying abscesses, these are conspicuous by circumscribed, echo-poor or echo-free areas.

CT

The picture of pyelonephritis is analogous to sonography: the kidney is **edematous swollen**, thus **enlarged and hypodense** in lateral comparison. If the entire kidney is affected, a kind of **wheel spoke pattern** may develop. Often the surrounding perirenal fat is also oedematously altered (imbibed). Perirenal abscesses present the typical picture of an accumulation of fluid, depending on the pathogen possibly with air inclusions and with a contrasting rim.

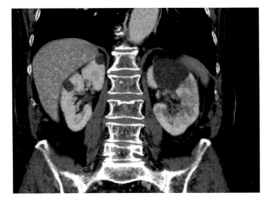

Fig. 19.6 Left pyelonephritis

Signs of **chronic pyelonephritis** in all imaging techniques are **scarring changes of** the renal parenchyma in the sense of circumscribed retractions, especially in the vicinity of the renal calices.

Cystic Masses

■ Clinic

Most often, renal cysts go unnoticed. If necessary, pressure pain, lower abdominal pain, urinary retention.

Uncomplicated Blanched Cysts

■ Diagnostics

CT/Sonography/MRI

These are **round**, have a **delicate (barely visible), smooth wall** that does **not** absorb **contrast**. Their content is **watery**. Accordingly, they are sonographically

anechoic with **dorsal sound enhancement**. In CT, they are imaged **fluid isodense** and thus have a density around **0 HU**. Similarly, on MRI, the signal is **hyperintense in T2 weighting** and T1-weighted **hypointense**—just as water should be. Such bland cysts are usually harmless incidental findings without relevance. Ultrasound is sufficient as a diagnostic tool. They do not require any further clarification or control.

Complicated Cysts

■ Diagnostics

CT/Sonography/MRI (■ Fig. 19.7)

These are those whose contents are **not clearly watery**, which have a **thickened wall**, show **septations** or are **partly calcified. In order** to assess the risk of malignancy, there is the **Bosniak classification**, the stages of which are also associated with corresponding diagnostic and therapeutic recommendations. The classification was originally intended for CT—however, it can also be used, at least in part, for sonography and MRI (■ Table 19.2).

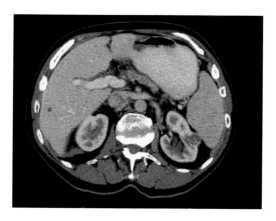

■ **Fig. 19.7**   Complicated renal cyst

■ **Table 19.2**   Bosniak classification

Type	Radiological Findings	Interpretation or Recommendation
I	– Watery – No septa – Gossamer or invisible wall – No solid shares – No contrast medium uptake	– Sitting cyst – No further clarification
II	– Content not water isodense—i.e. >20 HU density (CT), not anechoic (sono) or hyperintense in T1 weighting (MRI)—but homogeneous – few, delicate septations – Small calcifications on septa or cyst wall – No contrast medium uptake compared to native images	Complicated but benign (e.g., hemorrhagic) cyst
IIF F like Follow up	– Slightly thickened cyst wall or septations – Thick or coarse-grained calcifications – No contrast medium uptake	– Complicated but probably benign cyst – Controls at three, six and ten months to exclude growth in size or other changes
III	– Irregular, small-nodular thickenings of the zsten wall or septations – Optional contrast medium recording	– A malignancy cannot be excluded, but benign geneses (e.g. infection or hemorrhage) are also possible – Resection if the surgical risk is acceptable
IV	– Irregular solid portions – Contrast enhancement	Most likely cystic malignancy. Resection

Cystic Kidney Disease

These are diseases in which harmless cysts can become a problem for the patient or his kidney function due to their number and size, as they displace or even destroy the healthy kidney parenchyma. There are different forms and manifestations of such diseases, which are essentially hereditary.

■ Clinic

Symptomatic changes may include arterial hypertension and hematuria and recurrent urinary tract infections. Increasing abdominal girth and flank pain may also occur. Sooner or later, when there is an increasing loss of function of the kidneys, the most diverse symptoms of terminal renal insufficiency can occur (edema, performance kink, pruritus, loss of appetite, nausea/vomiting, dyspnea …).

■ Diagnostics (◘ Fig. 19.8)

CT/Sonography/MRI

In the adult form (autosomal dominant polycystic kidney disease = ARPKD), **in** addition to **multiple kidney cysts, cysts are** also found in **other organs** (pancreas, spleen, liver). Cerebral aneurysms are also frequently found in these patients.

❯ In patients with polycystic kidney disease, cerebral aneurysms should be excluded by MR or CT angiography.

Medullary sponge kidney is a congenital but not hereditary defect of the collecting ducts with cystic dilatations of the same. Thus, the (mostly small) cysts are found mainly in the pyramidal region and less in the cortex.

This is often accompanied by urolithiasis and urinary tract infections with corresponding symptoms.

Solid Masses of the Kidney

For the clarification of renal masses (and of course also complicated cysts), cross-sectional imaging techniques are moving to

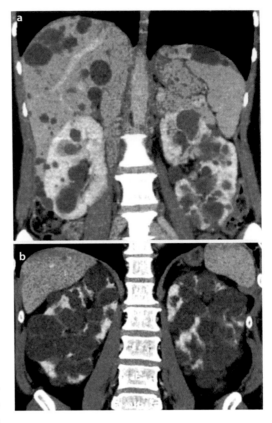

◘ **Fig. 19.8   a,b** Polycystic kidneys

the forefront. First and foremost CT—provided that the patient's age permits this.

■ Clinic

Initially non-specific and depending on the etiology, possibly hematuria, flank pain, B-symptoms.

■ Diagnostics

CT

Depending on the problem, different contrast agent timings may be important. In native CT, calcifications or hemorrhages in complicated cysts can be well delineated; in addition, in combination with a contrast-enhanced phase, it helps to detect or exclude any contrast medium uptake. The arterial contrast phase (approx. 15 s after intravenous contrast administration) facilitates the assessment of the feeding vessels, which can be important for preoperative planning, for example. It also facilitates the search for highly perfused (hypervascularized) liver metastases—should it be a malignancy. In what is usually referred to as the venous phase (approximately 60–80 s after contrast administration), there is still a marked difference in contrast between the cortical kidney and the cortical medulla in most patients (it is therefore also called the corticomedullary phase in connection with the kidney), which can mask space-occupying lesions. If a renal mass is suspected, it is worth waiting until the contrast medium is homogeneously distributed (after approx. 100–150 s after injection of KM). If involvement of the urinary tract is suspected, it may also make sense to image it with contrast. As a practical matter, the contrast agent is usually eliminated renally–so you just have to wait long enough for it to get there. The first test scan (imaging a slice to see if the ureters are contrasted) is usually worth doing without further preparation after 5 min at the earliest, depending on the patient and kidney. Then it should be considered to admit the patient again after 20–30 min. Or—if it is known in advance that a urographic phase will be needed—the excretion of contrast medium can be accelerated and intensified with low-dose loop diuretics, if necessary in combination with preceding hydration.

In most cases, the further clarification serves for a more precise assessment of a complicated cyst or for staging in the case of a concrete suspicion of malignancy, since many solid masses cannot be clearly assigned to a benign or malignant origin.

Angiolipoma

Angiomyolipoma (◘ Fig. 19.9) is an exception: as the name suggests, it is characterized by the fact that it contains fat—fat, however, is very rarely found in renal cell carcinoma. Therefore, if fat tissue is detected (by negative density values in CT or by a signal drop in fat-suppressed sequences in MRI) and there is no other evidence of malignancy

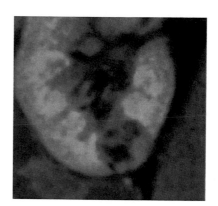

◘ **Fig. 19.9** Angiomyolipoma

(metastases, infiltration in surrounding structures, etc.), an angiomyolipoma may be present.

In all other cases, a definitive diagnosis from images is difficult or impossible.

❯ Solid masses of the kidney are always suspicious for malignancy—unless fat can be detected. If there is no further evidence of malignancy (no infiltration, no metastases), it is most likely an angimyolipoma.

Oncocytoma

Oncocytoma (◘ Fig. 19.10) sounds dangerous, but it is a benign, slow-growing tumor. On CT, it is **homogeneously contrast-enhancing** and often has a **radiating wheel-spoke pattern converging on a central scar**. Unfortunately, this is not a sure sign of benignity, on the contrary: oncocytoma and renal cell carcinoma look very similar, so that the finding requires histological confirmation—which in the vast majority of cases results in a (possibly partial) nephrectomy.

Lymphoma

Lymphomas can also settle in the kidney. However, an isolated lymphoma of the kidney is rare, since in the examination one always looks at the whole person or the entire imaging area, the view sooner or later

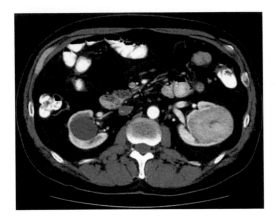

■ **Fig. 19.10**   Oncocytoma

falls on paraaortic or mediastinal lymph node packages. Lymphomas can take many forms within the kidney (as everywhere else): for example, in the form of **focal findings**, which are then usually **homogeneously contrasted**, but **absorb** somewhat **less KM** than the healthy renal parenchyma. But **diffuse infiltration** is also possible, which ultimately leads to an enlargement of the organ.

Metastasis

Metastases often occur in groups. Whether a diagnosis must be forced histologically depends on the oncological therapy plan or on the patient's diagnosis. In individual cases, a diagnostic puncture may be necessary. In a palliative situation, assessment of the response to chemo/radiotherapy in the next staging is often sufficient. Overall, a metastasis cannot be distinguished from an NCC image morphologically.

Renal Cell Carcinoma (NCC)

Renal cell carcinoma (■ Fig. 19.11) is the most common renal tumor in adults and can vary widely in appearance, depending on its histology.

■ **Diagnostics**

Sonography

On ultrasound, for example, it can be **hypo-, iso- or hyperechogenic** to the healthy

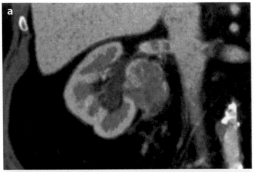

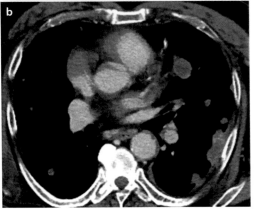

■ **Fig. 19.11**   **a** NCC on the right with thrombi in the renal vein. **b** NCC with diffuse pulmonary and pleural metastasis in the same patient in the soft tissue window

renal parenchyma. And since it can also show cystic parts, **anechoic areas** are also possible. An important diagnostic criterion, as can already be seen in the Bosniak classification, is **contrast sonography**. In **contrast sonography**, a **more rapid flow of contrast medium** and an even **more rapid washout can** sometimes be observed.

CT

On CT, it is usually somewhat **hypodense** compared to the healthy renal parenchyma and usually also accumulates **somewhat less contrast medium** than the rest of the renal parenchyma—but **hypervascularized areas** are also possible and the image becomes inhomogeneous at the latest in the case of **central necrosis** or **cystic portions.** For therapy/resection planning, an assessment of the **adjacent vascular and renal pelvic struc-**

19

tures is important. The hypernephroma—as the NCC is often called—often grows into the respective renal vein and therefore often results in thrombosis of the renal vein or the V. cava. In addition, filiae (most frequently in locoregional lymph nodes, lung and skeleton as well as skull) should of course also be excluded in the best case. Staging therefore includes a CT of the abdomen from 3 cm tumor diameter supplemented by a chest CT and a cranial MRI.

MRI

If questions remain (e.g. unclear bone lesions or liver foci that cannot be clearly classified, or questionable infiltration into surrounding vessels), a targeted MRI can provide clarity.

Nephroblastoma

Nephroblastoma is the most common malignant renal tumor in childhood (synonym: Wilms tumor) and occurs mainly in young children (before the age of four). Since it is often first noticed by a unilateral painless swelling of the abdomen, it is often already extended at the time of diagnosis and displaces adjacent structures.

- Diagnostics (◘ Fig. 19.12)

Sonography

Initially, sonography is usually performed, which reveals an **echo-rich mass** originating from the renal parenchyma with a **pseudocapsule** corresponding to the compressed surrounding renal parenchyma. Large tumors in particular cannot always be assigned with certainty to an organ by sonography—for example, differentiation from a neuroblastoma (malignant tumor of the sympathetic nervous system in childhood) may be difficult.

MRI

As further (objective because not examiner-dependent) imaging, an MRI is recommended, in which the mass is **inhomogeneous** both T1- and T2-weighted—with an equally **inhomogeneous contrast image**. In addition, the surrounding lymph node

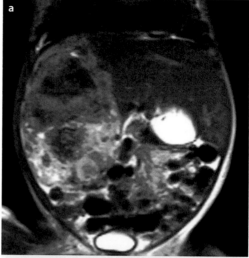

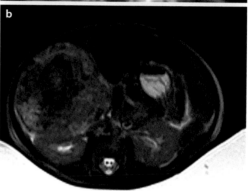

◘ **Fig. 19.12** Nephroblastoma t2-weighted. **a** Coronary, **b** Axial

stations and the liver should be assessed here (as already in sonography).

Conventional X-ray

Further staging includes the exclusion of lung metastases—an X-ray of the lung is required for this.

Vascular Stenoses and Occlusions
Renal Infarction

Renal infarction—like infarctions of other organs—is often preceded by arteriosclerosis. However, cardiogenic dissemination of an embolus, e.g. from a thrombus in the atrial ear in atrial fibrillation, or a septic embolism, e.g. in valve endocarditis, are also possible.

■ Clinic

In the acute stage, a renal infarction can be associated with severe pain.

■ Diagnostics

CT

If a renal infarction is suspected, the search usually begins with a CT scan or CT angiography. Conveniently, other causes of abdominal or flank pain can also be assessed here. In an arterial contrast phase or CT angiography, the condition and, if necessary, the occlusion of the afferent renal artery can be assessed. In the venous or nephrographic contrast medium phase, on the other hand, a **lack of contrast medium accumulation of** the affected (usually wedge-shaped) part of the parenchyma or, in the worst case, of the entire kidney is pathognomonic.

Sonography

The reduced blood flow can also be visualized by duplex sonography.

DSA

If an interventional therapy (e.g. a local thrombolysis via an intra-arterial catheter) is possible, one or the other procedure can be followed by a DSA in readiness for intervention with the aim of preserving the entire organ or its function as far as possible.

Old renal infarcts can be delineated as scarring retraction of the renal parenchyma (◘ Fig. 19.13).

Renal Artery Stenosis

Renal artery stenosis is often conspicuous by refractory (renovascular) hypertension and/or by a restriction of renal function. The possibilities of radiological diagnostics are manifold. Duplex sonography and MR angiography are at the forefront of diagnostics—if only because of the lack of radiation dose.

■ Clinic

Mostly unspecific, possibly symptoms of hypertension (dizziness, headache, nervousness, nausea, …)

■ Diagnostics

Sonography

Duplex sonography does not require the administration of contrast media—it does, however, require a patient who is "good at sound" **and** a motivated and/or experienced examiner.

MRI

With MRI, the amount of contrast agent required is low and not nephrotoxic, making MRI a good adjunct if renal function is reasonably preserved.

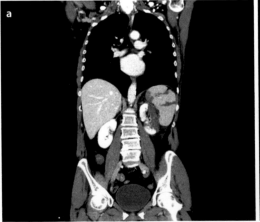
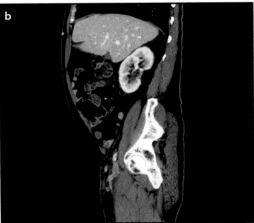

19

◘ **Fig. 19.13**   Renal infarction. **a** Fresh, **b** Old

CT

Of course, CT angiography is also possible for the detection of vascular stenoses. If a stenosis is detected, it can be repaired with (stent) dilatation in the course of conventional angiography. Here, too, however, the main concern is to preserve renal function. Arterial hypertension is usually fixed and does not regress even with revascularization.

Investment Variants
Renal Agenesis

If the kidney should not be paired, this is in many cases the result of a surgical intervention—but a missing kidney as an anatomical norm variant is also possible. The solution is usually found quickly on the basis of an anamnesis. If the patient does not provide any information, a look at the respective flank will help in the search for a suitable scar.

Malrotation

In the course of embryonic development, the kidney moves up from the pelvis to the lumbar region and also rotates its axis during this process. If this rotation does not occur, it is called malrotation (■ Fig. 19.14). Then it may (rarely) happen that a kidney is

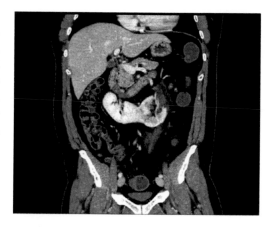

■ **Fig. 19.15**   Horseshoe kidney

found in the pelvis, for example. Or (more frequently) that the renal pelvis is not oriented medially, but ventrally.

Horseshoe Kidney

This is a fusion of both kidneys at their lower poles (■ Fig. 19.15), either complete with continuous renal parenchyma or in the form of a punctate connective tissue bridge.

Accessory Vascular Supply

This is a relict from embryonic development—as is usual for annex variants—which normally obliterates during the ascent from the pelvis and is replaced by the renal artery. These vessels become important, for example, when planning endovascular vascular prostheses, e.g. as part of an aneurysm repair, as "overstenting" of these vessels can lead to a relevant renal infarction (■ Fig. 19.16).

19.2.5 **Injuries to the Kidneys and Urinary Tract**

The question of a kidney injury is usually preceded by a corresponding history of "blunt" (fall/stroke) or "sharp" (stab wound/gunshot) violence. Depending on availability, the first imaging is usually sonography or a (polytrauma) CT.

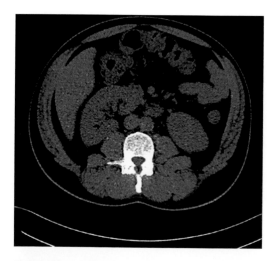

■ **Fig. 19.14**   Painting rotation

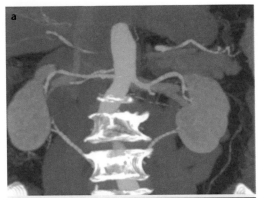

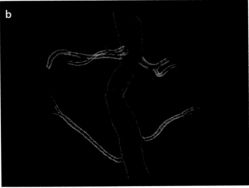

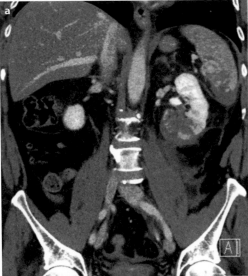

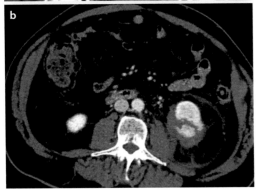

◘ **Fig. 19.16 a** Coronary MIP reconstruction and VRT of a 5-fold renal artery apposition. **b** VRT of a 5-fold renal artery apposition

Kidney injuries are classified based on their severity and the structures involved, such as the American Association for the Surgery of Trauma, AAST (◘ Fig. 19.17, ◘ Table 19.3).

19.2.6 Adrenal Gland

See also ► Chap. 22 (Adrenal adenoma, -carcinoma).

The healthy adrenal gland cannot be assessed in sonography. In cross-sectional imaging it is visible as a narrow Y-shaped structure in the upper retroperitoneum.

◘ **Fig. 19.17   a,b** Kidney trauma grade IV

Pheochromocytoma

The suspicion of a pheochromocytoma (primary benign mass with the potential for malignant degeneration) is usually based on the clinical symptoms and the examination of a 24 h collection urine for catecholamia or its degradation products and, if necessary, further laboratory tests. However, in order to plan appropriate (surgical) therapy, the surgeon must know where to find it.

◘ Table 19.3 Classification of kidney injuries

Organ contusion possibly with bleeding into the parenchyma or below the renal capsule	**Cortical parenchymal tear less than** 1 cm deep Perirenal (i.e. crossing the renal capsule) hematoma	**Cortical parenchymal tear more than** 1 cm deep and perirenal hematoma	**Parenchymal injury** into the cavity system (the urinary **tract**) Arterial or venous vascular injury	**Extensive parenchymal injury** (comminuted kidney) Vascular rupture Kidney stalk Mass bleeding

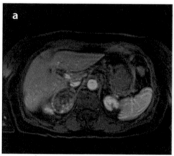 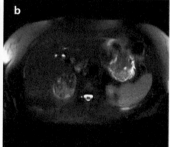 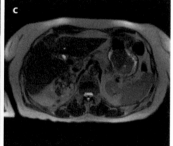

◘ Fig. 19.18 Pheochromocytoma. **a** T1-weighted. **b, c** T2-weighted

■ Clinic

Seizure-like high blood pressure (paroxysmal hypertension), permanent increase in blood pressure (persistent hypertension, often in children).

■ Diagnostics (◘ Fig. 19.18)

Sonography

Sonographically, the detection is only successful in large tumors and sometimes they occur in several localizations at the same time—not only within the adrenal glands, but also along the marginal cord.

❯ Pheochromocytomas are hormone-active and react to mechanical stimulation—e.g. in the course of a biopsy—with a hormone release if this is not inhibited in advance by medication. A diagnostic puncture is only indicated in exceptional cases when a pheochromocytoma is suspected—but should then be performed under appropriate premedication and circulation monitoring.

CT CT is helpful for localization of the tumor(s), which then includes the predilection sites borderline cord and adrenal glands (thorax and abdomen). Pheochromocytomas are **round-oval** shaped, **smooth bordered** and accumulate **contrast agent vigorously and early.**

MRI On MRI, pheochromocytomas are **fluid isointense**—that is, **hyperintense in T2 weighting** and **hypointense in T1 weighting**. This is particularly impressively visible on the basis of fluid- or edema-sensitive sequences such as a T2 weighting with fat saturation.

Adrenal Metastases

They are usually detected on CT as part of the staging of a primary tumor (bronchial carcinoma or melanoma) and are then still small (less than 3 cm in diameter). In the CT morphology they are **blurred** and absorb **contrast medium inhomogeneously.** Fat cannot be detected. If a definite diagnosis or histology is necessary, the mass of an adrenal gland can be biopsied with CT guidance.

19.2.7 Prostate

The healthy prostate is the size of a chestnut (about 3 cm in diameter) and surrounds the urethra, which arises from the urinary bladder. It tapers caudally, which is why its lower end is called the apex, while the broader, cranial part is called the base. In addition, the prostatic parenchyma is divided into several zones: the peripheral zone, the transitional zone, the central zone and the periurethral glandular region, which is tiny and not so important from the radiological point of view.

Prostatic Hypertrophy

Prostate hypertrophy is one of the most common diagnoses in the world of urology—and fortunately benign (BPH = benign protastahypertrophy). It develops during life due to an increase in the central zone around the urethra.

- Clinic

The compression of the urethra by the surrounding tissue proliferation ultimately leads to the typical complaints with pollakiuria, thin (dribbling) urine stream and residual urine formation.

- Diagnostics

Sonography/MRI (⬛ Fig. 19.19)

   Image morphologically, the prostatic hypertrophy is characterized by an **increase of the central poratata parts**, which have an **inhomogeneous internal structure in** sonog-

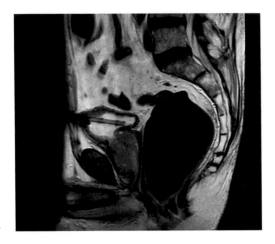

⬛ **Fig. 19.19**   Benign prostatic hyperplasia

raphy as well as in MRI. The obstruction of the urethra leads to an **increased trabecularization of** the (mainly ventral) bladder wall, in the sense of a so-called **barred bladder** as well as **increased bladder diverticula**. In the transabdominal sonography usually only an enlargement of the organ with elevation of the bladder floor can be seen.

Prostate Carcinoma

The **prostate carcinoma** develops mainly in the dorsally located peripheral zone. Therefore, it leads to obstruction symptoms much later. Sometimes, the clinical findings are already clear: a rough (like a knuckle) palpable nodule on rectal examination and PSA elevation. Then a transrectal, sonographically guided puncture by the treating urologist usually leads to a definitive diagnosis.

- Clinic

s. Hyperplasia, possibly hematuria.

- Diagnostics

MRI

   If the symptoms are unclear, e.g. if the PSA value is elevated and there is no correlation either by palpation or endosonography, MRI is required. A prostatic carcinoma is then apparent as a T2w-hypointense **area** in the peripheral (rarely in the central) zone. Diffusion imaging can visualize the **cytotoxic edema** triggered by the tumor. In addition, dynamic series can be used to assess **contrast flooding**, in which, as is so often the case, the tumor is evident by **rapid flooding** and **washout**. For the classification of such findings, a classification analogous to the BIRADS system of mammography, the PI-RADS classification, has become established. Another development is the **MR-guided biopsy of** tumor-suspicious lesions that cannot be reliably detected by sonography. This is done with special transrectal biopsy coils, so that specific suspicious regions can be biopsied.

CT

CT is not helpful for the diagnostic evaluation of the prostate itself. A distinction between malignant and benign enlargement is not initially possible. However, in staging, it is used to assess any transmural growth and to allow the detection of any metastases (lymph nodes, lung, bone). Osseous metastases of prostate carcinoma are typically osteoblastic—i.e. more sclerotic and initially often localized in the pelvis and lumbar spine.

Prostatitis

The question of **prostatitis** is extremely rare in radiology.

- Clinic

It is already clinically noticeable by fever, pain and dysuria. In the clinical examination it is also enlarged palpable and the palpation is very painful for the patient. In the laboratory, the PSA concentration is usually also elevated.

- Diagnostics

Sonography

Sonographically also an **enlargement of the organ** is visible, with a **reduced echogenicity** due to the edema (=water).

A chronic prostatitis cannot be distinguished from a carcinoma of the prostate

even with the help of the best images—the question can therefore only be clarified histologically.

19.2.8 Testis and Epididymis

The testis and epididymis are connected to each other by the ductuli efferentes testis. Usually, two such testicular and epididymis packages per man are built together in one scrotum.

Radiology may also involve examination of the testis and epididymis. Due to the high radiation sensitivity of the reproductive organ, one will avoid X-ray examinations of this organ as far as possible and try to progress as best as possible with sonography and MRI.

Hydrocele

One speaks of a **hydrocele** when the scrotum has stored fluid that surrounds the testis and epididymis. This is not infrequently an incidental finding of a CT of the abdomen or an MRI of the pelvis that has been "pulled down" a little too far.

Testicular Torsion

Testicular torsion is a condition that usually occurs in children and adolescents.

- Clinic

When the testicles twist around each other, they also wrap their inflow and outflow vessels around each other—with the result that there is first an obstruction of the venous outflow with painful swelling and reddening of the testicle and in the worst case later also with an occlusion of the arterial inflow—this results in an infarction or the loss of the testicle.

- Diagnostics

Sonography

The diagnosis is an emergency that requires immediate surgical care to avoid the aforementioned infarction of the testicles.

The quickest way to make a diagnosis is to take the transducer in hand: Duplex sonography is the quickest way to visualize the reduced or dried-up blood flow.

Inflammatory Changes of the Testis

Epididymitis is an inflammation of the epididymis, which rarely also leads to **orchitis,** i.e. an inflammation of the testicle.

■ Clinic

Clinically, the picture is similar to that of testicular torsion: painful swelling and redness of the scotum. In contrast to torsion, patients with epididymitis are more likely to be older gentlemen.

■ Diagnostics

Sonography

Duplex sonography may reveal **increased blood flow**. In addition, the testis and epididymis are **enlarged** and **echo-poor** due to the accompanying **edema**.

Varicocele

In the case of **varicocele,** the radiologist can sometimes take more than just pictures: it is virtually a matter of varicose veins (i.e. dilated, tortuous veins) in the pampiniform plexus within the testicle.

■ Clinic

Mostly no symptoms, but risk of infertility.

■ Diagnostics

Sonography

A varicocele can be diagnosed by duplex sonography. With a **phlebography,** the entire course of the vessel can be visualized even more precisely. In order to bring the contrast medium specifically to the site of the event, a catheter is first inserted via the groin into the renal vein in order to probe the confluence of the spermatic vein from there. In this way, the spermatic vein can be imaged all the way to the scrotal venous convolute by means of retrograde contrast medium distribution and then also closed interventionally—by means of an embolus or a sclerosing agent.

Testicular Retention

Testicular retention is defined as the absence of descent of the testes into the scrotum during the first three months of life. Depending on where the testis is located, it is named: Abdominal testis or Inguinal testis. If it oscillates between different locations, it is called a sliding testis.

■ Clinic

Mostly asymptomatic, but risk of infertility.

■ Diagnostics

MRI

If the sonographic search for a missing testis remains unsuccessful, a sectional image is requested. MRI is the only method that can be used for this purpose; it is usually successful in localizing the testis, even if the object of the search is still hidden in the retroperitoneum.

Testicular Tumors

Testicular tumors are diseases of the young man (age peak between the 20–40 years). The diagnosis usually already takes place at the urologist. Since the majority of cases are malignant tumors, the patient requires staging to detect any metastases (lymph nodes—initially parailiac and retroperitoneal, lung) with the aid of an appropriate CT of the abdomen or trunk.

Seminal Vesicles

Seminal vesicles are sometimes visible on abdominal imaging, both ultrasound and MRI and CT. For the sake of completeness, they should also be mentioned here. Diseases of the seminal vesicles are extremely rare. Issues involving the seminal vesicles, except perhaps in homes with major urology, (virtually) never occur. However, the attentive eye may notice calcifications of the seminal vesicles or the vasa deferens, which usually affect patients with diabetes mellitus.

19.3 Diagnostics

19.3.1 Diagnostic Radiology

Christel Vockelmann

Sonography

As already described in the previous chapter, sonography is also the most easily available imaging method in the diagnosis of the urogenital system, which can be used both as a screening method and for clarifying complaints. It is used both as a screening method and for the diagnosis of complaints. The main focus is on spatial damage in the renal parenchyma and dilatation of the renal pelvis as an indication of urinary retention. The urinary bladder can also be assessed very well when full. Sonography is also used to determine the residual urine. For this purpose, the volume of the bladder after emptying is determined sonographically.

Both the male and female genital organs can be well assessed sonographically. Not only transabdominal ultrasound is used for this purpose. With special transducers, transvaginal or transrectal sonography can also be performed. In Germany, these are generally performed by urologists or gynecologists. In other countries, e.g. France, this is also part of the examination spectrum of radiologists.

Conventional X-ray Diagnostics

Conventional radiology no longer has any relevant significance in the context of urogenital imaging. The intravenous excretory urogram has been completely superseded by computed tomography in the diagnosis of kidney stones. Nevertheless, in the diagnosis

of the abdomen, even in conventional images, attention should of course always be paid to calcifications in the course of the draining urinary tract. Roundish, somewhat cloudy calcifications in the pelvis of older women usually correspond to calcified uterine fibroids, a benign lump of the uterus.

❯ The question of ureteral stones should be clarified with low-dose computed tomography of the urinary tract.

Fluoroscopy/Angiography

The indications for fluoroscopic examinations or diagnostic angiographies of the urogenital system have also become very limited in recent years. A typical indication is cystography to exclude a urinary bladder injury after surgical interventions in the small pelvis.

A similar examination, namely a micturition cysturethrogram (MCU), is a typical examination in pediatrics. Here, the urinary bladder is also filled with contrast medium. In addition, a micturition of the small patients should then be performed. The indication for this is the suspicion of a vesicoureteral reflux, which leads to inflammation of the renal pelvis. This reflux occurs mainly with high pressure in the urinary bladder, which arises primarily during micturition.

For reasons of radiation hygiene, lateral images should be avoided as far as possible in children. The imaging frequency and fluoroscopy time should also be reduced to a minimum.

Computed Tomography

The method of choice is computed tomography in the detection of ureteral stones. These are usually calcium dense and can thus be excellently detected in computed tomography, even natively and in a low-dose technique. Depending on the CT device, the necessary radiation dose corresponds approximately to an X-ray examination of the abdomen in two planes.

In the diagnosis of renal tumors, computed tomography is well applicable. In this context, the diagnosis of the kidneys is usually performed within the framework of a CT abdominal scan. If there is a specific question about a renal tumor, a native examination of the kidneys should be performed if necessary to evaluate a contrast image. In addition to an arterial coil, a second series of examinations is performed in the nephrographic contrast phase approximately 100–150 s after contrast administration. CT urography can be added for questions of the urinary tract (◘ Fig. 19.20). For this purpose, the excretion of the contrast medium into the ureters must be waited for 7–10 min after contrast medium administration. Low-dose administration of furosemide, a loop diuretic, can be helpful here.

In the diagnosis of the genital organs in the small pelvis, computed tomography only plays a secondary role. Here, too, the uterus or prostate are also assessed in every CT examination performed for other reasons. In the case of sonographically detected malignant tumors, CT is performed for staging and the search for distant metastases. A classic example is the question of peritoneal carcinomatosis of an ovarian carcinoma.

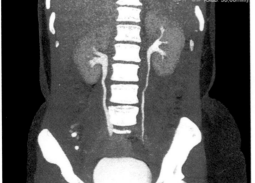

◘ **Fig. 19.20** Thick-slice MIP reconstruction of a CT urography without pathology

Magnetic Resonance Imaging

In contrast to computer tomography, magnetic resonance imaging also allows local staging of tumors of the internal genitals.

Sagittal sequences are useful for differentiating endometrial or uterine carcinomas; here, the tumor can be delineated hypointense to the myometrium after contrast medium administration. The depth of infiltration and, in particular, infiltration into neighboring organs must be assessed, as this can influence the therapeutic procedure.

Unlike most other tumors that are hyperintense delineable on T2-weighted imaging, prostate carcinoma is characterized by hypointense signaling on T2-weighted images. Therefore, thin-slice T2 imaging is necessary for the detection of prostate carcinoma, which, unlike benign hyperplasia of the prostate, grows in the outer gland of the prostate. This is usually performed axially as well as coronally and sagittally. The imaging is improved by the additional use of an endorectal coil for body array.

In addition, the prostate carcinoma can be detected with the help of spectroscopy. Here one uses the fact that the prostate carcinoma has more choline and less citrate than healthy prostate tissue. However, this technique is certainly only used in a fraction of patients with prostate carcinoma. In the majority of patients, urological-sonographic diagnostics are sufficient for the therapy decision.

19.3.2 Nuclear Medicine

Ursula Blum

Renal Scintigraphy

- **Renal Perfusion DTPA (Diethylenetriaminepentaacetic Acid)**

Diethylenetriaminepentaacetic acid (DTPA) is purely glomerular filtered. Thus, DTPA allows a perfusion study as well as the determination of the glomerular filtration rate (GFR). GFR is a measure of renal function

(■ Table 19.4). Indications for testing include suspected impaired renal function, possibly prior to chemotherapy or radiation therapy, and chronic renal insufficiency. The GFR depends on the age and sex of the patient.

■ Kidney Function

Renal function scintigraphy is frequently used. It can easily—and with low radiation exposure—provide reliable information on blood flow, the position of the kidneys, any anomalies that may be present, the side-separated function and the drainage conditions. It is also possible to visualize any reflux (backflow of urine from the bladder into the ureter or kidneys). Due to the low radiation exposure, the examination is also performed relatively frequently in children and adolescents.

Available tracers are ^{123}I-OIH (ortho-iodhippuric acid) and ^{99m}Tc-MAG3 (mercaptoacetyltriglycine). Due to its better availability, ^{99m}Tc-MAG3 has gained acceptance in clinical routine.

■ Postmicturition Images

In case of incomplete drainage from the renal pelvicocaliceal system or the ureter, static images should be performed after appropriate bladder emptying and a change of position (at least 15 min in an upright position).

These can take place directly after bladder emptying, but in addition, if possible, always 50–60 min p. i. as static recordings over 2 min.

■ Examination with Furosemide Exposure

If the baseline examination shows a delay in urine flow, the additional administration of furosemide is possible. Among other things, furosemide prevents the reabsorption of water in the kidney, so that the urine can no longer be concentrated. Contraindications are a known hypersensitivity to furosemide and low blood pressure (clinically relevant), a relative contraindication is a kidney stone.

The examination can be performed following a baseline examination or directly as an examination with furosemide exposure in the case of known urinary flow disorders.

Dosage:
- Infants: 1 mg/kg bw i. v.
- Oneyear to 18 years: 0.5 mg/kg bw, maximum 20 mg i. v.
- From 18 years: 0.5 mg/kg bw, maximum 40 mg i. v.

Time of Injection:
- F + 20: 20 min after radiopharmaceutical (e.g. after basic examination)
- F - 15: 15 min before the radiopharmaceutical
- F0: Simultaneous with the radiopharmaceutical
- F + 2: 2 min after the radiopharmaceutical

■ **Table 19.4** Normal values GFR. (Modified according to Dtsch Arztebl Int 2009)

Babies and Children	
Premature births	>0.5 mL/min/kg
Newborn	>10 mL/min/m^2
Week 2–8	16.3–44.6 mL/min/1.73 m^2 KOF
3rd–12th month	>70 mL/min/1.73 m^2 KOF
1–20 years	>80 mL/min/1.73 m^2 KOF

Adults (mL/min/1.73 m^2 KOF)		
Age [years]	Men	Women
20–29	77–170	71–165
30–39	70–162	64–149
40–49	63–147	58–135
50–59	56–130	51–120
60–69	49–113	45–104
70–79	42–98	39–90
80–89	35–81	32–75

The examination is otherwise performed in the same way as the basic examination. The evaluation is primarily visual. Here, it is best to distinguish between "normal" and "absent". According to the guideline, all findings in between should be reported as a percentage of the maximum activity before and after the administration of furosemide, as well as any post-micturition images that may be available.

■ **Examination After ACE Inhibitor Administration**

An (atypical) arterial hypertension can be caused by a renal artery stenosis. In this case, an activation of the renin-angiotensin system leads to an increase in blood pressure. The therapy of this high blood pressure is carried out, at least in the short course of the disease, by eliminating the cause, namely the renal artery stenosis. Often, however, the hypertension is already fixed.

The following medications should be suspended for the study if possible:

- ACE inhibitors depending on their half-life (3–7 days before)
- Diuretics: A few days before the examination

As part of a one-day protocol, the baseline scintigraphy is performed first according to the normal examination protocol. The patient is then administered 25–50 mg captopril p. o. Blood pressure is monitored every 10–15 min because an ACE inhibitor can lower blood pressure very dramatically. If there is a symptomatic drop in blood pressure, fluid should be infused. After 60 min, a new renal scintigraphy is performed, if necessary with increased activity (up to 200 MBq).

In a two-day protocol, the examination is performed first with ACE inhibitor administration. A normal result argues against renin-angiotensin-acting renal artery stenosis, the baseline examination would then be invalid.

The following parameters should be determined:

- Time until the occurrence of the maximum
- Quotient of activity after 20 min/activity at maximum (norm <0.3)

The following changes may occur with renal artery stenosis:

- Shift of the maximum >2 min or >40% to the baseline examination
- Change in 20 min/max quotient >0.15
- Reduction of the relative uptake >10%.
- Change in the time-activity curve with significantly delayed or undetectable drop over the affected kidney
- Decrease in calculated GFR >10

■ **Static Renal Scintigraphy (DMSA)**

Static renal scintigraphy is mainly performed on children. Here, the focus is not on the function per se, but the examination serves, among other things, to detect kidney tissue and, if necessary, to detect changes in the kidneys. In this way, small functional defects can also be detected, which can occur, for example, after repeated inflammations of the renal pelvis.

Even in the case of significantly impaired kidney function, it is possible to determine the percentage of the side, in this case e.g. before a planned surgical measure. The radiation exposure of such a renal scintigraphy is 1.2 mSv.

19.3.3 Valence

Christel Vockelmann

◘ Table 19.5 shows the use of the respective therapeutic options depending on the problem

◘ Table 19.5 Value of the therapeutic procedures

	Sonography	Conventional	Fluoroscopy/ Angiography	CT	MRI	Nuk	PET
Ureteral stone (urolithiasis)	P*	N	N	P	N	N	N
Renal function determination	N	N	N	N	N	P	N
Kidney tumor	P	N	N	W	W	N	N

N Not indicated, *P* Primary diagnosis, *W* Further diagnosis

P* Every patient with flank pain as an indication of renal colic is primarily examined sonographically. However, the actual stone can rarely be detected sonographically

19.4 Therapy

19.4.1 Interventional Radiology

Christel Vockelmann

Ultrasound/Nuclear Magnetic Resonance Imaging

For the treatment of uterine fibroids, in addition to the classic surgical therapy with a myoma enucleation or a hysterectomy, there is a very new procedure called HIFU (High Intensity Focused Ultrasound). Here, the target tissue is strongly heated (70–100 °C) within a few seconds by means of high-intensity focused ultrasound. The ultrasound can reach the target area very precisely and surrounding tissue is spared. In order to treat the target tissue precisely, the treatment is carried out in an MRT. This requires an upgrade of a normal MRI with the ultrasound including the control units. Due to the very precise therapy with sparing of the surrounding tissue, there are also developments to use the procedure in other areas (prostate carcinoma, pancreatic carcinoma and many more). The development of the next few years will show whether the procedure can establish itself permanently.

Angiography

Angiographic procedures are also used in the treatment of uterine fibroids. Indication for this is mostly the rejection of surgical therapy. For embolization, probing of both internal iliac arteries is necessary. Iliacae internae is necessary. The uterine arteries are then probed and embolized with particles. After the procedure, the patients regularly show a post embolization syndrome with severe pain and often fever, which requires in-patient pain therapy.

19.4.2 Radiotherapy

Guido Heilsberg

Urinary Bladder Carcinoma

Urinary bladder carcinoma (◘ Fig. 19.21) is irradiated adjuvantly as radiochemotherapy for organ preservation to the bladder 54–60 Gy with $5 \times 1.8/2.0$ Gy per week.

The patient is positioned in the supine position, the legs are padded with a standard positioning aid.

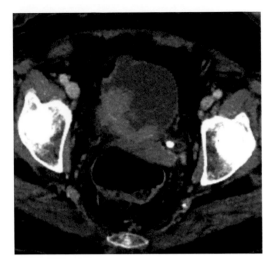

□ Fig. 19.21 Carcinoma of the dorsal and right lateral bladder wall. Incidental finding of urinary bladder diverticulum ventrally

Prostate Carcinoma (Carcinoma of the Glandular Tissue of the Prostate Gland)

Primary radiotherapy: in the case of **low risk,** only radiotherapy is performed; in the case of **intermediate risk,** radiotherapy is combined with six months of HAT. In the case of **high risk,** radiotherapy is performed in which, if necessary, the pelvic lymph drainage is also irradiated and hormone ablative therapy (HAT) is additionally given over 2–3 years. On the prostate analogue >72 Gy with 5 × 1.8/2.0 Gy per week as IMRT.

Adjuvant radiotherapy: On the former tumor bed 60 Gy and in case of biochemical recurrence 66 Gy.

Biochemical recurrence: In case of PSA increase (e.g. three blood samples in a row increased) radiotherapy is performed.

The patient is instructed to arrive at his radiation appointment with a well-filled bladder and, if possible, to empty his bowels beforehand.

The patient is irradiated in the supine position, with his arms on his chest so that they do not lie in the irradiation field in the case of obliquely incident fields.

Side effects: Diarrhea, dysuria, cystitis (bladder infection), proctitis, urinary urgency, urethral strictures, impotence, and incontinence.

Testicular Tumors (Seminoma, Non-Seminoma)

Classical seminomas are among the most radiosensitive tumors and are irradiated adjuvantly.

In stage one seminoma (localized involvement) adjuvant radiotherapy 20 Gy to the para-aortic lymph nodes at 5 × 2.0 Gy per week. In stage 2 (retroperitoneal LK metastases): 30 Gy for small metastases (up to 2 cm, stage 2A), 36 Gy for larger metastases (up to 5 cm, stage 2B) with 5 × 2.0 Gy per week as a so-called "hockey stick" on the para-aortic and pelvic lymph nodes.

Before any therapy: cryopreservation (the "freezing")

The irradiation is carried out in the supine position, the arms will be placed at the side of the body but also above the head in a tray.

Side effects: Nausea

Little Kevin (5 years) suddenly turned pale while playing in the playground and complains of severe pain. It is only after asking more closely that the mother finds out that Kevin has pain in the scrotum. As the boy cannot be calmed down, Mrs. Huber decides to drive directly to the nearest hospital. There the general surgeon Dr. Messer examines Kevin. His suspicion: a torsion of the testicle. Dr. Messer knows that it has to be done quickly if there really is a torsion of the testicle. Therefore, he personally registers Kevin with the radiologist Dr. Kremser for an ultrasound. Dr. Kremser examines the abdomen for orientation in order to establish a little contact with Kevin, who has been given a painkiller in the meantime. Then Dr. Kremser switches to the higher frequency linear transducer to examine the scrotum. First the healthy side is examined, here the testicle can be homogeneously delineated with good vascularization. Then Dr. Kremser examines the painful side and finds the testicle somewhat more echo-poorly distended, but above all: There is almost no blood flow. This makes it clear that Kevin does indeed have testicular torsion. Dr. Kremser therefore calls Dr. Messer: Kevin is operated on immediately. The operation succeeds quickly and the testicle is supplied with blood again. Kevin can go home again after a few days and has digested the whole shock quite quickly.

Practice Questions

1. A 20-year-old young man presents to you with renal colic. What tests do you perform?
2. Name typical image features of renal cysts in ultrasound, CT and MRI!
3. How can you distinguish benign prostatic hypertrophy from prostatic carcinoma?
4. What treatment options for prostate cancer are you aware of?
5. How can the radiologist diagnose diabetes mellitus?

Solutions ▶ Chap. 27

Musculoskeletal Diseases

*Mirja Wenker, Christel Vockelmann, Ursula Blum
and Guido Heilsberg*

Contents

© Springer-Verlag GmbH Germany, part of Springer Nature 2023
M. Kahl-Scholz, C. Vockelmann (eds.), *Basic Knowledge Radiology*,
https://doi.org/10.1007/978-3-662-66351-6_20

This chapter provides an overview of the diagnosis of musculoskeletal disorders. An introductory section covers a brief review of anatomy, followed by common clinical pictures, such as dislocations, fractures, tumors, and degenerative diseases.

20.1   General

Mirja Wenker

Diseases of the musculoskeletal system lead the list of causes of chronic pain worldwide. In addition to rheumatic diseases, this large group of diseases also includes arthroses, fractures and slipped discs. Almost every German has a musculoskeletal disease at some point in his or her life.

Musculoskeletal diseases are also the most frequent cause of days off work and the second most frequent cause of early retirement in Germany. This means that musculoskeletal diseases not only have a considerable impact on the quality of life of those affected, but are also a cost factor for the healthcare system.

An estimated 7,000,000 Germans suffer from diseases of the musculoskeletal system. The Federal Statistical Office estimates treatment costs at around 24 billion euros per year.

Prevention, diagnosis and therapy of these diseases are therefore a "societal task".

20.2   Anatomical Structures

Mirja Wenker

The skeleton provides stability to the body and protects the internal organs from injury.

The skeleton is an important mineral store, especially calcium and phosphorus, and inside many bones is the production site of blood cells. Humans have over 200 bones. A distinction is made between tubular bones (e.g. femur), short bones (e.g. carpus), flat bones (e.g. skull bones) and sesamoid bones. The latter are embedded in muscle layers and are located in places where tendons are exposed to high stress (a classic example and also the largest sesamoid bone in the human body is the patella). Tubular bones are divided into three zones, the centrally located diaphysis, the metaphysis adjacent on both sides, and the epiphysis, which forms the joint and is covered by a layer of cartilage.

Between the epiphysis and metaphysis is the epiphyseal groove, which becomes bony after the end of puberty when the growth hormone level drops and completes the growth in length.

20.2.1   Bone Structure

The essential components of the bone are the compacta or cortex, which forms the outer layer, and the cancellous bone, which is made up of delicate bone bellows on the inside. This contains the blood-forming **red bone marrow** and the **yellow bone marrow, which** consists primarily of fat. Hematogenously metastasizing tumors, such as breast or prostate carcinoma, primarily attack the red bone marrow, which is particularly well supplied with blood. Inflammation-causing bacteria also enter the bone marrow via the blood and lead to infection there.

The **vertebral bodies** consist mainly of cancellous bone, bounded by compacta in the base and top plates and the posterior parts of the vertebrae. Bones are attachment points for tendons and ligaments. Joints form their movable connection with each other.

Three types of **bone cells** are involved in the formation, remodeling and breakdown of bone. **Osteoblasts** are responsible for bone formation and subsequent mineralization and calcification of bone. They secrete calcium, phosphates and carbonates into the interstitial space, wall themselves and are then called **osteocytes.** This hardens the bone so that it becomes resilient. Damaged or overaged bone is broken down by the **osteoclasts.**

In adults, bone formation and decomposition are balanced. Approximately 20% of the bone mass is renewed annually in healthy adults. Pathological processes can disturb the balance. Oestrogen deficiency in older women, for example, leads to decreased blast activity and thus to reduced formation. In children, metabolism is increased in the epiphyseal fossa as the site of length growth (◘ Fig. 20.1).

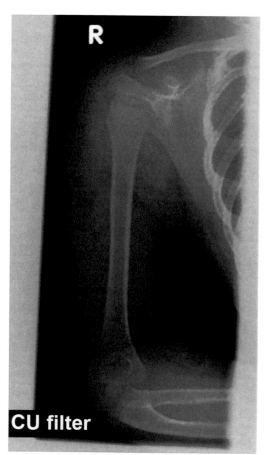

◘ **Fig. 20.1** Infantile humerus

20.3 Clinical Pictures

20.3.1 Fractures

■ Definition

A fracture is the interruption of the continuity of the bone with the formation of two or more fragments, usually as a result of direct or indirect force. Repeated overloading can lead to a so-called **fatigue fracture** (e.g. marching fracture). If a fracture occurs without adequate application of force in the presence of underlying pathological bone processes (e.g. in the presence of osteoporosis or osseous metastases), it is referred to as a **pathological fracture**. Fractures can be classified using the AO classification, but many fracture classifications also have their own names (e.g. Neer classification for fractures of the proximal humerus or Pauwels classification for femoral neck fractures).

Long Bong Bones, Short Bones

■ Clinic

Definite fracture signs: Axial malalignment, open fractures with bone fragments protruding from the wound, steps or gaps in the bone course, crepitation.

Uncertain fracture signs: pain, swelling, redness, hyperthermia, limited mobility (functio laesa).

■ Diagnostics

X-ray Image (◘ Fig. 20.2)

– Dislocated fractures are very easy to recognize by the displacement of the fragments against each other and a partly gaping fracture gap.

– Non-displaced fractures are characterized by sharply demarcated lightening lines and cortical steps.

❯ If a fracture is suspected, X-rays should always be taken in two planes, as a fracture in one plane can also be overlooked. In addition, a second plane provides information about any dislocation or

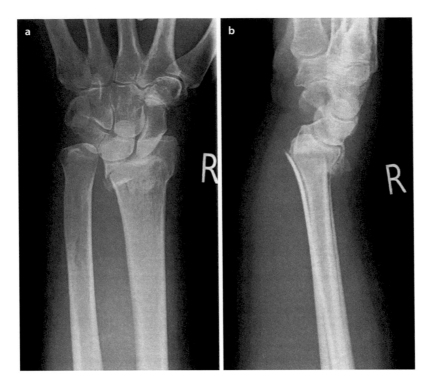

◘ Fig. 20.2   Distal, dorsally tilted radius fracture

axial deviation of fragments, which can be important for the trauma surgeon.

Particularly in the case of radial head and OSG fractures, it may even be necessary to take images in other planes (radial head target image, OSG oblique images) in order to prove a fracture.

CT   CT can be used to detect fractures that cannot be visualized on X-ray. Non-displaced fractures, particularly of the femoral neck and pelvis, may escape normal radiographic detection but are readily detectable on CT (◘ Fig. 20.3). An interruption of the cortical bone is usually seen, but submerged fractures may also result in a line of compression with interruption of the normal trabecular structure. CT is often also requested by the trauma surgeon for surgical planning in order to be able to accurately assess the individual fragments and their position in relation to each other as well as joint involvement.

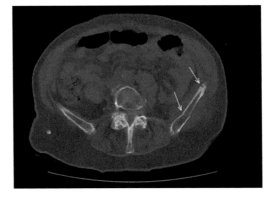

◘ Fig. 20.3   Fractures of the os ilium not visible in conventional radiographs due to intestinal gas overlays

MRI (◘ Fig. 20.4)   MRI is rarely used to detect fractures of the long bones or short bones. It is used in cases where a fracture is suspected despite a negative X-ray (occult fracture) and to visualize concomitant injuries of the capsular ligamentous apparatus. Fracture lines show up in the T1 weighting

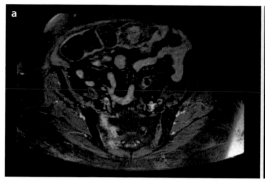
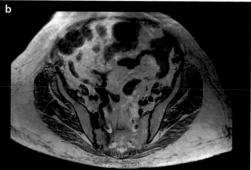

□ Fig. 20.4   a STIR, fracture of the massa lateralis right os sacrum. **b** T2, fracture of the massa lateralis right os sacrum

as a band-shaped signal reduction, and in the T2 weighting as a band-shaped signal increase (**□** Fig. 20.4b). In the STIR sequence, signal enhancement due to bone edema can be detected in fresh fractures (**□** Fig. 20.4a).

Vertebral Body

■ Clinic

Symptoms of a vertebral body fracture can vary. They can range from severe pain and neurological deficits to no symptoms in stable fractures. Sintering of the vertebral body can lead to increased kyphosis of the thoracic spine.

■ Diagnostics

X-ray

Conventional radiography may show a **reduction in the height of the vertebral body. Sharp-edged steps of** the leading edge suggest a more recent fracture (**□** Fig. 20.5). If a fragment breaks off, usually from the leading edge, a **fracture gap** can be demonstrated. In cervical fractures, widening of the prevertebral soft tissue shadow may indicate a fracture.

CT (□ Fig. 20.6)

A fresh fracture is shown on CT by **sharply delineated lightening lines** and **sharp-edged step formations.** CT is used in particular to assess the involvement of the posterior edge of the vertebral body. If this is affected, the fracture is unstable and

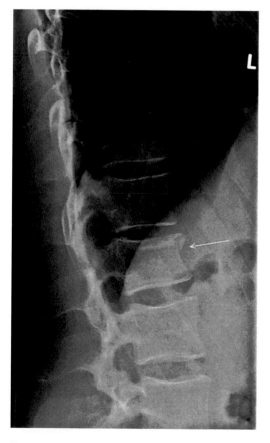

□ Fig. 20.5   Sharp step formation of the anterior edge, fresh ventrally accentuated impression fracture LWK 1

must be treated surgically. The sagittal reconstruction is particularly helpful for assessment.

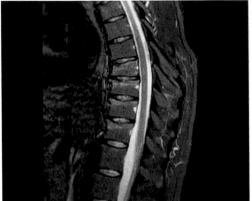

Fig. 20.7   STIR, fresh deck compression fractures BWK 8 to 11 with oedema

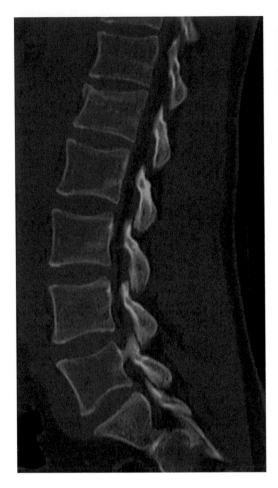

Fig. 20.6   Same fracture on CT

MRI (■ Fig. 20.7)

Particularly in patients with already known vertebral fractures, such as in osteoporosis, MRI can provide evidence of a fresh fracture or fresh fracture component in the case of an already known fracture via the detection of bone edema. The changes in T1 and T2 weighting correspond to those seen in fracture of the long tubular bones. Tears of the ligamentous apparatus and intraspinal hematomas can be detected.

Cranial Bones

■ Clinic

Symptoms vary depending on the affected area: cranial dome, facial skull, skull base.

They can range from pain to neurological symptoms to leakage of cerebrospinal fluid from the auditory canal. Fractures of the skull bone usually occur as a result of external force in the form of an accident, fall or blow.

■ Diagnostics

X-ray

Intracranial hemorrhage or, in the case of craniofacial trauma, fractures may occur as a result of violence, which cannot be seen in conventional X-rays. Therefore, X-rays to exclude fractures in these areas are **now obsolete**.

CT (■ Fig. 20.8)

The method of choice for imaging fractures in the region of the bony skull is CT. It can also be used to detect fractures that escape conventional X-rays, as well as intracranial processes (bleeding, intracranial pressure).

Central midface fractures are divided into three categories according to Le Fort (■ Table 20.1).

❯ If intracranial air pockets are found in the course of a skull fracture, this must be reported to the attending physician. This is then an open skull fracture, which must be covered with antibiotics.

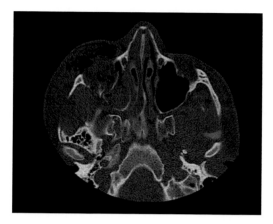

☐ **Fig. 20.8** Complex fractures of the right facial skull with fractures of the orbit, maxillary sinus and zygomatic arch, accompanying hematosinus on the right side

☐ Table 20.1	Le-Fort classification
I	The fracture line runs over the hard palate through the maxilla
II	In this form, the upper jaw is fractured in the form of a pyramid. The fracture runs through the ethmoid bone, the floor of the orbit and the anterior wall of the maxillary sinus
III	The Le Fort III fracture is characterized by the complete detachment of the facial skull from the base of the skull with the involvement of the orbita

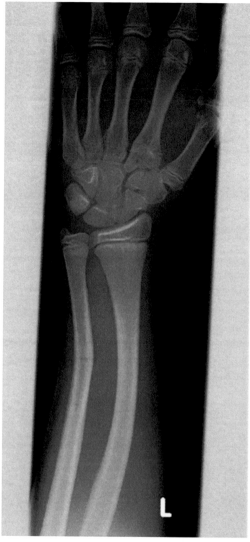

☐ **Fig. 20.9** Bowing fracture of ulna and radius left

Child Fractures

The child's bone is softer and more elastic, the periosteum more elastic than that of an adult, which is why children show different fracture forms. A distinction is made between green wood fractures and bulge fractures.

Greenwood Fracture

Subdivision into typical, compressed and curved ("bowing fracture") greenwood fracture. The long tubular bones are affected.

X-ray Typical greenwood fractures show an open cortical bone on the convex side with preserved periosteum, the concave side is broken. In compressed greenwood fractures, the cortical bone is preserved on both the concave and convex sides. Bowing fractures (☐ Fig. 20.9) show only the bending of the bone; a fracture gap cannot be demonstrated conventionally radiologically.

Bead Breakage

X-ray   This is a fracture of mostly long bones with preservation of the periosteum. Due to compression, the cortical bone at the site of the fracture is raised and a bulge is formed (◘ Fig. 20.10).

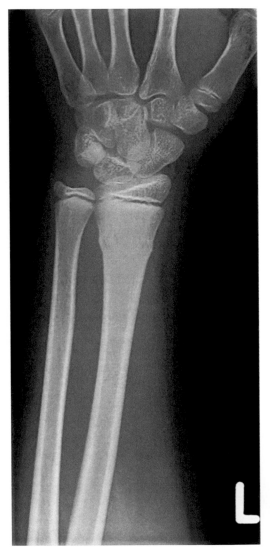

◘ **Fig. 20.10**   Bead fracture distal radius left

Injuries to the Epiphyseal Fossa

These are important because length growth is not complete until the epiphyseal joints are closed. If an injury to the epiphyseal joint occurs beforehand, this can lead to premature closure of the growth plate with restriction of length growth. Involvement of the joint with formation of a step in the articular surface may result in early arthrosis. Injuries to the epiphyseal joint are classified according to Aitken or Salter and Harris.

Sonography   Fractures in infancy can also be visualized by ultrasound (◘ Fig. 20.11). **Bulging and buckling of** the bone can be demonstrated. The displacement **of fragments in** relation to each other can also be imaged. Sonography can also be used in the course assessment to demonstrate **callus formation.**

20.3.2 Luxation

▪ Definition

This refers to dislocation in a joint with complete or incomplete loss of contact

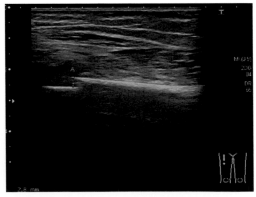

◘ **Fig. 20.11**   Radius fracture with cortical step formation

20

between the joint-forming surfaces. In the latter case, one speaks of a subluxation. This results in a malposition of the joint. The most common form is shoulder dislocation.

■ Clinic

Pain, swelling, functio laesa, visible malposition in the joint, recognizable empty socket, springy fixation in the joint

■ Diagnostics

X-ray

Two planes are always obtained to exclude dislocation, as dislocation can be missed in one plane (■ Fig. 20.12). Evidence

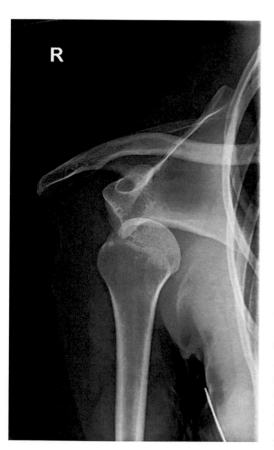

■ **Fig. 20.12** Ventrocaudal shoulder dislocation with empty glenoid cavity

of an **empty glenoid cavity**, clear **offset of the involved bones** against each other and **additional bony injuries** can be visualized.

CT and MRI

CT and MRI may be used in cases that are difficult to assess.

Sonography

Infantile luxations can also be diagnosed by ultrasound.

20.3.3 **Inflammatory Diseases**

Spondylodiscitis/Spondylitis

■ Definition

These are infections of the spine. In adulthood, the process is called **spondylitis.** Secondary development of **spondylodiscitis** may occur after infestation of the disc space per continuitatem. In children, primary hematogenous discectitis or spondylodiscitis is possible because of the still existing vascular supply of the intervertebral discs. At any age, a primary discectitis with secondary spread to the vertebral body as spondylodiscitis can develop postoperatively or postpuncturally. If the vertebral body and intervertebral discs are affected at the same time, it is no longer possible to clearly determine the beginning of the infection pathway, which is why the terms spondylodiscitis and spondylitis are often used synonymously. Pathogens can be bacteria (most commonly *Staphylococcus aureus*), fungi and rarely parasites.

■ Clinic

At the beginning there are often unspecific symptoms (subfebrile temperatures, night sweats, fatigue, unspecific back pain). Diagnostic clarification is often difficult at this time. A delayed diagnosis of about six months after the first appearance of the disease symptoms is to be expected. If the course is progressive, there may be load-dependent pain with concussion, tapping and pressure pain of the spine over the affected area. Fever is possible. Elevated inflammatory signs (CRP and ESR) and neurological deficits with compression of nerve roots and spinal cord by inflamed pannus are also possible signs.

■ Diagnostics

X-ray

In the early phase, skeletal changes are usually still absent. **Reduction in the height of an intervertebral space** and **increasing blurring of the adjacent base and top plates** are possible (◻ Fig. 20.13). In the further course, **destruction of the base and top plate of** the vertebral body, which increasingly scleroses in the healing stage.

CT (◻ Fig. 20.14)

Detailed recording of bony structures and their destruction. In the acute phase, **collapses of the vertebral bodies with moth-eaten appearance** on base and cover plates. In the course **sclerosis** with increase of bone density. The administration of a contrast medium makes it possible to distinguish abscesses in the spinal area, which also allows the simultaneous image-guided insertion of a drain.

MRI

Method of choice. Pathologies can be detected at an early stage with high soft tissue contrast and very good anatomical resolution, and their extent can be visualized.

The affected vertebral bodies and intervertebral discs show **edema** in STIR and T1. **Blurred end plates** are seen in T1. **Inflamed tissue clearly absorbs contrast medium** (◻ Fig. 20.15). In T2, there is iso- to hyperintense visualization of abscesses with **marginal contrast enhancement.**

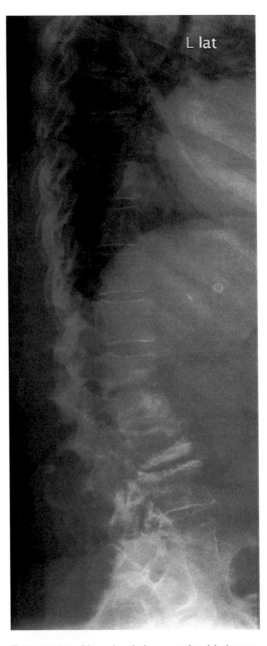

◻ **Fig. 20.13**   Blurred end plates, partly with destruction

Osteomyelitis/Osteitis

This is an infection of bone and bone marrow. The onset is in the bone by hematogenous pathogen seeding in primary osteomyelitis or as secondary osteomyelitis when soft tissue infections spread to the bone. The localization is often at the metaphysis of the long tubular bones.

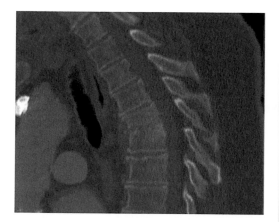

Fig. 20.14 Arrosion of the end plates BWK 5 and 6, height reduction BWK 5

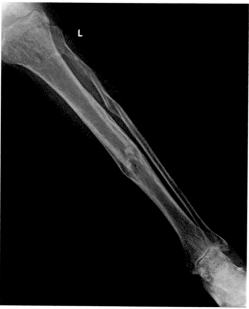

Fig. 20.16 Bone consolidated tibial fracture with chronic osteomyelitis in the tibia

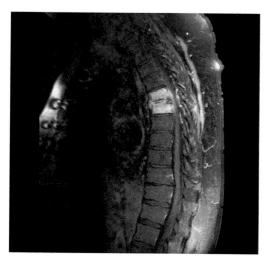

Fig. 20.15 T1-FS after KM, clear enhancement of the vertebral bodies and the associated intervertebral discs

■ Clinic

▬ **Acute osteomyelitis**: general symptoms (fever, chills, local pain). Local swelling, redness, hyperthermia. Elevated inflammatory parameters.

▬ **Chronic osteomyelitis**: frequently post-traumatic or postoperative. Redness, swelling, hyperthermia in the surgical area with disturbance of wound healing, pressure pain and restriction of movement. Elevated inflammatory parameters, fever.

■ Diagnostics

X-ray Image (■ Fig. 20.16)

The X-ray shows the following abnormalities:

▬ Bone destruction
▬ Unsharp-edged lesions
▬ Lamellar periosteal reaction
▬ Compacted soft tissues

On healing, new bone formation occurs, ranging from marginal to extensive sclerosis. In chronic osteomyelitis, the changes can only be assessed to a limited extent in the context of the surgical or traumatic changes.

Sonography

It is indicated in infancy and allows good visualization of soft tissue swelling. A **detachment of the periosteum** by a fluid fringe is seen, which may develop into an abscess in the course of time. Sonography allows visualization of cortical destruction. In adults, ultrasound diagnostics is limited to supplementary imaging of the soft tissues.

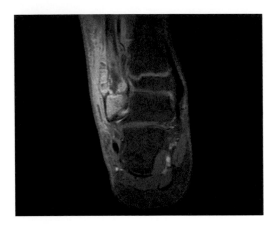

□ **Fig. 20.17** T1-FS after KM, marginal enhancement distal fibula, subperiosteal abscess

CT

This allows a detailed recording of bony destructions and sequestra.

MRI (□ Fig. 20.17)

In proton-weighted sequences with fat saturation, small, circumscribed, signal-rich lesions with hypointense presentation in T1 are often found. **Marginal edema** is always present. In T2 and STIR, there may be evidence of abscesses with marginal hypointensity and contrast uptake.

❯ Necrotic sequestra show no signal in T2 and STIR.

Rheumatoid Arthritis (RA)

▪ Definition

This is a systemic autoimmune disease affecting the synovium. In the course of the disease, destruction of the adjacent joints may occur. The incidence is 2% and the peak age at diagnosis is in the 4th to 5th decade of life.

▪ Clinic

Non-specific general symptoms occur before the first joint inflammation (prodromes: fatigue, weight loss, aching limbs). In the case of joint inflammation, acute swelling and pain of several joints as well as morning stiffness may occur, later joint malposition and subluxation. A laboratory-chemical detection of rheumatism factors is useful.

▪ Diagnostics

X-ray

There is symmetrical bilateral involvement, especially of the finger and toe joints with **soft tissue swelling, osteoporosis near the joint, transient joint space widening** due to joint effusion and **proliferation of the synovium,** later **joint space narrowing, erosions, subchondral cysts, ulnar deviation of the fingers, buttonhole and swan neck deformity of** the fingers. The final state is destruction of the joint with ankylosis.

CT

This is used to assess stability (e.g. in the case of cervical spine involvement) and for preoperative imaging.

MRI

Here, an infestation pattern as in conventional X-ray is shown. In fat-saturated T2 sequences bone marrow isointense signal changes correspond to potentially still reversible changes. Erosions in T1 hypointense. Signal enhancement in T2 in tendovaginitis. Contrast enhancement of synovium in synovitis.

Sonography

This allows detection of soft tissue swelling, joint effusion and tenosynovitis, visualization of erosions depending on the affected joint. Assessment of blood flow is also possible, as synovial hyperemia is an indicator of disease activity.

20.3.4 Degenerative Diseases

Herniated Discs

▪ Definition

This is a degeneration of the intervertebral disc with tears of the annulus fibrosus and protrusion of parts of the disc. In the case of dorsal, intraforaminal or lateral protrusion, depending on the extent, neural structures are affected. Mostly affected are L4/5 and L5/S1.

In terms of localization, a distinction is made between median, paramedian, intraforaminal and lateral disc herniations.

■ Clinic

Back pain, in case of affection of nerve roots dermatoma-related pain, loss of sensibility and paralysis, bladder and rectum weakness.

■ Diagnostics

X-ray

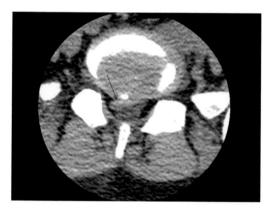

◘ Fig. 20.18 Right dorsoparamedian disc protrusion

Not indicated, as only the bony structures are imaged. However, it may indicate a different genesis of the symptoms, e.g. fracture with posterior edge involvement.

CT

This is reserved for patients in whom, for example, an MRI cannot be performed due to a pacemaker. The intervertebral disc presents as a soft-partisodense structure. Protrusions into the spinal canal or intraforaminal can be visualized (◘ Fig. 20.18).

MRI (◘ Fig. 20.19)

This is the method of choice and is usually performed in T2 hypointense annulus fibrosus with signal elevated nucleus pulposus; in the course of degeneration increasing hypointensity also of the biliary nucleus. A well-defined protrusion of the intervertebral disc with possible compression of the myelon or constriction of the neuroforaminae can be detected. Possible contact of the intervertebral disc with the nerve roots can be visualized. In the case of sequestration, disc tissue luxating cranially or caudally is shown with or without contact to the residual disc.

Arthrosis

■ Definition

This is a degenerative change in the joints that can occur increasingly over the course

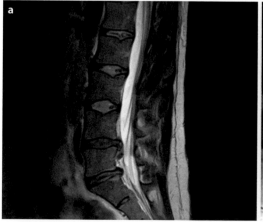
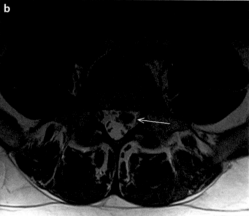

◘ Fig. 20.19 T2, left paramedian disc sequestrum folded over caudally

of a lifetime due to wear and tear. In younger years, it becomes manifest post-traumatically, especially with predisposing factors, e.g. hip dysplasia. Frequent localization is the knee and hip joint.

- Clinic

Pain, limited mobility, morning stiffness, worsening under load. Later also swelling and joint effusion. Ankylosis.

- Diagnostics

X-ray Image (◘ Fig. 20.20)

Important features include: **Joint space narrowing, subchondral sclerosis** of adjacent articular surfaces, **subchondral debris cysts, osteophytic marginal attachments, deformity** of articular components.

CT (◘ Fig. 20.21)

The features are similar to those seen on conventional radiographs (including visualization of free joint bodies).

MRI (◘ Fig. 20.22)

Cartilage and meniscus damage are clearly visible. There are **subchondral** oede-

matous **changes.** Reactive inflammations are conspicuous by enhancement after application of contrast medium.

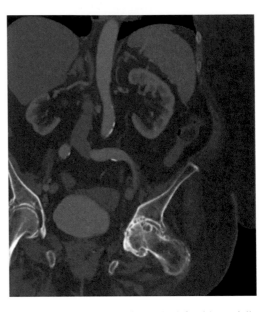

◘ **Fig. 20.21** Coxarthrosis on the left with partially abolished joint space and subchondral debris cysts

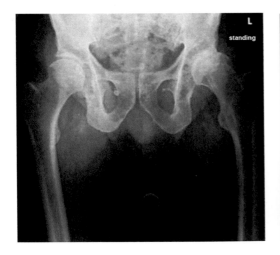

◘ **Fig. 20.20** Coxarthrosis on the left with already incipient deformation of the femoral head

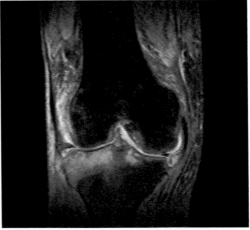

◘ **Fig. 20.22** Gonarthrosis with subchondral edema of the medial tibial head and inner meniscus lesions

20.3.5 Tumors and Tumor-like Lesions

In **benign bone tumors** and tumor-like lesions, the findings range from leave-me-alone lesions, which are usually incidental findings due to their asymptomatic nature, to lesions that require treatment due to symptoms or the occurrence of pathologic fractures.

Sarcomas are malignant tumors of the musculoskeletal system and occur rather rarely compared to carcinomas. A distinction is made between bone and soft tissue sarcomas.

Malignant bone tumors are rather rare overall. In adults, they account for 1% of all primary malignant bone tumors. In children, the figure is 5%. Osseous metastases of other tumors are significantly more frequent, but rarely occur before the age of 40.

Primary bone sarcomas arise in bone sections with particularly large growth. Risk factors may include Paget's disease or chronic osteomyelitis. Ionizing radiation after radiotherapy or prolonged diagnostic use can also induce bone sarcoma.

If a bone change is detected in the X-ray, the following criteria should be included in making a possible diagnosis:
- Type of lesion (osteolytic, osteoplastic, mixed, "moth-eaten", permeative)
- Border of the lesion (smooth, blurred)
- Changes in the cortical bone (thinning, destruction)
- Periosteal reaction (solid, Codman triangle, "onion skin", spicules, sunburst phenomenon)
- Codman Triangle
- Onion skin pattern
- Sunburst phenomenon
- Assessment of the matrix (bone, cartilage)
- Growth rate as an expression of aggressiveness
- Localization

Together with the patient's medical history and symptoms, an initial tentative diagnosis can be made and, if necessary, further examinations can be initiated.

Examples of Benign Tumors and Tumor-like Lesions
Juvenile Bone Cyst/Single Bone Cyst
- Definition

This is a benign cystic cavity formation which is mostly localized in the metaphysis of the long tubular bones. It belongs to the tumor-like lesions with an age peak between the 1st and 2nd decade of life.

- Clinic

It is an incidental finding as it is usually asymptomatic. In some cases, it may become conspicuous due to a pathological fracture.

- Diagnostics

X-ray Image (◘ Fig. 20.23)

The following features are conspicuous: **sharply edged lightening, centrally located, usually with sclerosis fringe, thinning of** the **cortex.** In the case of pathological fracture, fragments may fall into the bone cyst and "float" there ("Fallen Fragments", ◘ Fig. 20.23).

CT

CT is suitable for the determination of the density of the cyst contents and for the detection of fluid or unilocularity.

MRI

MRI is used to detect fluid in the lesion, which presents as signal-rich in T2. There is a marginal contrast enhancement.

❯ Differentiation from the aneurysmal bone cyst: This is multi-chambered as it is divided by septa. Due to blood in the cyst contents, fluid levels within the lesion occur because of the different density, which can best be detected with fat-saturated T2 sequences. Cortical destruction with soft tissue involvement may occur.

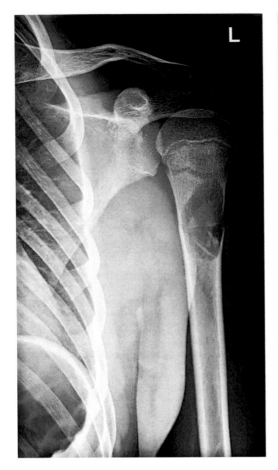

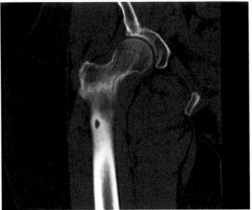

Fig. 20.24   Nidus in the proximal femur

Fig. 20.23   Pathological fracture in juvenile bone cyst, "Fallen Fragments" in the interior

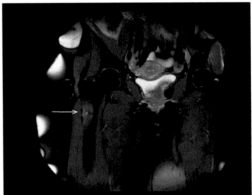

Fig. 20.25   T2-Spair, hyperintense nidus

Osteoid Osteoma

■ Definition

This is a benign osteogenic tumor of small size, often localized to the tibia and femur. The age peak is in the 1st to 3rd decade of life, the prevalence is 2–3% of all primary bone tumors.

■ Clinic

There is severe pain, especially at night, which responds very well to acetylsalicylic acid.

■ Diagnostics

X-ray

Within a sclerosis, a typical **central osteolysis**, the so-called **nidus**, is seen. Often an intracortical location is found.

CT

This is the method of choice with good visualization of the nidus even in conventionally radiologically not well visible areas. An early contrast image of the nidus is typical (**Fig. 20.24**).

MRI (**Fig. 20.25**)

The nidus presents with little signal in T1. The signal intensity in T2 varies depending on the extent of calcification.

Examples of Malignant Bone Tumors
Classic Osteosarcoma

- Definition

Osteosarcoma is a highly malignant, intramedullary tumor, which is mostly found on the metaphysis of the long tubular bones and is the most common malignant primary bone tumor with 40%. The peak age is between 15 and 25 years.

- Clinic

Increasing pain and swelling in the affected area.

- Diagnostics

X-ray

Osteosarcoma has a highly variable appearance, often **osteosclerotic** is found **next to osteolytic parts**, a **fuzzy border** and **periosteal involvement** with formation of **spicules. Codman triangle**.

CT

The characteristics are similar, but a **better differentiation between tumor mass and reactive changes** is possible.

MRI

Signaling is dependent on the degree of sclerosis. Information about **intramedullary spread, skip metastases, soft tissue and joint involvement** is possible.

Chondrosarcoma

- Definition

Chondrosarcoma is a malignant cartilage tumor and with 20% the second most frequent malignant primary bone tumor. Frequent localization is the pelvis and femur. The age peak is found in the 6th decade of life.

- Clinic

Pain and swelling that increase over weeks and months.

- Diagnostics

X-ray

There is **circumscribed osteolysis with destruction of the cortical bone**, the margins may be sharp or blurred. An accompanying periosteal reaction is possible. In about 50% irregular spotty calcifications occur.

CT (◻ Fig. 20.26)

The presentation is similar, but distension and destruction of the bone can be shown better.

MRI (◻ Fig. 20.27)

MRI allows good visualization of the cartilage cap and soft tissue component.

Osseous Metastases

- Definition

Osseous metastases are the most common secondary bone tumors caused by the spread of other tumors to the bones, e.g. breast carcinoma, prostate carcinoma, bronchial carcinoma. They can occur in all bones, but the preferred site is the axial skeleton. Osseous metastases rarely occur in the first three decades of life.

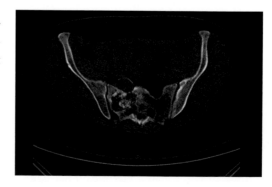

◻ **Fig. 20.26** Chondrosarcoma of the right lateral massa with marked destruction, presacral margin calcified soft tissue component

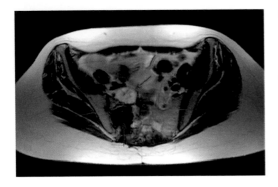

◻ Fig. 20.27 Bone cement inserted into chondrosarcoma of right lateral massa with signal effacement, presacral hyperintense soft tissue component

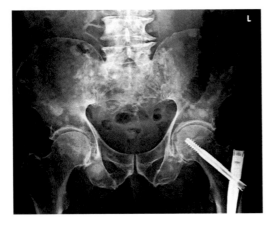

◻ Fig. 20.28 Diffuse osteoplastic metastasis of a prostate carcinoma

- Clinic

Dull pain. General symptoms in the context of the tumor disease (weight loss, fatigue). Can be noticeable due to pathological fracture.

- Diagnostics

X-ray Image (◻ Fig. 20.28)
- Osteolytic metastases (bronchial, renal, thyroid carcinoma): **circumscribed lighteningwithout marginal sclerosis, arrosion of** the cortical bone with possible spread into the adjacent soft tissues.

- Osteoblastic metastases (prostate, breast carcinoma): **fuzzy-edged compression of** the bone, can be small and patchy, but can also affect the whole bone.
- Mixed osteolytic-osteoblastic metastases (breast, prostate, bronchial carcinoma): **coexisting osteolytic and osteoblastic foci** that may confluence.CT

The image is similar, but clearly superior to the conventional X-ray image in detection.
  MRI (◻ Fig. 20.29)
Osseous metastases show low signal in T1, high signal in T2 with fat saturation as well as STIR. They show contrast enhancement.

20.3.6 Congenital Disorders of the Skeletal System

Congenital Hip Dysplasia

- Definition

This is a congenital developmental disorder of the acetabulum and the most common congenital skeletal maldevelopment. Girls are affected six times more often. In 1/4 of cases there is a bilateral manifestation. In the absence of treatment, dislocation of the femoral head with subluxation to luxation occurs.

- Clinic

Asymmetry of the gluteal folds, abduction inhibition, leg length discrepancy. Positive Ortolani test.

- Diagnostics

Sonography
  This is performed as part of the U3 examination, and often also as part of the U2 examination in children, and is used to visualize the cartilaginous preformed femoral head, cartilaginous acetabular notch

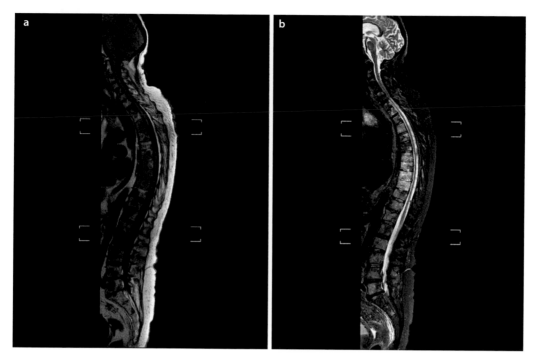

◘ Fig. 20.29 **a** T2, diffuse osseous metastasis, hypointense changes. **b** T1-FS after KM administration, enhancement of osseous metastases

with labrum acetabulare, and bony and cartilaginous acetabular roof in defined sectional planes. Sonography can be used to visualize the bony shape of the acetabulum and acetabular notch as well as the overlap of the femoral head by the cartilaginous acetabular roof. The classification is according to Graf.

X-ray

The procedure is performed from the 9th month of life with measurement of the hip with regard to the acetabular roof geometry and the centring of the femoral head in the acetabulum and determination of the acetabular roof angle according to Hilgenreiner (AC angle). This becomes smaller with increasing ossification of the acetabulum.

MRI

MRI is used for preoperative planning in therapy-resistant hip dysplasia. Obstacles to reduction can be detected. A femoral head necrosis can be excluded after forced reduction.

Congenital Foot Deformities

- Definition

This is a congenital deformity of the feet with malposition of the bones and typical changes in the arches of the feet. With a prevalence of 0.1%, clubfoot is the most common congenital foot deformity and the second most common congenital skeletal deformity after hip dysplasia. Early diagnosis and initiation of treatment are crucial for prognosis.

- Clinic

Usually at birth there are already visible deformities of the foot.

For example:

- Clubfoot (Pes equinovarus): complex foot deformity with pointed foot, varus position of the heel, sickle foot with inward rotation of the metatarsus and hollow foot.
- Flatfoot (talus verticalis): Malformation with a vertically standing talus and luxa-

tion of the os naviculare to the cranial side.

— Other examples are sickle foot (Pes adductus), hollow foot (Pes excavatus), heel foot (Pes calcaneus) and pointed foot (Pes equinus).

■ Diagnostics

X-ray

It is used to evaluate the axes and angles of the tarsal bones in the dorsoplantar and lateral rays.

MRI

Because the bone nuclei are still cartilaginous in infancy, MRI is **the method of choice** for visualizing the malposition in three planes.

CT

With advanced ossification of the foot skeleton, a good spatial view of the extent of the deformity can be obtained with 3D reconstruction.

20.3.7 Diseases of the Infantile Skeleton

Perthes' Disease/ Legg-Calvé-Perthes' Disease

■ Definition

This is an idiopathic necrosis of the femoral head. The peak age is between the 4th and 8th year of life. Boys are affected four times more often than girls.

■ Clinic

Pain with claudication. Restricted movement of the affected hip.

■ Diagnostics

X-ray Image (■ Fig. 20.30)

Changes in the conventional radiograph depending on the stage.

Risk factors for an unfavorable course are the so-called "head-at-risk" signs:

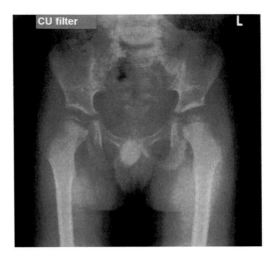

■ **Fig. 20.30** Perthes' disease on the right with flattened epiphysis

— Gage sign: Lightening at the lateral epiphysis and the adjacent metaphysis in the form of a recumbent "V"
— Calcification lateral to the epiphysis
— Diffuse metaphyseal reaction: either in the form of ligamentous lightening close to the joint or in the form of cystic defects
— Lateral subluxation
— Horizontal epiphyseal fissure.

Sonography

It is used to detect the joint effusion.

MRI (■ Fig. 20.31)

In the initial stage, MRI can detect the disease by bone marrow edema in the pineal gland with still inconspicuous X-ray findings. There is a drop in signal from the epiphysis in T1. Signal irregularities of the cartilage, possibly also cartilage thickening, an effusion and inflammation of the synovia can be detected. Incipient femoral head deformities can be delineated.

Epiphysiolysis Capitis Femoris

■ Definition

The epiphysis of the femoral head loosens and slips, usually in a medio-dorso-caudal

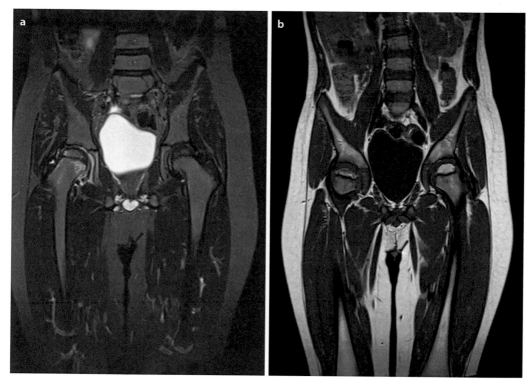

◘ Fig. 20.31 **a** STIR, Perthes' disease with edema in epiphysis and metaphysis. **b** In lateral comparison, clearly flattened and hypointense epiphysis on the right

direction. The peak age is between the 10th and 15th year of life. Boys are more frequently affected than girls. Bilateral involvement occurs in about 50%. Obesity predisposes to the disease.

■ Clinic

Painful restriction of movement. Limping. Restricted internal rotation.

■ Diagnostics

X-ray

It is recommended to take an a.p. and Lauenstein image (◘ Fig. 20.32). Anteriorposteriorly there is a **widening of** the **epiphyseal fossa**. The **epiphysis** appears **narrowed** by the dorsal tilt. A tangent applied to the superolateral femoral neck does not intersect the epiphysis. A good representation of the tilting of the epiphysis is possible in the Lauenstein image.

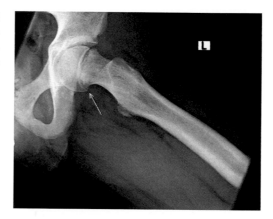

◘ Fig. 20.32 Lauenstein image, step formation between metaphysis and epiphysis with slipping of the epiphysis

Sonography

Here, the **step formation** between the femoral neck and the epiphysis is a sign of slippage.

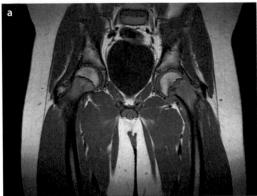
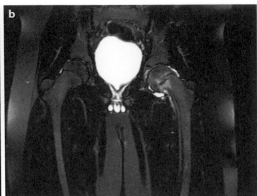

■ **Fig. 20.33** **a** Epiphysiolysis capitis femoris left with slippage of the epiphysis. **b** Lateral comparison of edema at epiphysis and metaphysis left and widened epiphyseal fossa

MRI (■ Fig. 20.33)

Here, an earlier image of the changes can be made than in the conventional X-ray image. MRI can be used in cases of clinical suspicion and inconspicuous X-ray findings. In T2, there is **signal enhancement and widening of the epiphyseal fossa**. Bone oedema may be detectable.

Coxitis Fugax

■ Definition

This is the so-called "hip rhinitis", a non-infectious inflammation of the hip joint that heals spontaneously. Coxitis fugax is often preceded by an infection of the respiratory tract or the gastrointestinal tract. The age peak is in the 3rd to 10th year of life.

■ Clinic

Schonhinken. Hip pain, often projected into the knee. Painful restriction of movement, especially internal rotation. Negative inflammatory parameters.

■ Diagnostics

Sonography

Here there is an **effusion of the joint**, the capsule is lifted from the bone.

X-ray

This can be done to exclude differential diagnoses, the symptoms are similar to Perthes disease and epiphysiolysis capitis femoris.

20.4 Diagnostics

20.4.1 Diagnostic Radiology Services

Sonography

Sonography represents the simplest option for the initial diagnosis of **muscular problems.** Increasingly, ultrasound is also used in **joint diagnostics.** Thus, a joint effusion can be easily detected sonographically. **Ligament structures** can also be viewed sonographically, at least in the first step. Ultrasound is used less frequently in fracture diagnosis, although sternal fractures or forearm fractures, for example, can be detected very well in pediatric patients.

Conventional X-ray Diagnostics

The basis of skeletal diagnostics is still conventional X-ray diagnostics. It can be used to detect **fractures.** The **healing process of** a fracture is assessed. Conventional diagnostics is also very well suited for diagnosing **luxations.**

Another important field of application is **functional diagnostics**, e.g. of the spine.

Conventional radiography is justified in soft tissue diagnostics for the **detection of foreign bodies.**

Fluoroscopy/Angiography

As a rule, fluoroscopic examinations of the skeletal system tend to be performed by orthopedic surgeons or trauma surgeons. This mainly involves intraoperative position checks and checks of osteosynthesis materials. In hospitals with a large spine or neurosurgery, however, **myelography** and **discography** are often performed as fluoroscopic examinations. Both examinations have their justification in the differential diagnosis of back complaints. Discography is nowadays mainly a provocation test. After puncture of the intervertebral disc via a fluoroscopically controlled dorsolateral approach, 1–2 mL of contrast medium is injected into the disc. The patient is asked whether the pain experienced is known and corresponds to that which now leads him to the doctor. In this case, the radiologist speaks of a positive discography, the affected disc contributes to the discomfort symptoms of the patient.

Myelography is used to detect spinal constrictions. Compared to MRI, which can of course also show a narrowing of the spinal canal very well, myelography has the advantage of functional diagnostics. Myelography can also be used to detect spinal canal stenoses that occur, for example, only when the lumbar spine is inclined.

Computed Tomography

Computed tomography is primarily used for the precise assessment of complex or conventionally questionable **fractures.** In the spine, computed tomography is used to accurately assess the posterior edge of the vertebral body, which is of central impor-

tance for stability in the event of a vertebral body fracture. CT diagnostics of intervertebral disc disease is only an exception in patients who are not amenable to an MRI examination.

Computed tomography of joints should, if possible, be performed in the neutral zero position, e.g. with the elbow extended. However, there are often limits here due to pain or also plaster casts.

In the context of fracture diagnostics, CT diagnostics plays an important role in the bony pelvis, since numerous fractures of the pelvis cannot be detected in conventional X-rays.

Plasmocytoma is a malignant disease of the bone marrow that can lead to multiple osteolysis throughout the skeleton. Until a few years ago, extensive conventional X-ray diagnostics, e.g. according to the Paris scheme, were performed for this disease. This included radiographs of the entire spine, pelvis, long bones, and skull. Despite these numerous images, a large number of the small osteolysis, often only 1–2 cm in size, could not be detected. Only the pathological fracture has often revealed the findings. Therefore, the primary diagnosis of plasmacytoma is nowadays performed by CT of the entire skeletal status.

Magnetic Resonance Imaging

Magnetic resonance imaging is the examination method of choice for the assessment of **intervertebral disc disease**. MRI also has the highest sensitivity in the detection of vertebral body metastases. The disadvantage compared to scintigraphy is the limited examination section and the lower availability.

In the diagnosis of ligament injuries and joint damage, MRI also shows the most accurate results. Another advantage of MRI is that medullary edema can be detected. This shows the involvement of the bone after a trauma, for example, even if there is no cortical interruption in the sense of a fracture.

In the case of primary bone tumors, an MRT examination is performed in addition to the indispensable conventional X-ray diagnosis.

20.4.2 Nuclear Medicine Diagnostics

Ursula Blum

Skeletal Scintigraphy

To prepare the ^{99m}Tc labeled bisphosphonates, the generator eluate is combined with an industrially prepared kit containing the inactive carrier and a reducing tin II salt in nitrogen inert gas atmosphere and freeze-dried form. To ensure reduction of the inert ^{99m}Tc O^{4-} into a reactive component, the generator eluate must be introduced into the kit under exclusion of air. The amount to be applied depends on age, weight and disease. The limit value is 500 MBq for benignity and 700 MBq for malignancy.

The labelled biphosphonates are taken up superficially into the hydroxyappatite matrix of the bone via osteoblast activity, depending on thickness, blood flow and bone remodeling.

Recording   The image is taken in the supine position, with the patient's arms lying next to the body and the legs symmetrically rotated inwards.

Assessment   Pelvis, WS and ileosacral joints accumulate physiologically increased as places of increased stress. Tubular bones absorb the activity more strongly than spongy bones.

Traumas   Fracture detection by skeletal scintigraphy is performed primarily in cases of occult fractures, unexplained complaints, child abuse, determination of fracture age, and detection of fatigue fractures.

❯ Only ten days after trauma are repair processes detectable by scintigraphy.

While a fresh fracture shows increased storage in the blood pool and mineralization phase, the activity enrichment of old events is only detectable in the mineralization. The positive finding should be confirmed by a control after four weeks.

Denture Loosening   3-phase skeletal scintigraphy can be used to assess the strength of an endoprosthesis and the resulting need for implant replacement. Cementless prostheses show band-like activity along the prosthesis shaft up to two years postoperatively, which is related to new bone formation on the prosthesis.

❯ Osteonecrosis
They show low storage in perfusion and blood pool, later with higher storage or normalized.

❯ Osteomyelistis
On 3-phase skeletal scintigraphy, osteomyelitis acute and chronic is notable for increased arterial perfusion, increased blood pool accumulation, and increased tracer uptake in the mineralization phase. The level of activity uptake gives an indication of the inflammatory activity of the process.

❯ Detection of Skeletal Metastases and Primary Bone Tumors
Because of its high sensitivity, the exclusion or detection of skeletal metastases is the most frequent indication for skeletal scintigraphy. Bone metastases in breast carcinoma, for example, can be detected six months before conventional radiological diagnosis, while those of prostate carcinoma can often be detected years earlier. 3-phase scintigraphy is also used for primary bone tumors (e.g. osteosarcoma).

◻ **Table 20.2**   Value of the diagnostic procedures

	Sonography	Conventional	CT	MRI	Nuk	PET
Fracture	N	P	W	W	W	N
Herniated Disc	N	N	N(*)	P	N	N
Ligament/Muscle Injuries	P	W	N	P	N	N
Metastases	N	N	W	W	P	W
Plasmacytoma	N	N	P	W	N	N
Primary Bone Tumor	N	P	W	P	W	W

N Not indicated, *P* Primary diagnosis, *W* Further diagnosis, * CT in contraindications for MRI

Inflammatory Scintigraphy of the Skeleton

Radioactively labeled anti-granulocyte antibodies or in vitro labeled autologous leukocytes can be used to detect bacterial inflammation after implantation of a joint prosthesis. They accumulate in the granulocytes and their precursors in the hematopoietic bone marrow. They are unsuitable in the trunk skeleton due to the physiological accumulations to be expected there.

[111]In or ^{99m}Tc-labelled leukocytes and ^{99m}Tc-labelled monoclonal anti-granulocyte antibodies are used to detect a granulocytic inflammatory reaction. Whole-body scintigraphy with non-specific antibodies is performed to clarify chronic inflammation, in chronic febrile episodes and to search for the fever-causing focus.

20.4.3 Valence

Christel Vockelmann

◻ Table 20.2 shows the use of the respective diagnostic options depending on the problem.

20.5 Therapy

20.5.1 Interventional Radiology

Mirja Wenker

Tumor Embolization

Osseous metastases of hypervascularized tumors lead to extensive blood loss during surgical therapy. To reduce these blood losses, such metastases are treated angiographically with particles and other embolization materials one to two days preoperatively. After superselective probing of the tumor-supplying vessels, embolization material is introduced until stasis in the vessel as evidence of vessel occlusion. A classic example of this is metastases of renal cell carcinoma.

Computed Tomography-Guided Bone Tumor Treatment

In particular, painful osseous metastases, regardless of the tumor entity, are nowadays approached interventional radiologically. There are two procedures: an injection of bone cement into lytic metastases or thermoablation, i.e. burning of the metastasis by

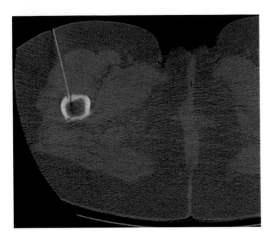

Fig. 20.34 Thermoablation of an osteoid osteoma, probe tip inserted into the nidus

electricity, which is also suitable for lytic or mixed osseous metastases.

Thermoablation is now the treatment of choice for osteoid osteoma (Fig. 20.34).

CT-guided therapies of osseous metastases can be used very well together with radiotherapeutic therapies and do not replace them as a rule. The advantage of CT-guided therapy is the very rapid reduction in pain symptoms.

Pain Management

Degenerative spinal diseases are one of the main reasons for sick leave in everyday working life.

In the case of diseases of the intervertebral discs with nerve root irritation or diseases of the facet joints, pain therapies controlled by computer tomography are used. A fine needle is inserted dorsally into the affected spinal segment and a local anesthetic and, if necessary, a corticosteroid are introduced into the facet joint, peripherally to the nerve root or epidurally under CT-controlled control. In recent years, however, there has been a decline in such interventions, especially in the outpatient sector, since health insurance companies and associations of panel doctors require a presentation to a pain therapist prior to therapy.

20.5.2 Nuclear Medicine

Ursula Blum

Radiosynoviorthesis (RSO)

RSO is an effective method for the local therapy of chronic joint inflammations. The aim is to remodel the connective tissue of the synovium. This is achieved with good results by injecting a radioisotope, which decays by emitting β^- radiation, into the joint space (e.g. ^{90}Y, ^{186}Re, ^{169}Er). The choice of radiopharmaceutical depends on the size of the joint. The smaller the joint, the shorter the range of the β^- radiopharmaceutical should be. The maximum/average range is 11 mm/3.6 mm for ^{90}Y, 3.7/1.2 mm for ^{186}Re, ^{169}Er 1.0 mm/0.3 mm.

The radiopharmaceutical is injected intraarticularly. At the same time, a cortisone preparation may be injected for transitional therapy.

Palliative Therapy of Bone Metastases

Osteoplastic metastases of prostate, breast or bronchial carcinoma can be treated palliatively with osteotropic radiopharmaceuticals if they do not respond to other available therapies. The goal of palliative bone pain therapy with short-range β^- radiotherapy is to improve the patient's quality of life or reduce pain medication. Nuclear bone pain therapy is contraindicated in cases of existing or impending spinal cord compression due to vertebral metastases or unstable fractures, existing bone marrow depression or renal insufficiency.

The following radiopharmaceuticals are applied via a venous catheter (Table 20.3).

The respective radiopharmaceutical is injected over one to 2 min, after which the venous catheter is flushed with 0.9% NaCl solution.

For radiopharmaceuticals containing a γ-component, a whole-body scintigram is obtained to document activity uptake six to 24 h after application.

◘ **Table 20.3** Venous catheter-applied radiopharmaceuticals

Radiopharmaceutical	Maximum Range	Medium Range	Physical Half-life	Amount of Activity to Be Applied
[89]Sr-Strontium chloride	6.7 mm	2.4 mm	50.5 days	1.5–2.2 MBq/kgKG
[153]Sm—HEDP	3.4 mm	0.6 mm	1.9 days	37 MBq/kgKG
[186]Re—HEDP	4.7 mm	1.1 mm	3.7 days	18.5 MBq/kgKG
[188]Re—HEDP	11 mm	2.7 mm	0.7 days	1295 MBq
[32]P	7.9 mm	3 mm	14.3 days	175–400 MBq
[117]Sn—DTPA	7 mm	2.4 mm	13.6 days	5–10 MBq/kgKG
[223]Ra—chloride	Few mm		11.4 days	50–100 kBq/kgKG

Blood counts are required every one to two weeks posttherapeutically for up to six weeks.

20.5.3 Radiotherapy

Guido Heilsberg

Soft Tissue Sarcomas

Soft tissue sarcomas are nowadays treated multimodally. Preoperative radiotherapy is given for very large tumors with a total dose of 50 Gy + boost treatment between six and 20 Gy, single dose at 2 Gy. The boost is usually irradiated percutaneously, but some clinics apply it during the operation (IORT intra operative radiotherapy), other clinics treat it with brachytherapy.

Storage is usually in a vacuum cushion.

Side effects: Skin reactions, fibrosis, lymphedema …

Bone Sarcomas

Chondrosarcomas are not chemosensitive. Chondrosarcomas and chordomas of the skull base are treated with protons or heavy ions.

Case Study

Benjamin is ten years old and a big fan of video games. He gave up playing football for it some time ago. Since then, he usually sits at home in the afternoon in front of the computer with a bag of chips (or two!). His left hip has been hurting him for a few days now, so he's been moving very carefully and hasn't participated in school sports either. When the pain doesn't improve, his father takes him to the doctor. The pediatrician, Dr. Menne, questions Benjamin in detail and examines the mobility in the hip joint. After the examination Dr. Menne suspects an epiphysiolysis capitis femoris. Because the complaints could also be from coxitis fugax or Pertes disease, Dr. Menne orders both a sonography of the hip joint and an x-ray of the left hip from the pediatric radiologist, Dr. Ass. The sonogram shows a small effusion in the left hip joint, which occurs in both coxitis fugax (also called hip flare) and epiphyseiolysis capitis femoris. The x-ray shows slippage of the epiphysis of the left femur, so Dr. Menne was right, it's not just the sniffles! Since epiphyseolysis capitis femoris can affect both hips, an X-ray of the right hip is also taken. Fortunately, this is not affected. Nevertheless, Benjamin has to be operated on, the left hip is stabilized with drill wires so that there is no risk of femoral head necrosis.

Practice Questions

1. Name safe and unsafe fracture signs! What should be considered when asking about fracture with regard to conventional X-ray diagnostics?
2. What criteria should be included in the assessment of a bone lesion?
3. What classification of herniated disc do you know?
4. What radiological interventional options do you know for musculo-skeletal diseases? Give examples.

Solutions ▶ Chap. 27

Cardiovascular Diseases

Mirja Wenker, Ursula Blum, and Christel Vockelmann

Contents

© Springer-Verlag GmbH Germany, part of Springer Nature 2023
M. Kahl-Scholz, C. Vockelmann (eds.), *Basic Knowledge Radiology*,
https://doi.org/10.1007/978-3-662-66351-6_21

21

Patients with cardiovascular diseases make up a large proportion of the patient population. At over 40%, they are one of the leading causes of death in Germany. In this chapter, the essential possibilities of radiological diagnostics and therapy of the heart and vessels will be presented. First, a brief overview of the anatomy is given. This is followed by a presentation of common diseases.

21.1 Anatomical Structures

Mirja Wenker

The heart and blood vessels together form the cardiovascular system. A distinction is made between a **large circulatory system** (systemic circulation: left ventricle—aorta—arteries—arterioles—venules—veins—v. cava—right atrium) and a **small circulatory system** (pulmonary circulation: right ventricle—pulmonary arteries—lungs—pulmonary veins—left atrium). The latter serves primarily to enrich the blood with oxygen and remove carbon dioxide.

The heart has the appearance of a three-sided pyramid with a base (basis cordis) and an apex (apex cordis). It is divided into the two atria (atrium sinistrum and dextrum) and ventricles (ventriculus sinistrum and dextrum) by the cardiac septa (septum interatriale, interventriculare and atrioventriculare). Blood flows through the mitral and aortic valves in the left heart and the tricuspid and pulmonary valves in the right heart.

The heart is covered by a network of vessels called the coronary arteries. The coronaries supply the myocardium with blood. The right coronary artery (A. koronaria dextra, RCA) runs across the posterior wall of the heart and supplies the wall of the right and left ventricle as well as the posterior section of the ventricular septum. The left coronary artery (A. coronaria sinistra)

divides into two branches, the R. interventricularis anterior (RIVA) and the R. circumflexus (RCX). The RIVA runs on the anterior surface of the heart and supplies the anterior wall of the right ventricle and the anterior and middle portions of the ventricular septum. The RCX runs on the left side towards the diaphragm and supplies the left atrium and the wall of the left ventricle.

Arteries are divided into those of the muscular and elastic type.

The veins have a narrower wall structure and are partially equipped with venous valves that prevent the backflow of blood.

21.2 Disease Patterns

Mirja Wenker

21.2.1 Heart

Acute Myocardial Infarction

- Clinic

Acute coronary artery occlusion leads to reduced perfusion of the dependent myocardium and, in the further course, to tissue destruction. Almost all cases are caused by arteriosclerotic changes. Acute myocardial infarction is fatal in about 1/3 of cases and remains the most common cause of death in industrialized nations.

Patients present with acute thoracic pain ("annihilation pain"), which may also move into the jaw and the left arm. In women, the symptoms may also be diffuse (nausea, malaise, etc.). Cold sweating and signs of heart failure are also symptoms.

- Diagnostics

X-ray

Conventional radiography often shows **no changes**. In extensive infarction, signs of **cardiac decompensation** with pulmonary venous congestion, pulmonary edema, and associated pleural effusions may be seen. Cardiomegaly may be seen.

Echography

Reduced ventricular function can be demonstrated with cardioechography. **Local wall motion abnormalities** are also seen. There may be evidence of thrombi.

CT

CT is used primarily to exclude other causes of acute chest pain. **Arteriosclerosis of** the coronary arteries can already be detected on normal chest CT. With coronary CT angiography, the coronary arteries can be examined in detail and stenoses can be detected. Thrombi and reduced perfusion in the affected myocardial area may be visible.

MRI

The cardiac MRI shows the **perfusion disturbance of** the infarcted myocardium in addition to the findings that can be delineated in the echography. A local edema provides a signal enhancement in the T2 weighting. The infarct area shows **delayed contrast enhancement** (◻ Fig. 21.1).

Angiography

Conventional coronary angiography is the method of choice for imaging the coronary vessels. In the course of the intervention, therapy can be performed directly by means of PTCA and, if necessary, stent implantation.

Cardiomyopathies

Cardiomyopathies are diseases of the heart muscle that are associated with a functional limitation of the heart. They lead to a thickening of the heart muscle and/or a dilatation of the heart cavities. The WHO distinguishes five forms of cardiomyopathy.

Dilated Cardiomyopathy (DCM)

■ Clinic

This is the most common form, there is dilatation of the left, sometimes also the right ventricle, the functional impairment appears as heart failure. In the primary form, the cause is unclear; in about one third of cases, there is a genetic predisposition.

■ Diagnostics

Echocardiography

The simplest and most cost-effective method of assessing the heart is echocardiography. It can quantify **impaired function** as well as **dilatation of** one or both ventricles.

Conventional X-ray/CT (◻ Fig. 21.2)

Conventional X-ray as well as CT often show only **global dilatation of** the heart. Depending on the stage of heart failure, pleural effusion may be present. Possibly a dilatation of the pulmonary vessels can be detected.

Cardio-MRI (◻ Fig. 21.3)

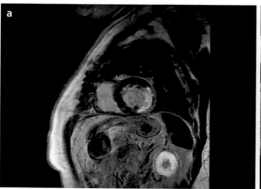
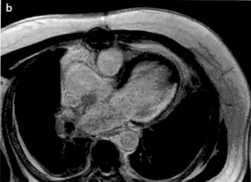

◻ **Fig. 21.1** **a, b** Posterior wall infarction with contrast image of the infarcted area

21

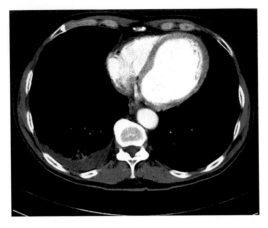

⬛ Fig. 21.2   DCM with dilated left ventricle

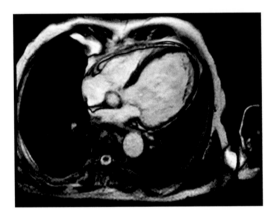

⬛ Fig. 21.3   DCM with dilated left ventricle

Cardiac MRI can most accurately depict cardiac **morphology** and **contrast behavior**. **Delayed contrast enhancement** results in patchy or striated focal KM images of the myocardium. In contrast to ischemic changes, these areas are localized subepicardially or intramurally.

Hypertrophic Cardiomyopathy (HCM)

- ■ Clinic

HCM is genetic, mostly autosomal dominant. There are structural changes in the contractile units. Hypertrophy of the myocardium is often asymmetric and may affect one or both

ventricles. If constriction of the left ventricular outflow tract occurs, this is called hypertrophic obstructive cardiomyopathy (HOCM).

- ■ Diagnostics

Echocardiography

Here, too, echocardiography is the first **tool of choice**. In addition to **myocardial hypertrophy**, impaired function can be demonstrated. The HOCM shows an anteior movement of the anterior mitral valve leaflet in systole, so-called SAM phenomenon ("systolic anterior motion").

Conventional X-ray

Conventional radiography may show a **raised left cardiac contour** as an indirect sign of hypertrophy. Only in advanced disease does an enlarged cardiac shadow and signs of heart failure become apparent.

Cardio-MRI (⬛ Fig. 21.4)

Cardiac MRI shows the same changes as echocardiography. In addition, a **delayed, non-segmental focal enhancement of** the myocardium is seen.

HCM with Hypertrophied Left Ventricular Myocardium

Synonym: Arrhythmogenic right ventricular cardiomyopathy (ARVC).

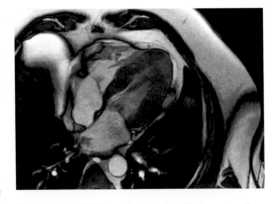

⬛ Fig. 21.4   HCM with hypertrophied myocardium of the left ventricle

- Clinic

This disease is defined by markedly reduced right ventricular function. The right ventricle is dilated and shows fatty or connective tissue remodeling of the myocardium.

- Diagnostics

Echocardiography

Echocardiography shows **dilatation of the right ventricle with thinning of the wall.** Due to the remodeling processes, individual wall sections may show A or dyskinesia, so-called microaneurysmata. The trabeculae show hypertrophy.

Cardio MRI

The cardio-MRI shows additional **fatty areas**, which appear hyperintense in the T1-weighting. These are localized subepicardially. Connective tissue dysplasias show a delayed enhancement after contrast medium application.

Restrictive Cardiomyopathy (RCM)

- Clinic

This is defined by diastolic dysfunction with normal systolic function. The ventricles are normal in size and the atria are dilated. High ventricular filling pressures occur due to endocardial fibrosis. RCM may be secondary to amyloidosis or sarcoidosis, for example, as part of storage or infiltration processes.

- Diagnostics

Echocardiography

Cardioechography demonstrates normal systolic and altered diastolic function. The ventricles are normal in size.

Conventional X-ray/CT

Conventional x-ray and CT show **enlargement of** the **atria** and signs of **pulmonary venous congestion** with accompanying pleural effusion.

Cardio MRI

Cardio-MRI is used in cases of suspected secondary cardiomyopathy. Here, depending on the underlying disease, an

altered signal behavior or an accumulation of contrast agent can be seen.

Unclassified Cardiomyopathies

These include isolated left ventricular non-compaction and Tako-Tsubo cardiomyopathy. These are also diagnosed mainly by echocardiography and cardiac MRI.

Myocarditis

- Clinic

Myocarditis is an inflammatory disease of the heart muscle. Viruses are the most common cause. The disease can be asymptomatic or mostly shows non-specific symptoms. Patients may present with cardiac arrhythmias, heart failure or cardiogenic shock, among other symptoms. Other cardiac diseases must therefore be excluded.

- Diagnostics

Conventional X-ray/CT

X-ray chest and CT are not infrequently unremarkable. In some cases there is a pericardial effusion. If the inflammation spreads to the lungs, pulmonary infiltrates and lymphadenopathy are seen.

Echocardiography

Echocardiography may also be unremarkable. If functional impairment occurs, diastolic and later systolic dysfunction is seen. In some cases, a pericardial effusion is seen. The myocardium may appear thickened.

Cardio MRI

The same findings as in echography can be detected in cardiac MRI. In addition, the affected areas show a T2 signal enhancement due to edematous and inflammatory-infiltrative changes. After contrast medium application an enhancement occurs.

Since there is no specific therapy so far, the treatment aims at symptom improvement. In most cases, the disease heals spontaneously. However, the disease can also lead to the development of DCM or even death.

Cardiac Tumor

Cardiac tumors are rare overall. They are benign in 75% (atrial myxoma, thrombi). 10% of all tumor patients have cardiac metastases.

Atrial Myxoma

Atrial myxoma is the most common primary tumor of the heart, accounting for approximately 50%. The often pedunculated tumor is benign and usually originates from the interatrial septum, but it can also be located at the heart valves. The majority are located in the left atrium, but in rare cases the right atrium may also be affected. The peak age is between 40 and 60 years.

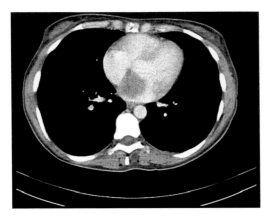

■ **Fig. 21.5**   Hypodense tumor in the left atrium

■ Clinic

Atrial myxomas can often remain asymptomatic and are frequently discovered as an incidental finding during echocardiography. If the tumor interferes with normal blood flow, symptoms range from arrhythmias and dyspnea to general symptoms such as fever and weight loss. Because thrombi may be superimposed on the atrial myxoma, washout can lead to peripheral emboli.

■ Diagnostics

Conventional X-ray

Conventional chest X-ray may show **dilatation of the affected atrium. Calcifications of** the tumor can be delineated. However, the findings are often unremarkable.

CT

On CT, the atrial myxoma is **inhomogeneous**. The tumor is mostly **hypodense** (■ Fig. 21.5) with partly cystic, necrotic or hemorrhagic parts. In a small percentage calcifications can be detected.

Echocardiography

On echocardiography the tumor may **appear broad-based** or pedunculated. It is usually **rich in echoes** and presents as **lobulated.** Thrombotic deposits may occur. A

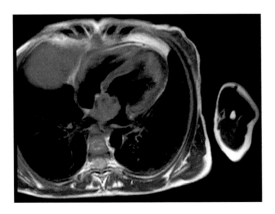

■ **Fig. 21.6**   Slightly inhomogeneous view of an atrial myxoma in the left atrium

location close to the valve may lead to valve insufficiency or obstruction.

Cardio-MRI (■ Fig. 21.6)

In addition to the CT and echocardiographic findings, the tumor shows **enhancement** on cardiac MRI. In T1-weighting it presents hypo- to isointense, in T2-weighting it mostly appears hyperintense.

> Contrast MRI is the important distinguishing feature from intraatrial thrombus.

Therapeutically, surgical excision and, if necessary, valve reconstruction are performed.

21.2.2 **Vessels**

Aortic Dissection

In aortic dissection, there is a proximal tear of the intima, allowing blood to enter the media. A second "false" lumen forms, which progresses distally and usually reconnects to the true lumen. The most frequent cause is arteriosclerosis.

■ Clinic

Aortic dissection presents as acute chest pain radiating to the back. Depending on the involvement of the aortic vascular outlets, neurological deficits, ischemia of the bowel and extremities, and, if the aortic valve is involved, aortic valve insufficiency may occur.

■ Diagnostics

CT Angiography

An aortic dissection can be depicted most quickly and best with CT angiography, as this also shows the outgoing vessels with the dependent organs well. The **aorta** is seen to be **dilated**. The dissection membrane can be easily demonstrated as a detachment of the intima from the vessel wall. Depending on the affected vessel section, aortic dissection is classified into three types according to DeBakey, simplified in the Stanford classification into two types.

The true lumen is usually smaller than the false lumen and shows a faster accumulation of contrast medium. If the false lumen includes vascular outlets, there is a reduced supply or complete lack of blood supply to the dependent organs with a threat of ischemia.

MR Angiography

MR angiography and **DSA** show the same changes as CT angiography, but are not the means of choice due to the fact that they are not available everywhere or take more time.

Stanford type A dissections require immediate replacement of the ascending

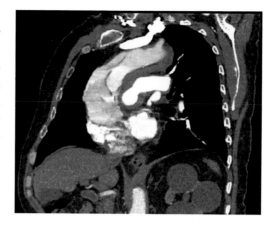

■ **Fig. 21.7** Aortic dissection with dissecting membrane in the ascending aorta

aorta and possibly also of the aortic valves. Stanford type B dissections are mostly treated endovascularly by means of an aortic prosthesis, but may also be treated conservatively in the absence of complications (■ Fig. 21.7).

Aortic Aneurysm

Aneurysms are localized bulges in the vessel wall of more than 50% of the normal vessel lumen. A distinction is made between three types of aneurysm.

1. In an **aneurysm verum,** all three layers of the vessel wall are affected. In the ascending aorta, an aneurysm is defined as having a width of more than 40 mm, and an abdominal aortic aneurysm is defined as having an infrarenal diameter of more than 30 mm. The main risk factor is aortic sclerosis. As the vessel becomes increasingly bulky, wall thinning occurs with the risk of rupture. Treatment is usually indicated when the vessel diameter exceeds 50 mm.

2. **Aneurysm dissecans**: see also Aortic **dissection** (section Aortic dissection).

3. In the case of a **spurium/falsum** aneurysm (false aneurysm), an injury to the intima and media results in a walled hematoma, whereby the adventitia remains intact. This can be caused by

21

blunt injuries or also by surgical interventions on the vessels (e.g. puncture in the course of an angiography).

■ Clinic

A large number of aneurysms are asymptomatic. They are often discovered as an incidental finding. Thoracic aneurysms can cause difficulty swallowing, hoarseness, coughing and difficulty breathing. An abdominal aortic aneurysm can cause abdominal pain, back pain, and urinary urgency. If it ruptures, there is a cutting pain.

■ Diagnostics

CT/MR Angiography (◘ Figs. 21.8 and 21.9)

CT and MR angiography show circumscribed or generalized **dilatation of the aorta**. Diameter and length can be well visualized on multiplanar reconstructions. Thrombosed portions and perfused lumen can be quantified. Involved arterial branches can be visualized.

Sonography

Sonography can be used for progress monitoring.

DSA

DSA is reserved for cases in which direct interventional treatment by stent graft is to

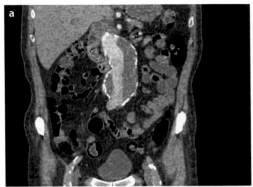
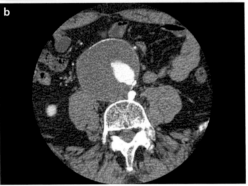

◘ **Fig. 21.9** a, b Aneurysm verum of the infrarenal aorta with markedly dilated lumen

be performed. Angiographically, only the perfused lumen can be visualized, not the extent of thrombosis.

Surgical or interventional treatment of an aortic aneurysm should be considered, depending on the location, when the aneurysm reaches a certain size or increases in size by more than 10 mm/year. A ruptured aortic aneurysm requires immediate treatment.

Traumatic Aortic Rupture

Traumatic aortic ruptures occur in the context of extreme shear forces. In most cases, the transition between the aortic arch and the descending aorta is affected.

■ Clinic

Complete ruptures lead immediately to death. In a covered rupture, bleeding is initially limited by the still intact adventitia.

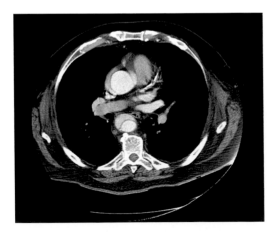

◘ **Fig. 21.8** Mural thrombosed aneurysm verum of the infrarenal aorta

■ Diagnostics

Conventional X-ray

Patients who have suffered a severe trauma (usually a traffic accident) are usually given a conventional chest X-ray in the shock room for initial assessment of potential injuries. On this image, a **widening of the mediastinum** due to hemorrhages can already be detected. The trachea shifts to the right, the left main bronchus to the caudal. Often a left-sided hematothorax is visible.

CT

The method of choice for the evaluation of a traumatic aortic rupture is CT, which is performed as a contrast-enhanced whole-body CT in the context of the trauma. Due to the capping of the rupture by the adventitia, a **pseudoaneurysm** forms at the rupture site. The contour may be very irregular due to wall hematomas. The detached portion of the vessel wall (flap) protrudes into the vessel lumen, it can be of varying thickness.

DSA

DSA should only be performed for endovascular therapy. Purely diagnostic DSA is not indicated.

A traumatic aortic rupture is treated with a stent graft or open surgery.

Acute Mesenteric Ischemia

Acute mesenteric ischemia is caused by occlusion of the arteries supplying the intestine, usually the superior mesenteric artery, or by thrombosis of the mesenteric vein. The non-occlusive form (NOMI) is due to reduced perfusion with reactive vasospasm. This leads to a circulatory disturbance of the corresponding intestinal segment with consecutive ischemia. Causes are e.g. cardiovascular diseases.

■ Clinic

Patients with acute mesenteric vessel occlusion initially present with severe cramping abdominal pain and possibly bloody diarrhea and symptoms of shock. In the latent stage, the pain symptoms subside, the so-called 'rotten peace'. In the late phase, the signs of irreparable intestinal ischemia from paralytic ileus to peritonitis and death become apparent.

■ Diagnostics

CT (◘ Figs. 21.10 and 21.11)

Acute mesenteric ischemia is an acute emergency and should be evaluated by CT as soon as possible. A contrast-enhanced examination with arterial as well as venous phase is recommended for the assessment of the arteries as well as the veins. The vessels can be assessed well and an occlusion can be directly visualized due to a **lack of contrast.** In addition, there is a **thickening of the intestinal wall** with accompanying distension.

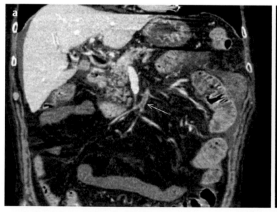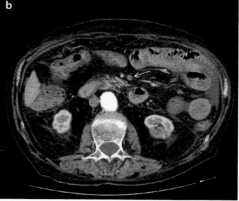

◘ **Fig. 21.10** **a, b** Acute mesenteric ischemia with thrombus in the superior mesenteric artery (arrows)

21

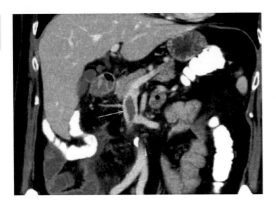

◻ Fig. 21.11 Mesenteric vein thrombosis with thrombus in the superior mesenteric vein (arrow)

The intestinal wall is **increasingly perfused**. Air pockets in the bowel wall (pneumatosis) also indicate bowel ischemia. In later stages free air in the abdomen or air in the portal vein system can be detected.

Doppler Sonography

Doppler/duplex ultrasonography may indicate vascular occlusion in the absence of signal, but imaging is often not possible in ileus.

MRI

The use of MRI is in principle possible for the clarification of mesenteric ischemia, but due to the time factor, CT should be given priority.

DSA

DSA should be performed if the CT results are inconclusive or if NOMI is suspected. Narrowed branches of the superior mesenteric artery as well as an **alternating image of vessel stenosis and dilatation** in the sense of a pearl cord-like pattern can be detected. **Delayed perfusion** also indicates reduced intestinal perfusion. At the same time, angiography can be used for therapeutic measures.

Interventional radiology may include aspiration embolectomy or intra-arterial lysis. An implanted stent can recanalize the affected artery. In the presence of NOMI, selective administration of vasodilators can be performed via a catheter. Mesenteric vein thrombosis can also be treated by local lysis. The irreversibly damaged parts of the intestine are resected surgically.

Peripheral Arterial Occlusive Disease (PAVD)

Disruption of arterial blood flow to the extremities is caused by plaque and calcium deposits with subsequent stenosis or occlusion of the vessel. In addition to smoking and diabetes, risk factors include disorders of lipid metabolism and hypertension. The risk increases with advancing age.

■ Clinic

Patients show the typical picture of intermittent claudication with load-dependent pain distal to the stenosis. In the advanced stage, pain at rest occurs, followed by necrosis or gangrene of the acras. The stages are classified according to Fontaine or Rutherford.

■ Diagnostics

CT Angiography (◻Fig. 21.12)

CT angiography shows both **calcifications** and **atheromatous plaques** along the iliac artery. In the lower leg, the arteries are often more difficult to assess because of their narrow diameter and decreased contrast compared with the iliac and femoral arteries. Collaterals indicate stenosis and occlusion. Multiplanar reconstructions and curved-planar reformations on which calcium is extracted should be performed for assessment. The disadvantage of CTA is metal artefacts, e.g. in the case of hip TEP, with consequently limited assessability of the vascular section running in this area.

MR Angiography

MR angiography after contrast agent application exclusively depicts the vessel lumen. Calcium is not depicted due to the lack of signal and is therefore more difficult to assess. As with CT angiography, the diagnostic quality of the arteries in the lower leg is limited. MIP reconstructions are used for

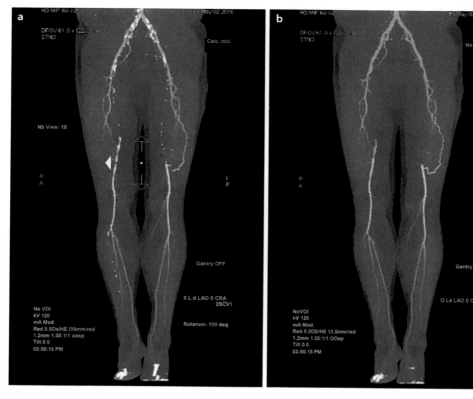

Fig. 21.12 **a** Long-stretch occlusion of the superficial femoral artery on both sides with pronounced collaterals, vessel reconstruction with lime. **b** Long-stretch occlusion of the superficial femoral artery on both sides with pronounced collaterals, vessel reconstruction after removal of the lime

better assessment. The advantage over CTA is the use of non-iodine contrast media and the lack of radiation exposure. However, the examination takes significantly more time and is more prone to motion artifacts.

DSA (▢ Fig. 21.13)

DSA also exclusively depicts the vessel lumen, calcium does not show up. Stenoses, occlusions and collaterals can be imaged well. By positioning the catheter tip in the superficial femoral artery, selective imaging of the arteries of the lower leg and foot can be performed. The advantage of DSA is a directly subsequent intervention.

Doppler Sonography

Doppler/duplex sonography can detect calcifications along the arteries. Within stenoses, there is flow acceleration with post-stenotic turbulence. The application is limited to the extremities, as the pelvic floor can often only be viewed to a limited extent due to intestinal gas overlays.

Interventional radiology can be used to perform lysis or thrombectomy for acute occlusion. In chronic disease progression, stent implantation can be performed in the pelvis and balloon angioplasty (PTA) with paclitaxel-coated balloons and, if necessary, subsequent stent implantation in the thigh. In the lower leg, PTA can recanalize the vessel in question.

Leriche Syndrome

Leriche syndrome is an occlusion of the infrarenal aorta with involvement of the aortic bifurcation. In chronic Leriche's syn-

21

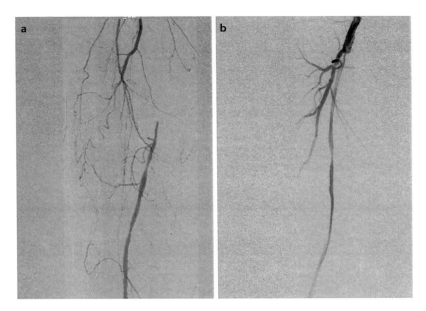

◘ Fig. 21.13 **a** Long-segment occlusion of the superficial femoral artery, collateral circulation. **b** Superficial femoral artery after PTA and stent implantation, recanalized lumen, collaterals no longer contrasted

drome, the occlusion develops slowly on the floor of pAVD, usually allowing strong collaterals to form to maintain perfusion of the lower extremity.

▪ Clinic

Patients present with intermittent claudication, sometimes with pain at rest, and bladder and rectal dysfunction and erectile dysfunction. Acute occlusion leads to the 6 P symptoms according to Pratt.
1. Pain
2. Pallor (pallor)
3. Pulselessness (loss of pulse)
4. Paresthesia (sensory disturbances)
5. Paralysis (inability to move)
6. Prostration (shock)

Acute occlusion is usually caused by an arterial embolic event.

▪ Diagnostics

CT/MR Angiography (◘ Fig. 21.14)

Acute Leriche syndrome represents a vascular surgical emergency and should be clarified as soon as possible by CT or MR angiography. The **occlusion of the infrarenal aorta including the aortic bifurcation and the iliac arteries** can be easily visualized. In chronic Leriche's syndrome, the usually pronounced collaterals supplying the periphery are also shown.

Doppler Sonography

Doppler/duplex ultrasonography reveals **aortic occlusion.** Collaterals can often only be depicted to a limited extent.

DSA

DSA can only be performed through an upper extremity access route. Depending on the placement of the catheter tip, collaterals and the distal outflow can be visualized.

Vascular surgery is indicated for therapy. In acute cases an embolectomy is performed. If this is unsuccessful or in chronic cases, an aortofemoral bypass (y-prosthesis) can be created.

Deep Vein Thrombosis of the Leg

This is a complete or incomplete occlusion of the deep leg veins, which can rise proximally to the pelvic floor. There is a risk of pulmonary embolism or post-thrombotic

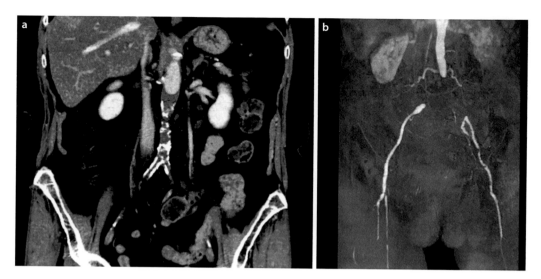

syndrome. Risk factors of thrombosis are insufficient exercise, e.g. after operations but also during longer air travel, coagulation disorders, smoking, taking certain medications.

■ Clinic

Patients report a feeling of heaviness in the legs, pain, increase in the circumference of the leg, redness of the affected limb. However, particularly in the case of thrombosis of the lower legs, the disease may also be silent. A pretest probability is first determined using the Wells test (■ Table 21.1).

Three or more points have a high pretest probability of deep vein thrombosis (75–85%), one to two points have a moderate probability (17–33%), and less than one point has a low probability (5–10%).

The D-dimers should also be checked. A lack of elevation and a medium to low pretest probability allow deep vein thrombosis to be ruled out by more than 95%.

Table 21.1 Wells score for suspected deep vein thrombosis

Malignancy active or <6 months	1
Paralysis, plaster	1
Bedridden (>3 days), surgery (<12 weeks)	1
Sensitivity along vein strand	1
Whole leg swollen	1
Calf circumference difference >3 cm	1
Impressible edema only on the symptomatic leg	1
Superficial collateral veins	1
Other diagnosis equally likely	−2

■ Diagnostics

Sonography (■ Fig. 21.15)

The method of choice for the imaging of a leg vein thrombosis is sonography.

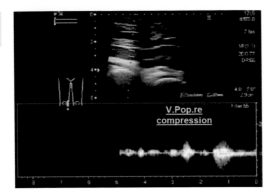

Fig. 21.15 Vena popliteal thrombosis, the vein cannot be compressed by the ultrasound probe

The **vessel lumen is clearly dilated** and the **vein cannot be compressed** due to the intraluminal thrombus. The thrombus may appear echo-poor to echo rich. A flow signal with respiratory modulability is absent.

Phlebography (■ Fig. 21.16)

Phlebography is often used in unclear cases or when the extremity cannot be seen (obesity, oedema, veins in the lower leg). Thrombi appear as **contrast medium cavities in** this case. Individual veins may also be completely non-contrasted or show collateral circulation.

CT/MRI (■ Fig. 21.17)

CT and MRI are mainly used to visualize the pelvic floor, which is otherwise often difficult to see. As in sonography, a **distension of the affected vein** is seen here, often with imbibition of the adjacent fatty tissue. In contrast to the perfused veins, the thrombosed vein shows a lack of contrast. Causative masses can be visualized.

Patients with DVT are initially treated with low-molecular-weight heparin, followed by secondary prophylaxis with vitamin K antagonists. Possible causes should be eliminated.

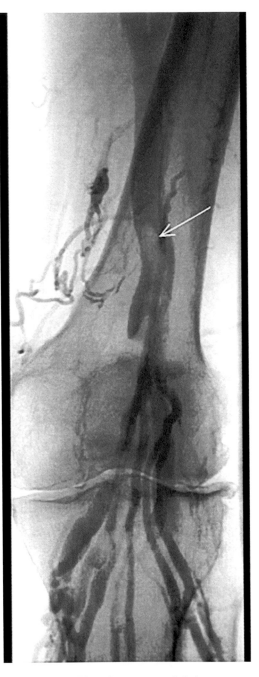

Fig. 21.16 Thrombus surrounded by contrast medium in the femoral vein (arrow)

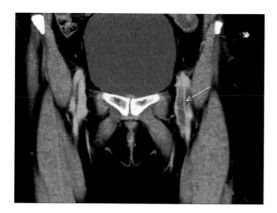

☐ **Fig. 21.17** Thrombus surrounded by contrast medium in the common femoral vein (arrow)

21.3 Diagnostics

Christel Vockelmann

21.3.1 Radiological Diagnosis

Sonography

Sonography is the basic building block in the diagnosis of the heart and blood vessels. In Germany, ultrasound examinations of the heart are performed almost exclusively by cardiologists. The same applies to the transesophageal echocardiogram (TEE). The ultrasound diagnosis of arteries and veins falls to radiology. This is carried out as color-coded duplex sonography in order to determine flow velocities. The degree of stenosis of the vessels can be derived from this. The assessment of the veins is supplemented by compression ultrasound. Since thrombus material cannot be compressed, a vein that cannot be compressed by the ultrasound probe can be diagnosed with thrombosis. Veins that can be freely compressed are not thrombosed.

Conventional X-ray Diagnostics

In the diagnosis of vascular diseases, conventional X-ray diagnostics has no significance. However, the X-ray thorax is still a basic examination for the assessment of the heart and cardiac output. This is supplemented by further examinations with ultrasound and especially MRI.

Fluoroscopy/Angiography

Phlebography as the basic diagnostic method for suspected leg or arm vein thrombosis has now been replaced by sonography. It is still performed for certain questions that cannot be answered by sonography alone or in the case of unclear sonographic findings.

Nowadays, diagnostic angiography has been increasingly displaced by sonography and cross-sectional imaging. Nevertheless, angiography is still considered the "gold standard" and is also used for diagnostic purposes, particularly in unclear cases. Due to the existing risk of bleeding when puncturing an artery, coagulation parameters (Quick/INR, PTT, platelets) should be checked before the procedure. As with any administration of contrast media, the renal retention parameters (creatinine, GFR) and the TSH value should be known.

Computed Tomography

Computed tomography is a very good method for non-invasive and rapid arterial and, to a limited extent, venous vascular diagnostics. The advantages of computed tomography compared to MRI are its availability everywhere and its rapid presentation, especially in emergencies.

A frequently performed examination is CT angiography of the iliac artery. The disadvantage of CT compared to DSA and MRI is that calcium plaques make it difficult to assess the vessels. They must first be extracted by further processing of the images. Nevertheless, CT angiography has its justification as a non-invasive procedure, especially with regard to the planning of interventional radiological interventions.

A newer field of investigation is CT coronary angiography, which can be performed in good quality with modern CT

21

equipment. Radiation exposure is comparable to diagnostic coronary angiography under optimal equipment and examination conditions. However, the examination is prone to artifacts. For example, an extrasystole can lead to the fact that the evaluation of the coronary vessels is not possible in the entire course of the examination.

Magnetic Resonance Imaging

Due to its high soft tissue contrast and the lack of radiation exposure, magnetic resonance imaging is suitable for vascular diagnostics. The vessels are made directly visible by the applied contrast medium. Due to the lack of signal, calcifications cannot be assessed.

In the context of cardiac diagnostics, MRI can detect findings that cannot be proven with any other imaging method. For example, in the case of myocarditis, intramural contrast enhancement in the myocardium can be detected, indicating scarring in the course of the inflammation. Cardiac muscle motion can be imaged more objectively and reproducibly than with ultrasound. The perfusion of the heart can be examined by means of stress MRI, which shows reduced perfusion of the heart muscle under stress.

21.3.2 Nuclear Medicine

Ursula Blum

SPECT Cardiac and PET Cardiac

Myocardial scintigraphy is primarily performed in patients with suspected stenosis of the arteries of the heart (coronary heart disease CHD) or if stenosis has already been detected.

Suitable SPECT tracers are **99mTc-Sestambi** and **99mTc-Tetrofosmin** (◻ Table 21.2). The previously used [201]thallium should only be used in exceptional cases due to the significantly higher radiation exposure.

In PET, **[18]F-FDG** (as a metabolic marker) is predominantly used. Rarely, ^{15}O-H$_2$O or [13]NH$_3$ are used as pure perfusion markers. In addition, lipid metabolism and sympathetic and parasympathetic innervation can be depicted with other markers.

The radiation emerging from the heart is weakened to varying degrees by the surrounding tissue. This attenuation can lead to an incorrect assessment of the blood flow conditions. There are several ways to mitigate these attenuation artifacts. Here, a change of position (examination in supine and prone position) or a low-dose CT in modern hybrid devices can be used. Another option for attenuation correction is the use of radioactive transmission sources. The use of a CT or transmission attenuation correction makes the examination more accurate, but increases the radiation exposure.

Usually, the examination is performed in two runs, once after **exercise** and once at **rest.** Both one-day and two-day protocols are used.

Exercise is either physical (bicycle ergometer, treadmill) or medicinal. Vasodilators (e.g. adenosine, regadenoson) or catecholamine derivatives (e.g. dobutamine) can be used for the medicinal stress.

The SPECT recording triggered by ECG is called **gated SPECT.** Gated SPECT allows statements to be made about the mobility of the left ventricle, and the following parameters are determined:
- End-diastolic volume EDV [mL]
- End systolic volume ESV [mL]
- Stroke volume [mL]: EDV—ESV
- Ejection fraction (LVEF) [%]: (stroke volume/EDV) * 100

In addition, statements can be made about the wall movement and the changes in the heart muscle in the individual parts.

Before a planned intervention on the coronary vessels, an assessment of the ben-

■ **Table 21.2** Cardiac SPECT with 99mTc-MIBI or -Tetrofosmin

Patient Preparation	Sober (at least 4 h) Discontinue medication if necessary – Ergometry: beta blockers, vasodilators – Medicinal: theophylline, dipyridamole; no caffeine, tea, chocolate (12–24 h before) Anamnesis Place and fix indwelling venous catheter Adjusting the ergometer to the patient Create ECG Measuring blood pressure and pulse Load according to the standard of the department
Activity:	One-day protocol: – 250 + 750 MBq 99mTc-MIBI or -Tetrofosmin Two-day protocol: – 400 MBq each 99mTc-MIBI or -Tetrofosmin
Application	i. v.
Acquisition:	Start of recording (15 min) 45–60 min p. i. Supine position, arms above head SPECT LEHR, 2- or 3-head, collimator tight adjustment 64 * 64 matrix, projections depending on camera system ECG-triggered
Evaluation	SPECT reconstruction: Filtered back projection or iterative reconstruction Reorientation along the heart axis Representation of the sectional views: – Short axis: From the tip of the heart to the base – Horizontal longitudinal axis: From bottom to top – Vertical longitudinal axis: From septum outwards EDV, ESV, LVEF, SSS, SRS Bulls eye view
Special Features:	In obese patients, adjustment of the dose if necessary
Radiation Exposure:	MIBI: 0.008 mSV/MBq Tetrofosmin: 0.007 mSv/MBq

efit should be made. Here, living (vital) or damaged (hibernating) tissue is distinguished from scarring changes. Only the function of vital or hibernating areas can be improved by the intervention.

The highest accuracy is provided by 18F-FDG-PET. Myocardial SPECT with 99mTc markers should be performed under special resting conditions (complete medication of the patient, in addition sublingual nitrate administration if necessary). Only very rarely is 201thallium used for this purpose, which allows vitality to be assessed 3–4 h p. i. (or 24 h p. i.) due to its reuptake into the heart muscle (redistribution).

Thallium protocols start a few minutes after exposure, in addition to a late exposure of 3–4 (possibly 24) hours.

Ergometric Load

Step test: Start with 25 (50)watts, increase every 1–2 min. Termination when target heart rate is reached or according to the termination criteria. After the injection, the load should be maintained for 1–2 min.

Target heart rate: 0.85 * (220 – age).

■ Termination Criteria

Absolute Termination Criteria

— ST-routes reduction >3 mm
— ST elevation >1 mm
— Blood pressure drop >10 mmHg with angina pectoris or ST depression
— Moderate to severe angina pectoris
— Severe respiratory distress
— Cyanosis
— Ventricular tachycardia >30 s
— Exhaustion of the patient
— Technical problems**Relative Termination Criteria**
— Elevated blood pressure (RR_{syst} > 230–260 mmHg, RR_{diast} > 115 mmHg)
— Blood pressure drop >10 mmHg without angina pectoris or ST depression
— Polymorphic extrasystoles, pairs (2 subsequent VES), volleys (>3 subsequent VES)
— Supraventricular tachycardia
— Bradyarrhythmia
— Occurrence of block patterns (AV block, thigh block)

■ Contraindications

Absolute Contraindications

— Acute coronary syndrome
— Unstable angina pectoris
— Symptomatic arrhythmias
— Decompensated heart failure
— Acute pulmonary embolism, myocarditis, pericarditis, aortic dissection

— **Relative Contraindications**
— Main stem stenosis
— Valve diseases
— Electrolyte disorders
— Arterial hypertension (RR_{syst} > 200 mmHg, RR_{diast} > 110 mmHg)
— Tachyarrhythmia, bradyarrhythmia
— Outflow tract obstruction, e.g. in hypertrophic cardiomyopathy
— Higher-grade AV block

— Left bundle branch block (if possible always pharmacological load)
— Physical and/or mental impairments
— Ventricular pacing rhythm

Pharmacological Exposure

Adenosine: 140 µg/kg/min i. v. via perfusor over (4-) 6 min, injection of the radiopharmaceutical after (3-) 5 min; allow adenosine to continue for at least 1 min afterwards. If necessary, combine with light ergometric exercise.

■ Contraindications

Absolute Contraindications

— Acute coronary syndrome
— Medium- to high-grade ventilatory dysfunction
— Bronchial asthma
— COPD requiring theophylline
— AV block II and III without pacemaker
— Sick sinus without pacemaker
— Low blood pressure (RR_{syst} < 90 mmHg)

Relative Contraindications
— Bradycardia (rate <40/min)
— Mild COPD
— Fresh cerebral infarction or fresh reduced blood flow

Regadenoson (Rapiscan®): Injection of 5 mL Rapiscan (=0.4 mg regadenoson) over 10 s, followed by 5 mL NaCl, after 10–20 s injection of the radiopharmaceutical. If necessary, combine with light stress.

Dobutamine: Infusion via a perfusor at 3-min intervals. Start with 5 µg/kg/min, increase to 10, 20, 30, 40 µg/kg/min until target heart rate is reached. If this is not reached, atropine is given (4 * 0.25 mg to max 1 mg i. v.). Injection 2 min before the end of the infusion, discontinuation criteria see ergometry.

Polar Tomograms

In the polar tomograms, the short-axis sections of the entire left ventricular myocardium are mapped onto a circle. This circle is divided into 17 (-20) segments.

This is followed by a semi-quantitative evaluation of the individual segments for both the stress test and the rest test (■ Table 21.3).

The normal collective should be created by yourself if possible.

■ **Table 21.3** Graduation of perfusion disturbance, modified according to guideline

Score	Perfusion		
	Description	Uptake in % of Maximum	Standard Deviation V. Normal Collective
	Normal	≥70%	<1.5
1	Slightly reduced	50–69	1.51–2.1
2	Moderately reduced	30–49	2.11–4.0
3	Significantly reduced	10–29	4.1–7
4	Missing	<10	>7

The Summed Stress Score (SSS) and the Summed Rest Score (SRS) are given. From this, the difference can be calculated, the **Summed Difference Score (SDS)**.

Especially on the basis of the SSS, an individual risk assessment for the respective patient is possible. The higher the SSS, the higher the risk of a cardiac event.

Especially on the basis of the SDS, an individual risk assessment for the respective patient is possible. The higher the SDS, the higher the risk of a cardiac event. The SDS is an aid in deciding, in the case of proven ischemia, whether the patient is more likely to benefit from drug therapy or intervention. With an SDS between 10–12, the patient is more likely to benefit from conservative therapy; with an SDS of 13 or higher, the patient is more likely to benefit from intervention.

21.3.3 Valence

Christel Vockelmann

(■ Table 21.4 shows the use of the respective therapeutic options depending on the problem.

■ **Table 21.4** Value of the therapeutic procedures

	Sonography	Conventional	Fluoroscopy/ Angiography	CT	MRI	Nuk	PET
TVT	P	N	W	N	N	N	N
Pulmonary embolism	N	N	N	P	N	W	N
pAVK	P	N	W	W	W	N	N
CHD	N	N	P	P*	W	W	N

N Not indicated, *P* Primary diagnosis, *W* Further diagnosis
P* Cardio-CT can be used as a primary procedure in certain risk constellations to exclude CHD. Another area of application is in the context of so-called triple rule-out diagnostics: This is used in patients who come to the clinic with very severe acute thoracic pain, in which the admitting physician cannot distinguish whether an aortic dissection, a fulminant pulmonary embolism or a myocardial infarction is present.

21.4 **Therapy**

Mirja Wenker

21.4.1 **Interventional Radiology**

Angiography

Angiography is an excellent procedure for the treatment of vascular diseases. This mostly involves vasodilator interventions. In the case of aneurysms or vascular injuries, however, vaso-occlusive measures are also taken.

Angiography is most often used for the treatment of peripheral arterial occlusive disease. Depending on the location of the stenosis, the puncture is performed antegrade or retrograde. The stenosis or vessel occlusion is probed with a wire and a catheter is advanced over the wire. After a contrast agent is administered to ensure that the catheter is back in the vessel lumen behind the occlusion, balloon dilatation or stent implantation is performed. In addition to these standard procedures, there are also newer methods such as atherectomy. This involves a catheter that peels and collects the plaque from inside the vessel so that the material can be removed along with the catheter. In the case of an acute arterial occlusion, a lysis catheter can be advanced into the thrombus. A thrombolytic agent is then applied via this catheter over a period of several hours.

> **Case Study**
>
> Mr. Topcak is 68 years old. When he retired, he got a dog. Lately, he has noticed pain in his right calf when walking the dog. These get better when he stops. In the meantime, however, he has to take a break every 100 m at the latest on his round with the dog. Therefore he turns to his family doctor. He suspects intermittent claudication because of the

symptoms. First, the family doctor examines Mr. Topcak and finds a missing foot pulse on the right side. He refers his patient to the angiologist. The latter determines with duplex sonography that Mr. Topcak has a short-segment occlusion of the distal superficial femoral artery on the right. The angiologist sends the patient to hospital for treatment. Here, an angiographic intervention is performed to recanalize the vessel and treat it with a drug-eluting balloon. Since the intervention, Mr. Topcak has been taking ASA 100 mg daily. In addition, the family doctor has improved his blood pressure and forbidden him to smoke. On the other hand, he is supposed to walk the dog extensively and thus exercise his vessels.

Practice Questions

1. What classifications of aortic dissection are you familiar with?
2. What is the procedure for suspected deep vein thrombosis?
3. What is the best procedure for imaging the aorta?
4. What interventional options are you aware of for treating lower extremity arterial occlusion?

Solutions Chap. 27

Endocrinological System

Martina Kahl-Scholz, Christel Vockelmann, Ursula Blum and Guido Heilsberg

Contents

This chapter deals with the essential possibilities of radiological diagnostics, nuclear medicine and radiotherapy for the diagnosis and therapy of the endocrinological system. An introductory section gives a brief overview of anatomy and function, and a concluding part contains some case studies from practice.

22.1 Anatomical Structures

Martina Kahl-Scholz

■ Thyroid Gland (Glandula Thyroidea)

The thyroid gland consists of two lobes (**lobus dexter et sinsister**), which are connected by a narrow connection (**isthmus glandulae thyroidea**). The isthmus is located at about the level of the 2nd-4th tracheal cartilage. A healthy thyroid gland weighs about 15–20 g in an adult.

■ Parathyroid Gland (Glandulae Parathyroidea)

The parathyroid glands are about the size of a lentil and are dorsally attached to the thyroid lobes.

■ Adrenal Glands (Suprarenal Gland)

The adrenal glands lie on the upper poles of the kidneys and are about 5 cm long, 3 cm wide and 1 cm thick. They are triangular or crescent-shaped and are also divided into cortex and medulla.

22.2 Disease Patterns

Martina Kahl-Scholz

22.2.1 Thyroid Goiter

Goiter describes an enlargement of the thyroid gland, which can be divided clinically into different degrees:

- Grade I: palpable goiter (Ia = not visible even with reclined neck; Ib = only visible with reclined neck)

- Grade II: visible enlargement with normal head posture
- Grade III: massive enlargement with compression and congestion

■ Clinic

The clinic depends on the size and the underlying disease (metabolic state).

■ Diagnostics

Sonography

Here, autonomous adenomas can be seen as **nodules of varying echogenicity** (■ Fig. 22.1).

Conventional X-ray

Conventional X-ray is of no value in this case, but a goiter may be detected on the basis of a different question (■ Fig. 22.2).

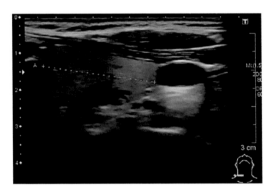

■ **Fig. 22.1**   Large struma node on the right in the B-scan

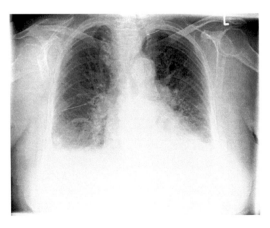

■ **Fig. 22.2**   Trachea displaced to the right (arrow) with left retrosternal dipping goiter with widening of the upper mediastinum

❯ X-ray contrast media should be avoided, especially in the case of hyperthyroid goiter, since the iodine contained in them can exacerbate hyperthyroidism and lead to a thyrotoxic crisis.

22.2.2 Thyroid Carcinoma

There is a subdivision into:
- Differentiated carcinoma (papillary thyroid carcinoma, follicular thyroid carcinoma)
- Undifferentiated carcinoma (anaplastic thyroid carcinoma)
- C-cell carcinoma

■ Clinic

Larger carcinomas may cause hoarseness, difficulty swallowing and difficulty breathing (in- and expiratory stridor). If a goiter grows rapidly in size and does not move the swallow, one should think of a carcinoma.

■ Diagnostics

Sonography

In sonography, above all an irregular, possibly destructive tumor structure should suggest a carcinoma. Furthermore, a fine needle aspiration or a punch biopsy can show whether malignant cells are present.

CT/MRI

CT and MRI are used for precise diagnosis of tumor extension, staging and follow-up if the suspicion is confirmed. Malignancy can only be detected in both procedures by means of the tumor growth crossing the organ; there are no other criteria for malignancy of a struma node.

Scintigraphy

Scintigraphy is the tool of choice for differential diagnosis.

❯ Here too: no administration of iodine-containing contrast medium. Various scintigraphic examinations to detect

metastasis can otherwise no longer be performed and radioiodine therapy is no longer possible for a period of two to three months after administration of a contrast medium.

22.2.3 Adrenal Adenoma

These are benign tumors that are usually hormonally inactive.

■ Clinic

Usually no symptoms.

■ Diagnostics

CT

On CT, adenomas appear **hypodense** and **absorb contrast.** However, differentiation from carcinoma is difficult.

MRI

On MRI, adenomas are **usually not very signal-intense** on T2 images, whereas **carcinomas** present **hyperintensely.**

22.2.4 Adrenocortical Carcinoma

■ Clinic

Carcinomas of the adrenal gland are usually clinically silent at first. In later stages, they may become conspicuous by infiltrating the neighboring organs.

■ Diagnostics

Sonography

There is an **inhomogeneous mass** which contains **echo-poor and echo rich parts.**

CT

There is a **strong contrast enhancement in** the tumor itself. Furthermore, the extension and destruction of other organ parts can be better assessed.

MRI

Since adrenal carcinomas have a **low fat content**, they present with a **high signal.**

22.2.5   Pituitary Adenoma

Adenomas of the pituitary gland are divided according to size into:
- Microadenomas (<10 mm) and
- Macroadenomas (>10 mm).

■ Clinic

About ¼ of the adenomas are hormone-active and can cause corresponding symptoms depending on the hormone produced. If the adenoma bleeds into the pituitary gland, headaches and visual disturbances may occur.

■ Diagnostics

Conventional X-ray

Here, a double contour of the sella and a displacement of the sella floor towards the caudal as well as destructions of the bony structures may be visible.

MRI

The tool of choice is MRI (◘ Fig. 22.3). **Indirect signs of** a mass (which could also be detected on CT) include:
- Impression of the Sella floor
- Elevation of the diaphragm sellae
- Pituitary stalk translocation

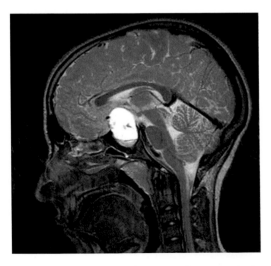

◘ **Fig. 22.3** Hemorrhagic macroadenoma of the pituitary gland in a sagittal T2 TSE sequence. Note the level at the base of the mass as a relative clear indication of hemorrhage

Classical for adenomas is that they accumulate **less contrast medium** than the rest of the pituitary tissue and show a **reduced washout effect** (on late images a higher intensity is shown, because the once absorbed KM is only slowly "washed out" again).

22.3   Diagnostics

22.3.1   Diagnostic Radiology

Christel Vockelmann

Sonography

Sonographically, the adrenal glands and thyroid are amenable to ultrasonography (◘ Fig. 22.1). During abdominal ultrasonography, the kidneys are positioned. Attention is paid to whether a mass can be demarcated at the upper pole of the kidney. Normal-sized adrenal glands cannot usually be visualized percutaneously by sonography.

The thyroid gland can be excellently assessed sonographically. The main focus here is on nodules. Cysts of the thyroid gland are also common, but are not hormone-active. Sonography is often performed in addition to thyroid scintigraphy in nuclear medicine. The purpose here is to differentiate cold nodules on scintigraphy, which may correspond to either a cyst or a mostly echo-deficient nodule. These cold, non-cystic nodules should then be histologically clarified, as thyroid carcinomas can be hidden underneath.

Conventional X-ray Diagnostics

Endocrinological diseases have no place in conventional X-ray diagnostics. Sometimes, however, a goiter can be seen on a conventional X-ray (◘ Fig. 22.2). This is when the thyroid gland is markedly enlarged and dips into the upper mediastinum. Then there is a tracheal shift to one side or even a compression of the trachea, in the worst case a so-called tracheomalacia. In this disease, the cartilage clasps of the trachea are softened so that the trachea can collapse. This becomes audible mainly through an inspiratory stridor.

Fluoroscopy/Angiography

In certain diseases of the adrenal glands, e.g. Conn's syndrome, it is necessary to take blood from the adrenal veins in a side-separated manner before surgical therapy for adrenal enlargement. This ensures that the affected adrenal gland is also responsible for the excessive production of the hormone aldosterone.

For selective venous blood sampling, a diagnostic catheter is advanced into the vena cava via the femoral vein. The right adrenal vein opens directly into the vena cava, the left one opens into the left renal vein, via which the adrenal vein is then probed. Blood is drawn selectively from both sides to then determine the aldosterone level in both samples.

Computer Tomography

Computed tomography can delineate adrenal space lesions very well. The assessment of the dignity is also successful in most cases. However, just like magnetic resonance imaging, computed tomography cannot contribute to hormone activity. Dignity can be proven by detecting fat in an adrenal mass. For this purpose, a native examination of the adrenal glands is sufficient in the first step. If the density of an adrenal mass is less than 15 HU, an adenoma is present. A dynamic CT scan with coils venous and after 10 min can be performed if the native coil detects a mass with a greater density. If the adrenal mass has a density of less than 37 HU venously and the contrast medium washes out by more than 50% in the late image, an adenoma is also present. In another constellation, at least a malignant tumor may be present. However, since nodular masses in the adrenal glands very often occur without clinical relevance, all findings with a size <3 cm are referred to as incidentalomas— i.e. incidental findings—provided that no underlying malignant disease is known in the patient.

The thyroid gland as another organ of the endocrinological system is often imaged in computed tomography. However, just as with magnetic resonance imaging, only a statement about the presence of nodes or cysts is possible. A malignancy can only be proven in the case of tumor growth that extends beyond the organ. Contrast enhancement is not indicative of this.

Magnetic Resonance Imaging

As with a computed tomographic examination, adrenal space findings can also be detected very well by means of magnetic resonance imaging. The advantage of the adrenal gland is that it is embedded in the retroperitoneal adipose tissue and can therefore be very well delineated in non-fat-saturated sequences. Actually, one sequence is also sufficient for the question of an adrenal space requirement. The question of fat content can be answered at the same time if a T1 in- and opposed phase sequence is acquired. If the adrenal space requirement shows a significant signal drop in the opposed phase, the evidence for fat is provided. Thus, an adenoma and no metastasis is present. However, magnetic resonance imaging cannot provide any information on hormone activity. More frequently, an MR examination is performed to clarify hypertension. MR angiography of the renal arteries is performed. It is always a good idea to include an axial planning sequence over the adrenal glands. Then the potential question of an adrenal space requirement, which arises in the next step, is answered at the same time and the patient does not have to be examined again.

Magnetic resonance imaging is a very good way to examine another organ of the endocrinological system: the pituitary gland. Here, not only macroadenomas, which could also be delineated on CT, can be detected, but also microadenomas. However, this requires an adaptation of the examination to the question "pituitary adenoma", a routine cranial MRI does not help.

The basis for the diagnosis of (hormone-active) microadenomas is the different contrast medium uptake of pituitary tissue and adenoma. The pituitary accumulates contrast agent rapidly and strongly, adenomas delayed. So we need a dynamic measurement over the pituitary. Coronary slices have proven best for this. Since the pituitary gland accumulates so much, the examination should be measured with a reduced contrast medium dose (50%).

22.3.2 Nuclear Medicine

Ursula Blum

Thyroid Scintigraphy

Thyroid function is scintigraphically depicted predominantly with ^{99m}Tc-pertechnetate. Classic indications are palpable or sonographically detectable nodular changes >10 mm, clarification of latent or manifest hyperthyroidism (focal/disseminated autonomy), unclear differentiation of an autoimmune thyreopathy or a Marine-Lenhardt syndrome, or as a therapy control after radioiodine therapy (less frequently after surgery). One domain of ^{123}I scintigraphy is the visualization of ectopic thyroid tissue (base of tongue, intrathoracic, struma ovarii), or if necessary in the case of connatal hypothyroidism.

^{99m}Tc-pertechnetate is taken up via the sodium-iodide symporter in the thyrocytes, but is not metabolized. After approx. 15 min a so-called steady-state (equilibrium of uptake and release) is reached. Iodine isotopes (^{131}sodium iodide and ^{123}sodium iodide), on the other hand, are actively transported into the thyroid tissue, bound to thyroglobulin and incorporated into the T3/T4 hormones. In routine diagnostics, the ^{99m}Tc-pertechnetate has become established. It is available as a generator product at any time, is a pure gamma emitter with a short half-life (sixhours) and is not bound in the thyroid gland. This results in a low radiation exposure of 0.01 mSv/MBq for adults (reference activity 70 MBq). For ^{123}I, the effective dose is 0.2 mSv/MBq (reference activity 10 MBq).

Saturation of the thyroid gland with non-radioactive iodine, e.g. after an examination with iodine-containing contrast media 6–8 weeks before the diagnosis, iodine-containing medications (especially amiodarone, iodine-containing eye drops) or extremely iodine-containing food interfere with thyroid scintigraphy. A correspondingly long waiting period should be taken into account. Thyroid therapeutics can also alter a scintigraphy and should be discontinued as long as possible beforehand, depending on the problem.

Fifteen to 20 min after application of 70 MBq ^{99m}Tc, the metabolic distribution pattern is recorded with a thyroid special collimator or a high-resolution low-energy collimator (LEHR collimator). To determine the position of the thyroid gland, a radioactive point source is used to mark the jugulum (and clavicle and palpable nodes if necessary) in the same position. To determine the technetium-thyroidal uptake (TcTU), so-called regions of interest (ROI's) are placed around the thyroid gland, in an underground region and, if necessary, around focal multiple accumulations.

$$\frac{SD\,impulse - UG\,impulse}{Netto\,Activity}$$

The percentage uptake of the injected activity depends on the iodine supply. With sufficient iodine supply in Germany, a TcTU with a normal TSH up to a maximum of 2% is considered normal. Ectopic thyroid tissue is easier to localize with ^{123}J because it is fixed in the organ and the scattered tissue and there is no overlap with the salivary gland region as with ^{99m}Tc-pertechnetate. Uptake can occur no earlier than 2 h p. i. ^{123}J is a cyclotron product and is only used for special, rare indications.

- Assessment of Quantitative Thyroid Scintigraphy

Normal Findings

Homogeneous distribution of the radiopharmaceutical in both thyroid lobes, the

TcTU is in the normal range. The salivary glands present with.

Pathological Findings

Globally elevated TcTU is found in iodine deficient areas, disseminated autonomy or Graves' disease. Thyrostasis can also lead to an increased TcTU. A focally increased uptake is found in autonomic areas. A distinction is made between so-called warm and hot nodules. Warm nodules are compensated autonomous areas, i.e. the healthy areas of the thyroid are still displayed. In most cases, the TSH is not yet completely suppressed. Hot nodules are decompensated autonomous areas that are no longer subject to the regulatory circuit. The healthy areas of the thyroid gland are no longer detectable by scintigraphy (suppressed), and the TSH is also usually reduced or no longer detectable.

- A globally reduced uptake is found in cases of acute inflammation of the thyroid gland (e.g. thyroiditis de Quervain), iodine contamination, thyroid hormone administration, after radioiodine therapy or radiation therapy of the neck region including the thyroid lodge, or possibly in the context of a chronic autoimmune thyreopathy.
- A focal under-enrichment (cold nodule) may correspond to a solid thyroid nodule (with increased risk of malignancy), a thyroid cyst, the Z. n after radioiodine therapy of an autonomous adenoma, or possibly a focal inflammation or metastasis.
- Ectopic thyroid tissue may occur intrathoracically, as well as predominantly along the median line from the larynx to the base of the tongue. Ectopic tissue lateral to the median line is rare, as is struma ovarii (usually benign teratoma of an ovary).

■ Further Investigations

Suppression scintigraphy: TSH production is suppressed by oral administration of thyroid hormones, then thyroid scintigraphy is performed again and the TcTU is determined. If the thyroid gland or node is subject to the control cycle, the TcTU decreases.

A relevant autonomy is assumed from a TcTU of 1–2%.

Thyroid puncture: Thyroid puncture is performed as a fine needle puncture. There is a technique with aspiration as well as without aspiration. The indication is based on the clinical findings. In the case of a suspected malignancy, puncture should always be performed; other indications may be a relief puncture of a large cyst, a node after radiotherapy in the neck region, possibly an elevated calcitonin value or unclear cervical lymph nodes. Contraindications are anticoagulation (with the exception of acetylsalicylic acid up to a maximum of 100 mg/die) and lack of patient cooperation or consistency of therapy. Usually, FNP is performed under sonographic control under aseptic conditions. The complication rate is low, with mild pain and bleeding being the most common. In aspiration, cannulas of about 22–23 G are used, and aspiration is performed by creating a negative pressure. In non-aspiration, cannulas of 25–27 G are used. Cytological examination can be performed either as a smear or by the thin-prep method. A minimum of six cell clusters, each containing at least ten thyrocytes, is considered sufficient material for examination. If the material is sufficient, molecular genetic examinations (in particular detection of BRAFV600E) can also be carried out on the basis of the FNP.

Hypofunctional areas in the ^{99m}Tc-pertechnetate scintigraphy and sonographically partly solid nodes are malignant with a probability of about 2% and therefore require further clarification. In this case, FNP should be performed as standard. If FNP is not possible due to contraindications, a scintigraphy with ^{99m}Tc-MIBI (2 methoxyisobutylisonitrile) can be performed. MIBI accumulates in the mitochondria of cells. Malignant tumors and metastases usually have a significantly increased cell division and are mitochondrially more active than healthy tissue. These changes can be visualized by imaging. The

22

scintigram is recorded 20, 60 and 120 min p. i., the recording parameters correspond to the ^{99m}Tc Pertechnetat study.

The increased metabolic activity of malignant thyroid changes can also be detected in the ^{18}F-FDG-PET. In the synopsis of the findings, further diagnostics or surgical resection can therefore be dispensed with if necessary.

❯ Thyroid scintigraphy and the determined ^{99m}Tc TU provide information about function, size, shape and location of the thyroid gland. In the presence of hot nodules, a suppression scintigram can be added to clarify the relevance of therapy. Hypofunctional solid nodules with suspicious findings show an increased risk of malignancy and should be further clarified by FNP.

Parathyroid Glands (Glandulae Parathyroideae)

■ Examinations of the Parathyroid Gland

^{99m}Tc Pertechnetate/^{99m}Tc MIBI Scintigraphy

Adenomas and hyperplasias of the parathyroid gland can be visualized by means of a combined ^{99m}Tc-pertechnetate and ^{99m}Tc-MIBI (methoxy-iso-butyl-isonitrile) scintigraphy. The mitochondria-rich, oxyphilic cells of parathyroid adenomas take up more ^{99m}Tc-MIBI (compared to thyroid tissue). In addition, the retention is more pronounced

Assessment of Quantitative Parathyroid Scintigraphy

The assessment is either a so-called subtraction scintigraphy: The ^{99m}Tc-pertechnetate scintigraphy is subtracted from the ^{99m}Tc-MIBI scintigraphy (acquisition in the same position and session). The second assessment is to compare the planar ^{99m}Tc-pertechnetate scintigraphy with the planar MIBI scintigraphies over time. While a rapid MIBI wash-out is seen in healthy thyroid tissue, retention is increased in parathyroid adenoma. It is possible to generate a 3-D image of MIBI scintigraphy using SPECT. The SPECT technique increases the sensitivity of the procedure (Deutsche Gesellschaft für Nuklearmedizin e. V. Leitlinien, Verfahrensanweisung für Parathyroid Scintigraphie).

❯ Especially adenomas that cannot be adequately detected preoperatively by sonography, CT and MRI, or those that could not be found intraoperatively, are submitted to ^{99m}Tc MIBI scintigraphy.

22.3.3 Valence

Christel Vockelmann

■ Table 22.1 shows the use of the respective therapeutic options depending on the problem

■ **Table 22.1** Value of the therapeutic procedures

	Sonography	Conventional	Fluoroscopy/ Angiography	CT	MRI	Nuk	PET
Goiter	P	N	N	N	N	P	N
Adrenal Space Demand	P	N	N	W	W	W	W
Pituitary Space Requirement	N	N	N	N	P	N	N

N Not indicated, *P* Primary diagnosis, *W* Further diagnosis
P* Cardio-CT can be used as a primary procedure in certain risk constellations

22.4 Therapy

22.4.1 Radiotherapy

Guido Heilsberg

Thyroid Carcinoma

In thyroid carcinoma, percutaneous radiotherapy is used only in a small group of high-risk patients: when surgery and radioiodine therapy could not achieve complete tumor cell destruction, in recurrence or in the palliative situation of skeletal metastases with risk of fracture, brain metastases, and upper influence congestion.

22.4.2 Nuclear Medicine

Ursula Blum

Radioiodine Therapy

Iodine is selectively stored in thyroid and thyroid tissue-like tumors and metastases via the sodium iodide symporters. This behavior is used in radioiodine therapy. The ^{131}J used here transitions to ^{131}Xe by emitting beta-minus radiation with an average range of 0.5 mm and a gamma component (energy 364 keV) that can be used for imaging and a half-life of 8.04 days. The most important benign indications for radioiodine therapy are functional autonomies, Graves' disease and euthyroid strumen. A corresponding indication for the therapy of malignant tumors is the still existing functional similarity to thyroid tissue. This is the case with papillary (approx. 70% of malignant thyroid tumors) as well as follicular (approx. 20% of malignant thyroid tumors), the so-called differentiated thyroid carcinomas.

Undifferentiated malignancies such as medullary or anaplastic thyroid carcinoma are not amenable to radioiodine therapy. They are treated postoperatively with external radiation or chemotherapy.

The dose applied during radioiodine therapy depends on the type of disease. The individual determination takes place within the framework of the so-called radioiodine test. Before starting, sufficient iodine abstinence must be ensured. Iodine contamination from medicinal iodine sources, food supplements, toothpaste or fish and seafood dishes must be avoided. If necessary, the therapy is carried out in a euthyroid metabolic state.

After administration of a small amount of radioiodine (1–5 MBq ^{131}J or 5–10 MBq ^{123}J), the absorbed activity is determined at different times with the aid of a measuring probe, the essential components of which are a 5 cm thick NaJ crystal and a suitable collimator (e.g. after 24, 48, 72 and 96 h, in Graves' disease 4–8 h). The volume to be treated is determined by sonographic and scintigraphic imaging, in case of tumor recurrence or metastases by CT- or MRI-based volumetry. The subsequent dose calculation is performed using the so-called Marinelli formula:

$$\text{Activity} = K \times \frac{\text{radiation dose}(\text{Gy}) \times \text{volume of the radiated organ}(\text{mL})}{\text{maximal enhancement}(\%,\text{Uptake}) \times \text{effective half} - \text{life}}$$

The quantity K is a constant with the value 24.67.

The effective half-life can be estimated empirically (approx. 7–8 days, in Graves' disease approx. 3 days) or determined individually, since the individual differences are only slight.

❯ Radioiodine therapy should be performed as soon as possible after the radioiodine test in order to have comparable conditions of radioiodine kinetics.

If a therapeutic ^{131}J capsule is administered, admission to an appropriately equipped ward is required in accordance with national regulations. A decay facility to collect the excreta, which are initially highly radioactive, shall be provided.

❯ Before radioiodine therapy of malignant thyroid diseases, surgical removal of the thyroid gland and affected lymph nodes is mandatory, not only for histology. If the thyroid gland were to be preserved, the dose would have to be significantly higher in accordance with the larger volume, which would be accompanied by an increased side effect rate.

Subsequent radioiodine therapy is directed at the residual thyroid tissue and any metastases that may be present.

The patient is discharged if the measured activity at a distance of 2 m does not exceed 250 MBq (guideline in radiation protection).

❯ The selective storage of ^{131}J in benign and differentiated malignant tumors and their metastases offers the possibility of a therapy closely related to the pathological process. While radioiodine therapy is performed following surgical removal of a differentiated thyroid carcinoma, it can be an alternative to surgery for benign tumors.

■ Acute and Chronic Adverse Reactions and Their Protective Therapy (◻ Table 22.2)

With increasing cumulative doses over the total lifetime, the risk of developing acute myeloid leukemia increases. In contrast, the risk of an increase in other malignant tumors as a result of high-dose radioiodine therapy of the thyroid gland is controversial. After 70 years of therapy experience in the field of benign thyroid diseases, an increased therapy-related cancer risk could not be proven.

■ Aftercare

In addition to history, hormone determination (TSH/Tg) and sonography of the thyroid lodge and soft tissues of the neck, depending on the risk profile ^{131}J whole body scintigraphies are performed three months, one year and if necessary in two year intervals after endogenous or exog-

◻ **Table 22.2** Overview of side effects

Gastritis	Administration of antacids or proton pump blockers
Sialadenitis	Under discussion
Gonadal load	Decrease due to administration of diuretics and laxatives
Intracerebral or intravertebral metastases for edema prophylaxis	Corticosteroids
Pulmonary Fibrosis	Dose restriction in pulmonary metastases, especially when combined with chemotherapy
Bone marrow depression in the treatment of osseous metastases	Continuous blood count control

enous rhTSH simulation. Further examinations may include CT, skeletal and MIBI scintigraphy and, depending on the molecular tumor entity, FDG-PET, DOTATOC-PET or octreotide scintigraphy.

PET examination is particularly indicated when iodine storage of the tumor or its metastases has been lost in the course of the disease, i.e. the tumor is poorly differentiated or de-differentiated.

The prognosis of consistently operated and radioiodine-treated differentiated thyroid carcinomas is consistently good, since this tumor form can be irradiated in isolation due to the selective radionuclide storage of malignant cells, while sparing healthy tissue (Deutsche Gesellschaft für Nuklearmedizin e. V. Leitlinien, Verfahrensanweisung Radioiodtest, RJT benigne Schilddrüsenerkrankungen, differenzierte Schilddrüsenkarzinome, Ganzkörperzintigraphie ^{131}J).

Case Study

Mr. Press, 35 years old, has recently developed high blood pressure. His family doctor sends him to hospital for clarification and optimal therapy adjustment. First, a sonography is performed. However, since this cannot reliably exclude adrenal space damage, an MRI of the adrenal glands is also performed and, in the same examination, an MR angiography. Renal artery stenosis as the cause of the hypertension can be excluded. However, a mass of the left adrenal gland is found, and the right adrenal gland is also somewhat enlarged. A pheochromocytoma is suspected. After laboratory and urine tests, a side-separated venous blood sample can be taken from the adrenal veins. In case of ambiguity, a MIBG scintigraphy can also be performed.

Practice Questions

1. What would be your tentative diagnosis if you find nodules of varying echogenicity on thyroid ultrasonography?
2. What are the features of an NN adenoma on CT?
3. What is the tool of choice to visualize and evaluate a pituitary tumor?
4. What is an important contraindication to thyroid scintigraphy?
5. What substances are used for labeling in adrenal scintigraphy?
6. When is radioiodine therapy used for the thyroid gland?

Solutions ▶ Chap. 27

Lymphatic System

Martina Kahl-Scholz, Christel Vockelmann, Ursula Blum, and Guido Heilsberg

Contents

© Springer-Verlag GmbH Germany, part of Springer Nature 2023
M. Kahl-Scholz, C. Vockelmann (eds.), *Basic Knowledge Radiology*,
https://doi.org/10.1007/978-3-662-66351-6_23

23

This chapter deals with the essential possibilities of radiological diagnostics, nuclear medicine and radiotherapy for the diagnosis and therapy of the lymphatic system. An introductory section provides a brief overview of anatomy and function, and a concluding section contains a case study from practice.

23.1 Anatomical Structures

Martina Kahl-Scholz

In addition to the **lymph vessels,** the lymph **node stations** (filter stations) and the lymph organs (e.g. thymus, spleen, tonsils and appendix) are part of this complex system. The lymph is drained into the venous system.

The **spleen** as an important lymphatic organ is located in the left upper abdomen in direct proximity to the stomach, kidney and large intestine. The spleen is about 4 cm thick, 7 cm wide and 11 cm long.

> "4711": Thickness (4), width (7) and length of spleen (11) in cm.

It shows a side facing the diaphragm (**Facies diaphragmatica**) and a side facing the abdominal organs (**Facies visceralis**), which is divided into the **Facies gastrica, colica** and **renalis.** At the mizhilus (**hilus** splenicus), the splenic **artery** and **vein** enter and leave the spleen, respectively.

The **thymus** as another important lymphatic organ is located in the upper mediastinum behind the sternum, extends to the pericardium of the heart and consists of two lobes. It is a primary lymphoid organ and significantly involved in the imprinting of lymphocytes and the development of immunocompetence. The thymus grows until infancy and maintains its size until puberty.

After puberty, the thymus begins to become fatty and the thymic tissue decreases more and more until the gland consists mainly of fatty tissue.

23.2 Disease Patterns

Martina Kahl-Scholz and Christel Vockelmann

23.2.1 Systemic Diseases

There are several diseases that affect a complex organ system or even the whole body. These systemic diseases are often accompanied by a co-reaction of the lymphatic system, most likely by enlargement (painful or asymptomatic) of the lymph nodes. Systemic diseases include leukemias, anemias, rheumatoid diseases, sarcoidosis, systemic lupus erythematosus and many others. Last but not least, cancers are also systemic diseases if lymph node metastases develop due to metastasis of the lymphatic channels.

- Clinic

The clinic depends on the underlying disease.

- Diagnostics

Sonography

Sonography is **the method of choice** in lymph node diagnostics. In addition to the size of the lymph nodes, the blood supply to the lymph node can also be assessed. And even a **disturbance of** the **architecture**, with the normal **fat hilus of** a lymph node as an indication of a lymph node metastasis, can be detected with high-resolution sonography—and a little patience—even with only minor changes.

> The standard value for an enlarged lymph node is 1 cm.

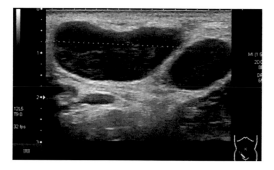

⬛ Fig. 23.1 Lymph node enlarged to 2.8 cm with absent fat hilus in confirmed lymphoma disease

In addition to the fatty hilus, the second very important criterion for distinguishing between normal and suspicious lymph nodes is their **shape**. Oval lymph nodes are more likely to be benign, **round lymph nodes** are always suspect.

Typical for pathological lymph nodes is the **absence of a fatty hilus**, which can be detected on ultrasound as a **central hyperechogenic zone** (⬛ Fig. 23.1).

CT/MRI This fine diagnosis makes ultrasound superior to computed tomography and in most cases also to magnetic resonance imaging. For this reason, mediastinal lymph node enlargements diagnosed by CT are often first assessed by endosonography.

Endosonography Endosonography means that the gastroenterologist or internist inserts an ultrasound probe into the oesophagus, comparable to an oesophago-gastro-duodenoscopy. In unclear cases, a mediastinal lymph node can then also be punctured endoscopically using ultrasound. EBUS is also an option. This refers to the endobronchial ultrasound examination. This is somewhat more complex than endosonography through the esophagus, because air does not conduct the sound waves and therefore a sound window must first be created in the bronchus.

23.2.2 Hodgkin's Disease

Hodgkin's lymphoma is a malignant tumor of the lymphatic system, which is characterized by a painless swelling of lymph nodes. The presence of a special type of cell (Sternberg-Reed cells) distinguishes it from non-Hodgkin's lymphoma.

■ Clinic

In addition to lymph node swelling, B symptoms may develop.

■ Diagnostics

CT

Computed tomography is the standard method for determining the status of the lymph nodes in cases of suspected diseases of the lymphatic system. In the staging of a possible lymphoma, not only the thorax and abdomen should be examined, but also the cervical lymph nodes. This serves to have an objective and in the course comparable imaging.

As with sonography, computed tomography can detect the fatty hilus as a fatty **isodense central zone** in the lymph node even in relatively large lymph nodes in the groin. This is indicative of **benignity of the lymph node**. An **absent fatty hilus** is a sign of **pathologic change**, such as malignancy or inflammation. The shape also plays an important role in the evaluation of the lymph node as in sonography. A further indication of malignancy or benignity results from the localization of the lymph node.

MRI

See CT

23.2.3 Non-Hodgkin's Lymphoma

The collective term non-Hodgkin's lymphoma (NHL) covers all malignant diseases of the lymphatic system (malignant lymphomas) that are not Hodgkin's disease.

- Clinic
▶ Section 23.2.2.

- Diagnostics
▶ Section 23.2.2.

23.2.4 Lymph Node Metastases

▶ Section 23.2.1.

23.2.5 Splenic Cysts

- Clinic

Splenic cysts are usually an incidental finding and accordingly often behave asymptomatically. An exception can be parasitic cysts.

- Diagnostics

Sonography

On sonography, the cysts appear **homogeneous** and echo-poor. They show a **smooth border** with a **dorsal sound enhancement.**

CT

Again, the cysts show **smooth bordered** and **homogeneously hypodense**. They do **not** take up **KM.**

> ❯ If it is an echinococcus cyst, multichamberedness is the key distinguishing feature.

23.2.6 Spleen Abscess

In the course of an infection (e.g. by mycoplasma), pus accumulates in the spleen tissue.

- Clinic

Nausea and vomiting, upper abdominal pain (capsular pain) and splenomegaly.

- Diagnostics

Sonography

An **echo-poor** and **blurred** structure is revealed.

CT

The density depends on how advanced the abscess is. A **rather hypodense** structure is often seen, which absorbs **KM in** the **marginal area.**

23.2.7 Splenic Infarction

Splenic infarction results from occlusion of the lienal artery or its branches with consequent tissue death.

- Clinic

Acute abdomen, vomiting and nausea, there may be fever and splenic pain.

- Diagnostics

Sonography/Duplex Sonography

Isoechogenic, later anechoic area, often **wedge-shaped** (supply areas of the artery), can be seen on sonography, There may be calcification subcapsular and retraction of the splenic tissue. Duplex sonography can assess the blood flow through the splenic arteries and for surgery.

CT

Again, **wedge-shaped hypodense** structures that do **not** accommodate **KM are** evident.

23.2.8 Splenic Rupture

Traumatic splenic rupture is one of the most common intra-abdominal injuries that should be controlled, especially in cases of polytrauma (with, for example, left rib fracture).

- Clinic

Pain in the left upper abdomen (possibly with sweeping sign = radiation into the left shoulder).

■ Diagnostics

Sonography

A splenic hematoma appears on ultrasound as an **echo-poor to -free sound-conducting zone** localized in or around the spleen. Smaller hematomas may not be seen.

CT

CT is the tool of choice. A hematoma is identified by **lower density values** that approach the isodense range after a few days.

23.2.9 Thymoma

Thymoma is the name given to tumors of the thymus, which account for about 15% of all mediastinal tumors (3/4 are benign, only 1/4 are malignant).

■ Clinic

Often the diagnosis is accidental, the tumors grow slowly and rarely cause symptoms.

■ Diagnostics

Conventional X-ray

There is an **unclear mediastinal mass**, which should be further clarified by CT/MRI.

CT/MRI

Thymomas and thymic carcinomas usually present as a **well circumscribed soft tissue mass in the upper anterior mediastinum.** Vascular infiltration or sheathing as well as pleural metastases are indicative of malignancy. Magnetic resonance imaging (MRI) of the thorax may be helpful in rare cases to assess vascular infiltration.

23.3 Diagnostics

23.3.1 Radiological Diagnosis

Christel Vockelmann

Sonography

Sonography is also the screening method of first choice in the diagnosis of lymphatic diseases. The cervical lymph node stations along the cervical-vascular nerve sheaths, axillary and inguinal can be excellently examined with a high-resolution transducer (■ Fig. 23.1). The abdominal lymph nodes paraaortally and the spleen can be examined with abdominal ultrasonography. This fine diagnosis makes ultrasound superior to computed tomography and, in most cases, to magnetic resonance imaging.

Conventional X-ray Diagnostics

Conventional X-ray diagnostics have no significance in the context of a targeted examination for suspected lymphatic disease. Nevertheless, lymphatic diseases and lymph node enlargements can of course also be diagnosed in the context of other reasons or clinical suspicions. Sarcoidosis or Boeck's disease, a granulomatous systemic disease, leads to a typical hilar plumpness on conventional radiographs of the lungs (■ Fig. 23.2), where a narrow fringe of lung can classically be delineated between the hilar and cardiac shadows (in contrast to a hilar bronchial carcinoma).

Fluoroscopy/Angiography

Fluoroscopy and angiography play no role in the diagnosis and therapy of diseases of the lymphatic system.

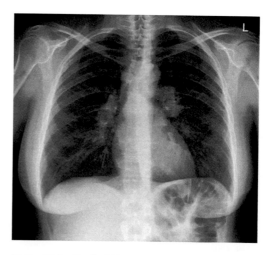

■ **Fig. 23.2** Typical hilar enlargement in sarcoidosis

Computer Tomography

Computed tomography is the standard method for assessing the status of the lymph nodes in cases of v. a. diseases of the lymphatic system (■ Fig. 23.3). In the course of therapy, the size of the lymph nodes and also of the spleen is assessed to evaluate the success of therapy. In addition, it is possible to detect organ manifestations of lymphoma better than with magnetic resonance imaging and sonography. In addition to lymph nodes and spleen, all organs can ultimately be involved in the disease.

A further indication of malignancy or benignity results from the localization of the lymph node. Thus, several lymph nodes are found mediastinally infracarinally in almost all patients. These are not to be considered suspicious per se. However, if these lymph nodes are found in front of the aortic arch, then at least a control examination should be recommended; depending on further findings, further diagnostics and clarification may also be indicated. Round lymph nodes with relatively strong contrast enhancement adjacent to a colon carcinoma in the percolated adipose tissue are equally suspicious for lymph node metastasis, even if the size of the lymph nodes is less than 1 cm. ■ Figure 23.4 shows a gastric carcinoma with several lymph node metastases.

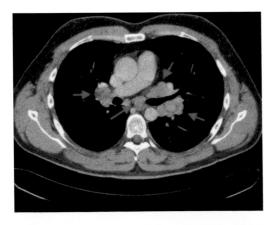

■ **Fig. 23.3** CT image showing mediastinal and bihilar lymph node enlargement in sarcoidosis

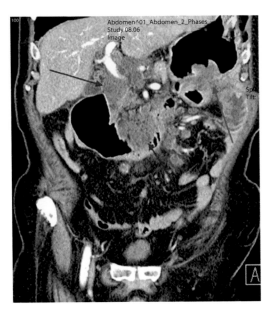

■ **Fig. 23.4** T4 gastric carcinoma with extensive lymph node metastases

The combination of CT and PET offers the advantage of combining morphological and biological information.

Magnetic Resonance Imaging

Like computed tomography, magnetic resonance imaging is very good at detecting the size of lymph nodes and also a fat hilus as a diagnostic criterion (■ Fig. 23.5). The disadvantage is the generally limited scope of the examination. In the case of circumscribed cervical lymph node enlargements in younger patients, however, magnetic resonance imaging is always an appropriate follow-up diagnostic method to sonography. The local lymph node status in rectal cancer can also be detected very well by MRI as part of local staging.

23.3.2 Nuclear Medicine

Ursula Blum

Sentinel lymph node scintigraphy can be used to detect the relevant lymph nodes (sentinel lymph nodes) and, if necessary,

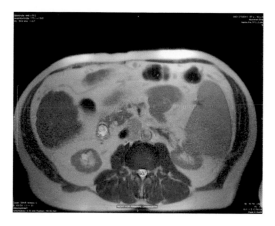

◻ **Fig. 23.5** Pathologically enlarged lymph node in HCC

lymphatic channels in primarily lympho-genic metastatic tumors.

Introduction to Sentinel Lymph Node Scintigraphy

The sentinel lymph node (SLN) is the lymph node(s) through which a malignant tumor is primarily drained. If these are free of tumor cells, lymphogenic metastasis can be excluded with a high degree of probability. The histological examination of the sentinel lymph node has a direct impact on the extent of resection and, if necessary, the subsequent therapy. Topographic anatomy using the example of breast carcinoma

Tumor cells can detach themselves from the cell structure and enter the lymphatic system, settle there under unfavorable conditions, divide and form metastases. First of all, there are usually metastases in the nearby regional lymph nodes, which, in the case of breast carcinoma, are located within the breast, in the axilla or parasternally, depending on the location of the tumor. Even more rarely, drainage into the contra-lateral axilla is found. The collecting vessel coming from the regional lymphatic drainage area can transport the tumor cells to the secondary, or tertiary lymph node stations. In the venous angle (thoracic duct) the lymphatic system enters the venous blood

system and thus in advanced stages tumor cells reach the bloodstream, the tumor now metastasizes hematogenously.

Sentinel Lymph Node Scintigraphy Using the Example of Breast Carcinoma

To visualize the SLN,[99m] Tc labeled colloids with a particle size of approximately 20 nm to 100 nm are injected. These are recognized by the lymphatic system as foreign bodies and transported away. The applied amount of activity must be so high that the lymph node can be found intraoperatively with an appropriate measuring probe. The injection can be intracutaneous, subcutaneous or per-itumoral. To date, no application method is superior to any other. According to the cur-rent guideline, 100–200 MBq are injected 24 hours before surgery, with a radiation expo-sure of the patient of 0.5–1.5 mSv.

The recording on a large field camera proceeds as follows:
- LEHR Collimator
- Matrix 256 x 256
- Early static images of the thorax and ipsilateral axilla from ventral 300 sec
- Late static images of the thorax and ipsi-lateral axilla from ventral and lateral over 300 sec
- The images are usually taken with the injection site shielded; acquisition should be performed without it.

The patient lies on his back, the arm of the side to be examined is spread at a 90-degree angle.

A surface phantom thinly covered with 57 Co lies under the patient. It is placed so that the contours of the axilla of the affected side are visible.

If no SLN can be visualized two hours p. i., the mamma should be massaged and warmed for 10 minutes. The SLN is then vis-ible in the following 10 minutes, otherwise a late image is acquired the next morning immediately before surgery. The detection rate depends on the injection, ranging from approximately 80% for peritumoral/intraparenchymal injection to 98% for intradermal injection in various studies. The SLN shown can be marked on the skin. The surgeon uses a special gamma probe to locate and remove the SLN. The lymph node is immediately examined histopathologically. In case of negative findings or micrometastasis (<2 mm), axillary dissection is currently not performed according to the latest guideline (AWMF, 07/2013).

> The enrichment of the SLN only serves to locate this lymph node, a statement on the dignity is not possible!

The following mistakes must be avoided:
- Incorrect indication
- Skin contamination
- Faulty injection
- Overlay of the SLN through the injection site
- Previous operations, manipulations, therapies or additional diseases
- Covering of lymph nodes close to tumors by lead shielding
- Premature termination of the investigation
- False negative result in case of complete metastasis of the lymph nodes
- Inadequate reporting of findings

Another possible application of sentinel lymph node scintigraphy is the visualization of the sentinel lymph node in malignant melanoma, head and neck tumors, penile carcinomas, vulvar carcinomas and other tumors. Here, the visualization of anatomical neighboring structures by fusion of SPECT with CT cross-sections can be helpful for easy intraoperative detection of the SLN.

PET in Lymphoma Diagnostics

Lymphomas are rapidly growing malignancies. As a rule, they have an increased energy requirement and absorb a corresponding increase in glucose.

A glucose analogue, fluorodeoxyglucose (FDG), is used to represent glucose metabolism. This is obtained by replacing an oxygen atom in glucose with 18 F. The latter decays via a β decay. This decays via a $β^+$ decay. The two resulting gamma quanta can be detected, i.e. made visible, by two opposing detectors in positron emission tomography (PET).

For lymphoma detection, the 18 F-FDG PET is injected i.v. Since there is a correlation between mitosis, proliferation rate, tumor aggressiveness and nuclide accumulation, the intensity of the accumulation provides information about the metabolic behavior of the malignancy.

If no current, diagnostic CT is available (not older than 14 days), this can be acquired in the same session.

Indication for PET

The 18 F-FDG PET is more sensitive than other morphologically diagnostic methods in both primary staging and restaging.

In the early diagnosis of lymphomas, the 18 F-FDG PET is used to clarify the spread – in the case of limited spread, a short course of chemotherapy or local radiation may be sufficient, while longer, more intensive treatment must follow if the tumor involves several regions of the body. After only two cycles of chemotherapy, the response to therapy can be evaluated, which may then lead to a reduction in the number of chemotherapy cycles in the case of negative or improved PET, or to an intensification or change in the chemotherapy protocol in the case of unchanged or worsened PET.

At the end of intensive chemotherapy, a negative PET can lead to the waiving of additional radiotherapy and thus to a reduction in toxicity. The waiver is only possible because in PET the morphologically detectable residual tissue can be reliably distinguished in fibrosis and the residual tumor.

The 18 F-FDG PET can provide a prognosis estimate. For example, the recurrence rate for positive post-therapeutic FDG PET is between 90 and 100%, and between zero and 17% for negative findings. In the case of positive findings, either a lack of remission or the occurrence of a recurrence can be assumed.

Radiotherapeutically, the 18 F-FDG PET can contribute to the exact target volume definition.

Special Features in Pediatrics

In children and adolescents, lymphoma is the third most common cancer.

Due to the high life expectancy of these patients, the focus here is on minimizing therapy-related late effects, including secondary malignancies, cardiovascular events, pulmonary fibrosis, and endocrinological changes.

The 18 F-FDG-PET is used pre-therapeutically and intratherapeutically for early clarification of treatment success, so that a possible attenuation of therapy can be discussed.

■ Dealing with the Child

Intravenous access should be established before the child arrives, this minimizes stress. A warm environment increases the well-being of the child and causes a reduction of the tracer in the brown adipose tissue, which can be additionally supported by medication. This preparation optimizes the later collection of findings. The activity is raised according to weight and is a minimum of 26 MBq in 2D mode and 14 MBq in 3D mode. Before starting the examination, the bladder must be emptied or the diaper changed. If the PET/CT examination is used for radiation planning, appropriate positioning must be carried out in consultation with the radiation therapist.

■ Dealing with Parents

The procedure of the examination must be explained in detail to the child and his parents (resting time, duration of admission, details of the examination procedure, necessity of sedation or anesthesia, presence of diabetes mellitus, administration of an iodine-containing contrast medium). Parents must be informed of the urgent need to abstain from food for four to six hours before the examination. Sweet drinks, chewing gum and sweets require special mention. If the parents are involved in the examination, the children usually cooperate better. If the examination is acquired during the child's normal bedtime, sedation may not be necessary.

Possible Sources of Error

❯ When growth factors are administered, the 18 F-FDG uptake in bone marrow and spleen may be increased. If cell proliferation occurs in the bone marrow after chemotherapy, the 18 F-FDG uptake in the bone marrow is also increased.

In children there is physiologically an increased FDG uptake in the thymus, furthermore of the lymphatic tissue in the nasopharynx. The chewing muscles can store more FDG after pacifier use or after breastfeeding, the larynx after crying or screaming.

23.3.3 Valence

◻ Table 23.1 shows the use of the respective therapeutic options depending on the problem

	Sonography	Conventional	Fluoroscopy/Angiography	CT	MRI	Nuk	PET
Lymphoma	P	N	N	P	W	N	W
Sentinel-node						P	

□ **Table 23.1** Value of the therapeutic procedures

N Not indicated, *P* Primary diagnosis, *W* Further diagnosis

23.4 Therapy

23.4.1 Interventional Radiology

Christel Vockelmann and Martina Kahl-Scholz

CT-Guided Biopsy

Radiological therapeutic interventions on lymph nodes are technically feasible, particularly in the form of thermoablation. In the overall context of oncological therapy, however, such an intervention may only make sense in selected individual cases. In contrast, a CT-guided biopsy (□ Fig. 23.6) is often necessary, especially of the paraaortic lymph node enlargements. These are often not accessible by endosonography. In addition, only fine-needle aspiration can be performed by endosonography. The tissue obtained in this way is often insufficient to allow a pathological differential diagnosis of lymphoma. Therefore, a CT-guided punch biopsy is usually obtained from the lumbar region. Frequently, a coaxial procedure is performed in order to obtain several samples. It is important to obtain sufficient material.

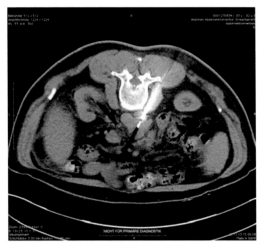

□ **Fig. 23.6** Biopsy of pathological lymph node aortointercaval with securing metastasis of HCC

23.4.2 Radiotherapy

Guido Heilsberg

Hodgkin's Disease

Early stages are treated with combined chemotherapy and radiotherapy, using the techniques:

- **Involved-field** (IF) = technique that includes only the affected lymph nodes

- **Extend-field** (EF) = technique that includes affected lymph node regions with adjacent, clinically unaffected regions.

Used with a dose between 20–36 Gy/ED 1.6–2 Gy/5×.

The side effects depend on the radiation localization.

Non-Hodgkin's Lymphoma (NHL)

Generally, NHL is treated by radiotherapy and chemotherapy with a total dose between 24 and 40 Gy.

Practice Questions

1. What features help to distinguish a malignant from a benign lymph node on sonography and CT?
2. What is the evidence for a multichambered, echo-poor structure in the spleen that does not pick up KM?
3. What features may indicate a thymoma?

Solutions ▶ Chap. 27

Case Study

Lars probably has Hodgkin's disease, i.e. malignant lymphoma. Since the ultrasound already suggests a typical malignant lymphoma of the neck, the diagnosis is quickly confirmed with a punch biopsy. To complete the staging, a PET-CT is primarily performed at the university. Here mediastinal lymphoma is still revealed. Lars undergoes a combined radio-chemo therapy as part of a study. Already after a few days the swelling on the neck goes down. After a few weeks, Lars has survived the therapy. He now has to go for regular follow-up care, but so far no recurrence has occurred.

Pediatrics

Esther Münstermann and Christel Vockelmann

Contents

© Springer-Verlag GmbH Germany, part of Springer Nature 2023
M. Kahl-Scholz, C. Vockelmann (eds.), *Basic Knowledge Radiology*,
https://doi.org/10.1007/978-3-662-66351-6_24

In the following, a brief overview of important pediatric clinical pictures (from the areas of thorax, GIT, urogenital tract, musculoskeletal diseases as well as oncology) as well as their radiological diagnostics and possible technical interventions is given.

24.1 Thorax

24.1.1 Respiratory Distress Syndrome (ANS)

Surfactant deficiency. Respiratory distress syndrome (RNS) can occur in premature infants <28 weeks gestation due to lung immaturity, in shock situations, and in infants of diabetic mothers, for example.

- Clinic

Apnea, cyanosis, tachypnea

- Diagnostics

X-ray Thorax (◻ Fig. 24.1)
ANS is divided into four stages:
- Fine granular lung pattern
- I + Beyond the heart contours
- II + Blurring or partial obliteration of the contours of the heart and diaphragm
- "White lung"

In the first 6 h of life the classification is uncertain because of still present lung fluid and after surfactant administration.

❯ Sepsis with B streptococci can simulate ANS in clinical and radiographic signs.

24.1.2 Meconium Aspiration

Intrauterine hypoxia leads, among other things, to vasoconstriction of mesenteric vessels and thus to hyperperistalsis and finally to premature meconium discharge, which inactivates surfactant.

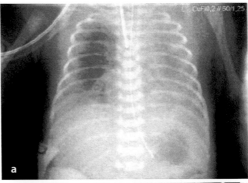

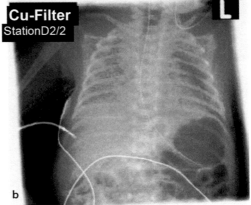

◻ **Fig. 24.1** **a** Respiratory distress syndrome grade II, **b Respiratory** distress syndrome grade III with fine-spotted compressions and positive aerobronchogram. Properly inserted gastric tube. Overlay by ECG electrodes

Meconium aspiration is more likely to affect dystrophic and transferred neonates.

- Clinic

Depending on the severity from tachypnea to asphyxia

- Diagnostics

X-ray Chest
Symmetrically distributed, dense, patchy, sometimes nodular pulmonary infiltrates. Pulmonary hyperinflation, flattened diaphragm, occasionally minor pleural effusion or pneumothorax.

24.1.3 Oesophageal Atresia

■ Clinic

OEsophageal atresia can be suspected prenatally sonographically by a missing gastric bubble and a polyhydramnios. In about 50% of cases other malformations are also present (e.g. VACTERL association: vertebral, anus, cardial, tracheal, esophageal, renal, limbs).

■ Diagnostics

X-ray Thorax and Abdomen (□ Fig. 24.2)

Esophageal atresia is divided into five different stages (type I to type IIIc). Type IIIb occurs in approx. 87% of cases.

> ❯ Placement of a gastric tube before performing a chest X-ray is mandatory in neonates and premature infants!

24.1.4 Catheter in the Thoracic Region

Wash-in Catheter

The intravenous catheter is placed over a suitable vein (e.g. V. mediana cubiti, V. basilica) under sterile conditions and should be positioned in *front of* the right atrium. The beginning of the catheter should always be imaged as well, since the catheter may have already coiled up at the beginning.

Umbilical Vein Catheter (NVK)

The umbilical vein catheter is placed via the umbilical vein through the ductus venosus Arantii into the inferior vena cava (□ Fig. 24.3) and is used, among other things, to enable exchange transfusion or measurement of central venous pressure. The catheter should end 1 cm above the diaphragm.

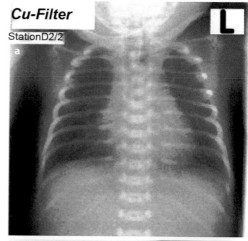
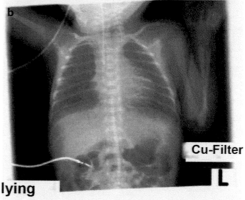

□ **Fig. 24.2** **a, b** Oesophageal atresia type IIIb with looping of the gastric tube in the blind sac and evidence of esophagotracheal fistula through the air in the included upper GI tract

Umbilical Artery Catheter

The umbilical artery catheter is used to measure pO_2 in ventilated preterm infants. The appropriate position should be above the diaphragm, at a safe distance from the outlet of the renal arteries.

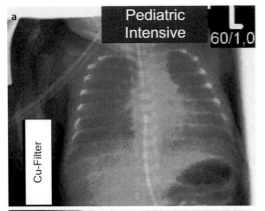

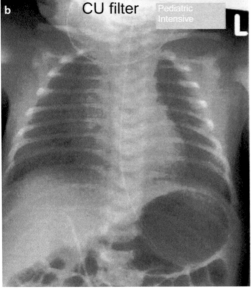

◻ Fig. 24.3   a Correct and **b** incorrect installation of a NPC

24.2   Gastrointestinal Tract

24.2.1   Necrotising Enterocolitis (NEC)

NEC is an acute inflammatory reaction with pervasive necrosis of the intestinal wall, which often leads to perforation. Premature infants are affected up to 90%.

■ Clinic
Often insidious symptoms, deterioration of the general condition, apnea, bradycardia, pressure-painful abdominal wall with venous markings, fresh blood in the stool.

■ Diagnostics
X-ray Abdomen
   NEC is divided into five stages:
— I: Suspicion of NEC with radiologically thickened intestinal walls
— IIA: Thickening of the intestinal wall with double contour due to edema formation (pneumatosis intestinalis)
— IIB: Pneumatosis intestinalis, hepatosplenomegaly, free fluid
— IIIA: IIB + Pneumatosis intestinalis over several intestinal loops, additionally air in portal vein
— IIIB: Pronounced pneumatosis intestinalis, free air subphrenic or prehepatic, indirect visualization of free air by visible lig. falciforme, central brightening

24.2.2   Duodenal Atresia

Duodenal atresia is defined by occlusion of the lumen by a membrane, complete disruption or circular compression from the outside by a pancreas anulare. Duodenal atresia is more common in syndromes and, for example, in trisomy 21.

■ Clinic
Bilious vomiting in occlusion below and clear vomiting in occlusion above the papilla vateri.

■ Diagnostics
X-ray Abdomen
   The so-called "double bubble" (◻ Fig. 24.4), an air bubble in the stomach and in the duodenum, is seen.

24.2.3   Invagination

This is an invagination of a part of the intestine into the following caudal part of the intestine. This results in constriction of

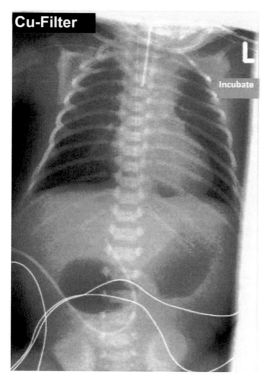

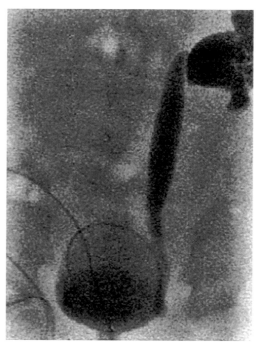

◻ Fig. 24.4 Distended stomach and distended duodenum, in the rest of the picture an airless abdomen. Incidental findings: non-central NPC, gastric tube, endotracheal tube and CVC via the right arm correct

the mesenteric vessels with oedema, stasis hemorrhage, intestinal necrosis due to ischaemia.

■ Clinic

Acute colicky pain and vomiting, rectal bleeding

■ Diagnostics

Sonography

Cocard form (shooting target phenomenon, target sign) of the intestinal part with invaginate

X-ray Abdomen

Visible during colonic contrast enema due to discontinuation of the contrast agent.

24.3 Urogenital Tract

24.3.1 Vesicourethral Reflux (VUR)

If vesicoureteral reflux is suspected (e.g. in cases of high fever urinary tract infection in the first year of life, recurrent UTIs), a micturition cystourethrogram should be performed. For this purpose, the urinary bladder is filled with water-soluble contrast medium and, during micturition or even before, the contrast medium flows back from the bladder into the refluxing ureter, which under certain circumstances can extend into the renal pelvis.

■ Diagnostics

Micturition Cystourethrogram (◻ Fig. 24.5)

There is a classification into five degrees:
- Grade I: VUR only in the ureter

◻ Fig. 24.5 Micturition cystourethrogram with reflux

- Grade II: VUR into the ureter and pyelon
- Grade III: VUR into the ureter and pyelon with pyelon dilatation
- Grade IV: VUR into the ureter and pyelon with pyelon dilatation and pressure atrophy of the parenchyma
- Grade V: Massive VUR with extensive destruction of the parenchyma.

24.4 Musculoskeletal

24.4.1 Child Abuse (Battered Child)

In cases of suspected child abuse, imaging (sonography, X-ray, CT, and MRI) reveals fresh fractures as well as older fractures. Diffuse CNS hemorrhages and subdural hemorrhages of various ages can be detected in shaking trauma.

24.4.2 Osteomyelitis

Osteomyelitis can be caused, for example, by a hematogenous septic spread of bacterial foci, but also post-traumatically or iatrogenically.

- Clinic
In addition to high fever, there is local pain with soft tissue swelling.

- Diagnostics
Conventional X-ray
  The X-ray is usually unremarkable in the acute stage. A lightening of the cancellous bone may be seen. Later, destruction, including of the cortical bone, and a periosteal reaction and sequestration become visible.
  MRI makes early diagnosis possible.

24.4.3 Hip Dysplasia

All newborns receive a hip sonography at U3 in order to enable an early therapy in case of hip dysplasia.

- Diagnostics
Sonography
  The classification is made according to Graf. For this purpose, the acetabular roof angle (= alpha angle between the extension of the os ilium and the tangent to the bony acetabular roof) and the cartilaginous roof angle are measured (= beta angle between the extension of the os ilium and the tangent to the cartilaginous labrum acetabulare).

24.5 Oncology

24.5.1 Neuroblastoma

Neuroblastoma is a malignant solid tumor that arises from degenerated immature cells of the sympathetic nervous system. Most commonly, neuroblastoma arises in the adrenal medulla and in the limiting cord along the spine, and approximately 70% is located in the abdomen at diagnosis. Metastases can be found in the liver, bone and bone marrow, and lymph nodes. Rarely, metastasis to the brain occurs.
  Newborns, infants and children under six years of age are most commonly affected.

- Clinic
Symptoms are varied and may include palpable abdominal tumor, bone pain, skin lesions.

- Diagnostics
In addition to a clinical and laboratory examination (catecholamine metabolites and NSE), sonography of the abdomen and

neck and an MRI of the affected region, as well as a MIBG scintigraphy are necessary for diagnosis. A bone marrow aspiration and a tumor biopsy (N-myc amplification) are also part of the diagnosis.

Neuroblastoma is divided into six different stages (INSS, stage I-IV-S), therapy is carried out according to the therapy optimization protocol.

- Conventional X-ray

Neuroblastomas often present inhomogeneously and with central calcifications and necrosis.

24.5.2 Nephroblastoma (Wilms' Tumor)

Nephroblastoma is a malignant solid tumor that arises from degenerated primitive tissue cells. Infants up to five years of age are most commonly affected and are usually asymptomatic at diagnosis. Nephroblastoma usually occurs unilaterally. Metastasis occurs early to the lungs, otherwise metastases to the liver, brain and bone are possible.

- Diagnostics

For diagnosis, in addition to the clinical examination, a sonography of the abdomen and an MRI of the tumor region is necessary. In addition, a chest X-ray is performed in two planes and, if pulmonary metastases are suspected, a CT of the lungs.

The staging is done according to the SIOP classification. Therapy is carried out according to the SIOP therapy optimization study.

❯ In 5% of cases a vena cava tumor thrombus occurs.

24.5.3 Medulloblastoma

Medulloblastoma is the most common malignant brain tumor in childhood and adolescence.

- Pathogenesis

The preferential location of the tumor in the cerebellar vermis in combination with the growth often leads to occlusion of the 4th ventricle, which results in intracranial pressure increase and consecutive hydrocephalus.

- Clinic

Symptoms may include morning vomiting, nausea, headache and lethargy. In addition, cerebellar signs such as ataxia, disturbed gait, nystagmus or dysdiadochokinesia may also occur.

- Diagnostics

MRI

For imaging, an MRI of the entire craniospinal axis must be performed. In the T2 image, the solid part of the tumor is predominantly hyper- to isointense to the cerebellar cortex and shows a heterogeneous appearance. The T1-weighted image shows a predominantly hypo- to isointense, heterogeneous tumor. The contrast image is non-specific and inhomogeneous. Metastases are best detected in the T1-weighted image after contrast medium administration.

24

Case Study

Little Lisa has just turned two years old. Now she has a stomach ache and fever. The pediatrician Dr. Rührig examines Lisa. The abdomen is soft and without guarding. However, in the ultrasound examination, the left renal pelvis appears somewhat distended. Since Lisa appears seriously ill, Dr. Rührig decides to obtain some urine through a one-time catheterization. This shows a massive leukocytosis as well as a slight erythrocyturia. A micturition cystourethrogram is performed because of the suspicion of reflux with accompanying inflammation, which is confirmed.

Practice Questions

1. What are the different types of catheters in children in the thoracic region and how do they differ?
2. In connection with which clinical picture do we speak of the "white lung"?
3. You detect a cocard form (shooting target phenomenon, target sign) of the intestinal part in the sonography—what is your suspected diagnosis?
4. What imaging is recommended for medulloblastoma and what are typical signs?

Solutions ► Chap. 27

Testing

Contents

MC Questions and Answers

Mirja Wenker, Christel Vockelmann, and Martina Kahl-Scholz

Contents

© Springer-Verlag GmbH Germany, part of Springer Nature 2023
M. Kahl-Scholz, C. Vockelmann (eds.), *Basic Knowledge Radiology*,
https://doi.org/10.1007/978-3-662-66351-6_25

In this chapter, 20 multiple-choice questions on the contents of the book are asked for practice. When answering the questions, it is explained exactly why the answers are correct or not correct.

25.1 MC Questions

1. Which statement about fractures is false?
   A. A CT should be performed to assess the stability of a vertebral body fracture.
   B. X-rays to exclude fractures should always be taken in two planes, even if the fracture is already visible in the first plane.
   C. Basic diagnosis of the skull fracture is the X-ray image.
   D. On MRI, fresh fractures show up as bone edema, among other signs.

2. Which statement regarding bone tumors is correct?
   A. Bone tumors can always be clearly assigned radiologically.
   B. The "sunburst" phenomenon describes a reaction of the soft tissues adjacent to a bone tumor.
   C. Primary malignant bone tumors are common overall.
   D. Rapid growth of a tumor indicates high aggressiveness.

3. Which answer is correct? In aortic dissection
   A. The true lumen is usually greater than the false.
   B. MR angiography should be given priority over CT angiography because of the lack of radiation exposure.
   C. Stanford B dissection can involve the aortic valve.
   D. May lead to organ ischemia due to involvement of the aortic vascular outlets.

4. Which answer is incorrect? The Leriche syndrome
   A. Refers to an occlusion of the infrarenal aorta involving the aortic bifurcation.
   B. Can occur acutely due to an embolic event.
   C. Can occur in chronic form. Then the collaterals can be suitably depicted with Doppler sonography.
   D. Can only be visualized angiographically from the arm.

5. Which answer is correct? The MR cardiography
   A. Is the method of choice for imaging cardiomyopathies.
   B. Shows delayed CM accumulation in the affected area during myocardial infarction.
   C. Can only represent morphology.
   D. Always shows abnormal findings.

6. Which statement about contrast media is false?
   A. Negative contrast agents include carbon dioxide (CO_2), nitrogen dioxide (NO_2), inert gas, air, water, methyl cellulose, paraffin suspensions, and sorbitol (or mannitol).
   B. Double contrast refers to performing fluoroscopy with a positive CM and a negative CM.
   C. The edema signal in STIR or TIRM sequences is masked by CM administration, so these sequences must be performed before contrast administration.
   D. Sonography is performed with contrast media containing oil.

7. Which statement is correct? The Löffler infiltrate
   A. Shows up in extensive pneumonia.
   B. Can be detected apically in pulmonary edema.
   C. Is typical in ascaridosis.
   D. Can occur as a result of radiation.

8. Which statement about fractures of the head and neck is false?
   A. Fractures of the skull base are divided into frontobasal (frontal sinus posterior wall, ethmoid roof, sphenoid sinus) and petrous fractures.
   B. Decreased sensation in the supply area of the infraorbital nerve, motility disorders of the bulb and difficulties in opening the mouth may accompany a zygomatic fracture clinically.
   C. Imaging of the NNH allows assessment of the nasal skeleton, orbital walls, and shadowing/mirroring (hematosinus) in midface fractures. A lateral image allows co-assessment of the maxilla, ethmoid cells and sphenoid sinus.
   D. In the case of zygomatic fracture, blow-out fracture may occur.

9. The sentinel lymph node scintigraphy
   A. Is mainly used for prostate carcinoma.
   B. Is performed with99m Tc labeled colloids.
   C. Is used to detect inflamed lymph nodes.
   D. Can only be performed preoperatively.

10. Which statement about thyroid cancer is false?
    A. Carcinoma variants include differentiated carcinoma, undifferentiated carcinoma, C-cell carcinoma.
    B. In sonography especially an irregular, possibly destructive tumor structure should suggest a carcinoma.
    C. Percutaneous radiotherapy is a frequently used treatment option.
    D. Since pertechnetate is available as a generator product at any time and, as a pure gamma emitter with its short half-life of six hours, results in a low radiation exposure when washed out more quickly, it is used for routine diagnosis of the thyroid gland for scintigraphy.

11. Rank the different examinations in ascending order of radiation exposure.
    A. MR abdomen – CT skull – X-ray forefoot – X-ray thorax – CT abdomen
    B. X-ray forefoot – X-ray thorax – CT skull – MR abdomen – CT abdomen
    C. MR abdomen – X-ray forefoot – CT skull – X-ray thorax – CT abdomen
    D. MR abdomen – X-ray forefoot – X-ray thorax – CT skull – CT abdomen
    E. X-ray forefoot – X-ray thorax – MR abdomen – CT abdomen – CT skull

12. Which statements about imaging in acute stroke are correct?
    A. The native CT of the skull reliably allows the exclusion of a hemorrhage.
    B. Native CT of the skull also shows ischemic stroke in the early phase.
    C. MRI diffusion imaging is positive no earlier than six hours after stroke onset.
    D. CT angiography can detect intra- or extracranial vessel occlusion.

13. In the case of a subarachnoid hemorrhage (SAB)
    A. …you can't use contrast material because of the vasospasm.
    B. A CT angiography must be performed immediately, especially if the blood is distributed in the basal cisterns, in order to detect an aneurysm as the cause of the SAB at an early stage.
    C. A delay in vascular imaging must be avoided at all costs, as vascular spasms develop rapidly due to SAB and adequate vascular contrasting is no longer possible as a result.

D. In most cases of aneurysm rupture, rapid interventional therapy by means of aneurysm coiling is necessary.

E. The ruptured aneurysm is treated electively in the interval.

14. Which statements are correct? For premature infants
A. The insertion of a gastric tube is obligatory before a chest X-ray to exclude esophageal atresia.
B. Hard-beam technique is used to image the thorax.
C. An MRI is contraindicated because brain maturation has to be completed first.
D. A common condition is respiratory distress syndrome due to lung immaturity, which can be detected by reduced radiolucency of the lungs on X-ray.

15. Radiotherapy is considered in the treatment of the following tumors:
A. Rectal Cancer
B. Carcinoid of the small intestine
C. Esophageal Cancer
D. Breast Cancer

16. Liver metastases
A. Can't be differentiated sonographically.
B. Can always be reliably distinguished from cysts on CT.
C. Can be treated with transarterial chemoembolization due to the leading arterial supply.
D. Can be very well delineated in primovist MRI of the liver.
E. Are not detectable in PET-CT due to the diffuse tracer uptake of the liver tissue.

17. If you suspect urolithiasis, you should
A. Do an intravenous pyelography.
B. ...and get a CT urography.
C. To avoid unnecessary loss of time, directly perform a low-dose CT without prior sonography or laboratory diagnosis of the urine status.

D. A renal scintigraphy, since a functional impairment of the kidney is to be assumed.

18. For the clarification of hyperprolactinemia
A. The target acquisition of the sella turcica in the lateral beam path is necessary.
B. A routine MRI of the skull is performed.
C. A contrast CT of the skull is sufficient, since a macroadenoma can be assumed.
D. A fine-layered examination of the pituitary gland with a contrast medium is necessary.

19. A Hodgkin's disease
A. Is another term for tuberculosis, named after the discoverer of Mycobacterium tuberculosis.
B. Is a malignant lymphoma that responds very well to combined radio-chemotherapy.
C. Can't be detected on PET-CT.
D. Can be confirmed without histological confirmation with typical imaging.

20. The following statements are correct:
A. The effective dose is expressed in sieverts (Sv) and is a measure of the biological effect of the radiation, since the parts of the body exposed to the radiation are included in the calculation.
B. The effective dose can be used to compare different radiation exposures such as a skeletal scintigraphy and a skeletal CT.
C. When procedural instructions for CT examinations have been established, it is not necessary to record the radiation exposure of the examination for each patient.
D. The incident dose is always equal to the surface dose.

25.2 **MC Responses**

1. **C is incorrect**, X-rays to detect a skull fracture are obsolete nowadays, CT scans are taken instead. Re A: Assessment of the posterior edge on CT for stability assessment. Re B: Fractures can be dislocated in one plane or deviated from the axis.

2. **D is correct**. A: Often several differential diagnoses are possible, ultimately clarifying is the histology. B: The sunburst phenomenon describes a reaction of the periosteum. C: Primary malignant bone tumors account for only 1% (adults) to 5% (children) of all tumor diseases.

3. **Answer D is correct**, a supply of aortic vascular outlets from the false lumen may result in absent or inferior perfusion of organs. A: The true lumen is usually smaller than the false one. B: Because of the urgency of rapid diagnosis, CTA should be given priority. C: Aortic valve involvement may occur with Stanford A dissections.

4. Answer C is wrong. Sonographically, the collaterals can usually be depicted only inadequately, CT and MRI are better suited.

5. Answer B is correct. A: Echocardiography is the method of choice because it is inexpensive and available everywhere. However, cardio-MRI is increasingly being used for clarification. C: The advantage of cardio-MRI is that it can image not only morphology but also cardiac function. D: Just like echocardiography, cardio-MRI may be unremarkable in myocarditis.

6. Answer D is incorrect. Contrast media containing oil are used in myelography, for example, and gas-filled microbubbles are used in sonography. The imaging of the contrast agent microbubbles in diagnostic sonography is based on excitation of the microbubbles in the sound field, whereby the microbubbles start to oscillate (oscillation).

7. Answer C is correct. In ascaridosis (roundworm infestation with Ascaris lumbricoides), X-rays show confluent spot shadows that "migrate" across the lungs. This migration is also known as Löffler's infiltrate (which can also occur with some medications such as penicillin). It is present when the infiltrate is no longer detectable after a maximum of 10 days, eosinophilia is present and relatively minor (pulmonary) symptoms are present.

8. Answer D is incorrect. In the case of an orbital fracture (not a zygomatic fracture), if the force is applied directly to the eye, a so-called blow-out fracture can occur, in which the orbital floor fractures and orbital contents can enter the maxillary sinus.

9. Answer B is correct. To visualize the SLN, 99mTc labeled colloids with a particle size of approximately 20–100 nm are injected. These are recognized by the lymphatic system as foreign bodies and are removed. The applied amount of activity must be so high that the lymph node can be found intraoperatively with an appropriate measuring probe.

10. Answer C is incorrect. In thyroid carcinoma, percutaneous radiotherapy is used only in a small group of high-risk patients, when surgery and radioiodine therapy have failed to achieve complete tumor cell destruction, in recurrence or in the palliative situation of skeletal metastases with risk of fracture, brain metastases as well as upper influence congestion.

11. **Answer D is correct.** MRI is a procedure without radiation exposure. X-ray images require very little radiation in the peripheral skeleton, and comparatively little radiation is also required in

Table 25.1 Radiation exposures

	Approximate radiation exposure
X-ray extremities	0.01 mSv
X-ray thorax	0.1 mSv
X-ray abdomen	0.7 mSv
X-ray lumbar spine two levels	1.1 mSv
CT skull	2–3 mSv
CT thorax	1–7 mSv
CT abdomen	8–16 mSv

the thorax because of the high radiation transparency of the lungs (■ Table 25.1). CT examinations require considerably more radiation, although the skull is associated with lower radiation exposure due to its smaller volume and less radiation-sensitive organs.

12. **Answer A and B are correct.** Diffusion imaging on MRI detects cytotoxic edema and thus the infarct area after only a few minutes. Native CT can only detect the infarct after a few hours.

13. **Answer A and E are incorrect. In** the case of a ruptured aneurysm, there is always a risk of recurrent hemorrhage, so that rapid diagnosis and therapy must be performed. Intracranial hemorrhage is not a contraindication for contrast administration.

14. Answer A and D are correct. An MRI is contraindicated only in the first trimester of pregnancy, as there is no evidence yet to what extent the strong magnetic field can harm the fetus. From the second trimester onwards, and thus also in premature babies, an MRI can be performed. X-rays of the thorax are performed in adults using the hard-beam technique to radiate through the ribs. In children, tube voltages adapted to the

body size or weight are used; the hard beam technique would lead to an absolutely overexposed image in premature babies.

15. **Answer B is incorrect.** The small intestine is very sensitive to radiation and, in addition, due to its high motility, is not always in exactly the same place in the body, so that exact therapy planning is not possible. In the case of rectal and oesophageal carcinoma, radiotherapy is used neoadjuvantly before surgical therapy, usually in combination with chemotherapy. In breast carcinoma, radiotherapy is given after breast-conserving therapy in order to reduce the risk of local recurrence.

16. B, C and D are correct. Primovist is a liver-specific contrast agent that is not absorbed by tumor-altered liver cells, in contrast to healthy liver tissue. Sonographically, metastases can usually be delineated in an echo-rich round shape. Necrotically decaying metastases or very small metastases cannot be reliably distinguished from cysts on CT; contrast sonography or MRI with primovist can then be used for further examination. If the metastases show sufficient storage of FDG depending on the primary tumor, liver metastases can be detected very well on PET-CT.

17. **Answer C is correct.** You should perform a low-dose CT of the urinary tract after prior sonography and laboratory diagnosis of urine status. Sonography is mandatory as primary imaging to confirm the suspected diagnosis of urolithiasis and to make differential diagnoses such as diverticulitis or appendicitis less likely.

18. **Answer D is correct.** Hyperprolactinemia raises the possibility of a pituitary adenoma, which is often a few mm in size. Therefore, a fine-slice targeted MRI scan of the pituitary gland with a contrast agent dynamic range is required. In the early contrast phases, the pitu-

itary gland already accumulates the contrast agent, and the adenoma stores the contrast agent with a slight delay. A conventional image of the sella turcica is obsolete.

19. Only answer B is correct. PET-CT is highly sensitive in the staging of lymphomas. Histological confirmation is essential for precise differentiation. As a rule, an entire lymph node is removed for this purpose if a lymph node that is easily accessible by surgery is affected. Tuberculosis is also called Koch's disease, named after Robert Koch.

20. **Statements A and B are correct**. Statements C and D are incorrect. For each examination with a radiation exposure, the individual value applied to patient xy must be stated. The effective dose does not have to be calculated, but e.g. for X-ray examinations the dose area product and for computer tomography the dose length product of the respective examination are documented. The incident dose is the dose which can be measured "free air" without scattering bodies. The surface dose is the dose that occurs on the patient's skin. Here, in addition to the incident dose, there is also the dose component that is scattered back to the surface in the patient.

Clinical Cases

Mirja Wenker, Christel Vockelmann and Martina Kahl-Scholz

Contents

© Springer-Verlag GmbH Germany, part of Springer Nature 2023
M. Kahl-Scholz, C. Vockelmann (eds.), *Basic Knowledge Radiology*,
https://doi.org/10.1007/978-3-662-66351-6_26

The following chapter presents typical cases that can occur in practice. Accompanying questions are asked, which serve to apply what has been learned.

26.1 Pulmonary Embolism or …

Mrs. Walter presents to the emergency department with pain at mid-thoracic level. With concomitant dyspnoea, a CT is initially performed to rule out pulmonary embolism. This is not confirmed, but the sagittal reconstruction shows a marked decrease in the height of the 6th spinal cord. The base plate of the 6th spinal cord and the cover plate of the 7th spinal cord are clearly out of focus and appear to be "pitted", and the intervertebral space is narrowed. In the meantime, the laboratory results are also available, which show an increase in the inflammation parameters.

 1. What is your tentative diagnosis?
2. How can the diagnosis be further clarified?

✅ 1. Your suspicion is spondylodiscitis.
2. Complementary MRI scans should be performed as a means of choice for visualizing spondylodiscitis; here, evidence of edema in the vertebral bodies and the intervertebral disc as well as of contrast enhancement can be obtained. MRI is also the most reliable way to demonstrate epidural abscessation, which may require neurosurgical intervention.

26.2 Swollen Hands

Mr. Menert presents to his family doctor. The 47-year-old complains of flu-like symptoms that have been present for several weeks. In addition, he has had swelling of the hands for several days. He finds it difficult to work on the computer at a large insurance company, especially in the morning, because his fingers are very stiff. In the course of the day the work becomes easier again.

❓ 1. What is your tentative diagnosis?
2. Which findings in the X-ray are typical?

✅ 1. They suspect rheumatoid arthritis.
2. Typical symptoms are: symmetrical bilateral involvement, especially of the finger and toe joints, soft tissue swelling, osteoporosis near the joint, transient joint space widening due to joint effusion and proliferation of the synovium, later joint space narrowing, erosions, subchondral cysts, ulnar deviation of the fingers, buttonhole and swan-neck deformity of the fingers. The final state is destruction of the joint with ankylosis.

26.3 Pain in the Lower Leg

Mr. Müller, 65 years old, presents to the emergency department with acute onset of pain of the right lower leg. Trauma is not remembered. The patient reports that he has already had a stent inserted in the left common iliac artery and the right internal iliac artery due to an arterial vein disease. Furthermore, the patient is known to have hypertension. On physical examination, the right lower leg is cold and white discolored. The inguinal pulse is palpable, the popliteal pulse is not.

 1. What's your tentative diagnosis?
2. What imaging techniques can confirm this diagnosis?
3. Which radiological therapy methods are possible?

✅ 1. Your suspicion is acute arterial occlusion.

2. Other imaging modalities would be: Sonography: lack of flow, CTA/MRA/DSA: lack of contrast distal to the occlusion, if possible CTA before DSA for treatment planning.

3. DSA with an attempt at lysis or thrombectomy is an option. If paresthesias and paresis are already present, surgical thrombectomy must be considered as an alternative, depending on the localization, since revascularization must then be achieved within a maximum of six hours.

26.4 Chest Pain and Circulatory Problems

Mrs. Tewes is not feeling well at all. This morning she suddenly got chest pains that radiate to her back. She also feels dizzy and has difficulty forming sentences. She has a known history of PAOD.

❓ 1. What is your tentative diagnosis?
2. What imaging techniques can confirm this diagnosis?

✅ 1. They suspect aortic dissection involving the supra aortic vascular branches with neurological symptoms.
2. Immediate CT angiography must be performed to assess the extent of dissection and involvement of the outgoing arteries, exclusion of other pathologies. The situation is life-threatening!

26.5 A Swollen Leg

Mr. Franke presents to the general practitioner's office. He reports that his left leg has been noticeably swollen for several days. In addition, his calf hurts at times. On physical examination, the left leg is clearly swollen

and slightly reddened compared to the side. When pressing on the calf and on the sole of the foot, the patient clearly states pain. The patient has a history of renal insufficiency and epilepsy.

❓ 1. What is your tentative diagnosis?
2. What is the further procedure?
3. What imaging techniques can confirm the diagnosis?

✅ 1. They suspect deep vein thrombosis.
2. First, the clinical scores for the probability of DVT are determined.
3. Sonography: lack of compressibility of the veins, lack of flow signal, CTA and phlebography, among others, not indicated in renal insufficiency.

26.6 Hematuria

Mr. Steinemann is 37 years old and apart from a discrete hypertension, for which, however, according to his family doctor he does not have to take any medication, he has no previous illnesses. This afternoon he had his wife drive him to the central outpatient clinic after he developed severe pains in the left flank, some of which also extend into the lower abdomen. There is intermittent improvement in between, but overall this discomfort has been going on for about two hours. Nausea and vomiting are denied. In the clinical examination—which is difficult because of the patient's bent posture due to pain—the surgical colleague on duty, Dr. Immerda, finds an overall soft abdomen without defensive tension, but there is a knocking pain in the left renal bed. Dr. Immerda orders a laboratory examination of blood and urine and performs an ultrasound of Mr. Steinemann's abdomen. Here he notices a dilated renal pelvis. The urine status, which has been evaluated in the meantime, also shows hematuria. Mr. Immerda picks up the phone and calls the radiologist on duty in order to initiate a clarification of the cause.

❓ 1. Given the above history, what is the most likely differential diagnosis?
2. What are the possible complications?
3. What diagnostic methods are available?

✅ 1. The colicky symptoms and hematuria are indicative of urolithiasis.
2. A frequent complication is urinary retention. This often leads to accompanying inflammatory reactions of the obstructed kidney. Injuries in the course of the ureter can later lead to scarred strictures. In the case of large occluding stones (>5 mm) (and forced diuresis), the congestion can lead to a rupture of the calyx. To assess the risk, imaging is necessary to provide information about stone size and localization.
3. The method of choice is a low-dose CT of the abdomen, as it provides a significantly higher information gain with a low radiation exposure (approximately two X-ray images of the abdomen).

examination the internist on duty notes a pressure pain over the bladder. In addition, the renal bearings are throbbing.

In the meantime, the first laboratory results are back: leukocytes and CRP are elevated. In the urine erythrocytes, leukocytes and nitrite have been detected.

The colleague wants to "play it safe" and asks for an ultrasound of the abdomen.

❓ 1. Do you already have a suspected diagnosis?
2. Why does it make sense to do an ultrasound? What are the complications?

✅ 1. Acute pyelonephritis is suspected in the context of an ascending urinary tract infection.
2. If a urinary tract infection, which is usually uncomplicated in a young woman, leads to an inflammation of the renal pelvis, this may be due to a disturbed urine outflow with corresponding urinary stasis. In addition, perinephritic abscesses may occur in the course of renal pelvic inflammation, which may require specific treatment and can be detected sonographically.

26.7 Frequent Urination

Mrs. Honeymoon is currently on her honeymoon in Europe with her newlywed spouse. Unfortunately, Mr. and Mrs. Honeymoon have to interrupt their trip for a stay in the central emergency room. The newlyweds are visibly unwell: she has a fever of 39.8 °C, back pain and she is vomiting several times. Until yesterday everything had been wonderful, they had breakfast in a small café in Strasbourg and then drove on towards Germany. Yesterday evening she already felt unwell. When asked, the husband remembers that they had to stop frequently to urinate during the journey. During the clinical

26.8 Riding Accident

Clarissa fell off her horse and has been complaining of weakness and stomach pains ever since. As a precaution, her parents take her to the outpatient clinic of the nearest hospital. There Dr. Immerda takes over the patient. The blood pressure is 110/90 mmHg, the heart rate 96/min. The doctor does an ultrasound right in the outpatient clinic. He sees free fluid in the abdomen and the right kidney looks "funny". He is not sure about the other organs. Clarissa continues to feel bad, her blood pressure is slowly dropping and her rate continues to rise. Dr. Immerda calls and asks for a CT—today he sounds very nervous on the phone. He has already alerted his senior physician on background duty.

❓ 1. According to this history, what injuries are to be expected?
2. In your opinion, is a CT indicated?
3. Do you need contrast media? If so, which contrast agent phases make sense?
4. What questions need to be answered before the examination?

✅ 1. A fall from a horse can, of course, result in a variety of internal and external injuries. Since the young patient landed on the grassy ground, she may have been spared fractures. The complaints and examination findings suggest an injury to an internal organ of the right flank. The kidney and, of course, the liver are possible candidates.
2. Yes, even if the patient is young and one would like to avoid radiation exposure, the examination findings seem to indicate an injury to abdominal organs that requires immediate treatment. On the one hand, the extent of the presumed kidney injury and further treatment can be assessed, and on the other hand, dangerous concomitant injuries, e.g. of the liver, the large abdominal vessels or the spinal column, can also be recorded.
3. You need contrast medium: on the one hand, to assess the feeding vessels, which may also be injured. After administration of contrast medium, the renal and hepatic parenchyma can be better assessed and any subcapsular hematoma can be clearly differentiated. In addition, it may be possible to detect the source of a hemorrhage by contrast leakage into the tissue. In order to detect injuries of the urinary

tract, it may make sense to prepare a urographic contrast medium phase.
4. In young women of childbearing age, pregnancy should normally always be ruled out. Allergies and renal dysfunction should also be clarified before a contrast agent is administered. In this particular case, the falling blood pressure and rising heart rate indicate a life-threatening situation that does not permit any delay. Only an anaphylactic reaction to contrast administration should stop you now.

26.9 Laceration to the Forehead

Mrs. Liesegang, a 69-year-old spry pensioner, has had to take blood-thinning medication for several years. Dr. Peters, her family doctor, has therefore prescribed her Marcumar. Mrs. Liesegang takes the weekly blood checks and the tablet intake seriously, the values are therefore mostly in the target range with an INR of 2–2.5. This morning Mrs. Liesegang tripped over the carpet on her way to the kitchen and sustained a laceration to her forehead. In addition, she has had a slight headache since then and therefore goes to the hospital. There, the head laceration is treated by the accident surgery resident Dr. Bruch. She also sends Ms. Liesegang for a CT scan to check for bleeding.

❓ 1. What is the expected bleeding after a fall in elderly patients?
2. How do you distinguish an epidural from a subdural hemorrhage?
3. What does the term "ICB loco typico" mean as opposed to atypical intracerebral hemorrhage?
4. Name causes of intracerebral hemorrhage.

✅ 1. V. a. Subdural hematoma.
2. The distinction is possible on the basis of shape and cranial outline.

3. The term describes hypertensive bleeding in contrast to atypical bleeding in which, for example, a tumor or vascular malformation is the cause.
4. Causes are:
   (a) Arteriovenous malformations
   (b) Cavernomas
   (c) Intracerebral tumors or metastases
   (d) Sinus vein thrombosis (bleeding in the vicinity of the thrombosed sinus).

26.10 Persistent Headache

Mr. Meyer, 58 years old, has had constant headaches for a few weeks. Until now he has always been healthy and maintains a very healthy lifestyle with lots of sport. He is very busy at work at the moment, so he initially blames the pain on stress. Now, however, he has noticed a twitching in his left arm that has stopped but still worries him. He goes to his family doctor, Dr. Hinnerk. He examines him thoroughly, also looking at the back of his eyes. He then refers Mr. Meyer for an MRI because of the headache. As Dr. Hinnerk is worried about the symptoms, he calls the radiologist Dr. Leucht to get the appointment for the examination that week.

Dr. Leucht finds a 5 cm lesion right parietal in the cerebrum, which shows T2-weighted hyperintensity with finger-shaped extension into the gyri. After contrast administration a garland-shaped enhancement is seen.

 1. What are Dr. Hinnerk's findings at the back of the eye?
2. How is the twitching of the left arm to be evaluated?
3. What type of contrast agent is used in MRI?
4. What's Dr. Leucht's diagnosis?
5. What are the treatment options for Mr. Meyer?

1. The reflection of the ocular fundus shows papilledema.
2. Twitching of the left arm is the manifestation of an epileptic seizure, often the first symptom of brain tumors.
3. MRI uses contrast medium containing gadolinium, which leads to a shortening of the T1 relaxation time.
4. The most likely diagnosis is glioblastoma, which is a highly malignant astrocytoma.
5. Treatment options include surgery with supplemental local chemotherapy, if necessary, and radiation therapy.

Solutions

Mirja Wenker, Martina Kahl-Scholz, and Christel Vockelmann

© Springer-Verlag GmbH Germany, part of Springer Nature 2023
M. Kahl-Scholz, C. Vockelmann (eds.), *Basic Knowledge Radiology*,
https://doi.org/10.1007/978-3-662-66351-6_27

In this chapter you will find the solutions to the practice questions asked in each chapter.

■ **Chapter 1**

1. **Photoelectric effect**: If photon radiation hits matter, the entire energy can be transferred to an electron of the atomic shell (photoabsorption). The shell electron is either raised to a shell of higher energy (excitation) or knocked out of the atomic shell (ionization). The latter occurs when the energy of the photon exceeds the binding energy of the electron to the nucleus. The remaining energy is transferred to the electron (photoelectron) as kinetic energy. The photoelectric effect is the basis of imaging in diagnostic radiology, which works mainly in the energy range up to 100 keV. The radiation emitted by the X-ray tube is attenuated differently by tissues of different density, such as bone, soft tissue, fat or connective tissue, so that the resulting radiation image has different gray scales depending on the attenuation. **Compton scattering:** In the so-called Compton effect, the photon emits only part of its energy to the shell electron of an outer shell and is scattered with its residual energy in a different direction. Secondary electrons of lower energy are emitted in lateral direction, those of higher energy in forward direction. Scattered photons lead to image degradation in radiological, diagnostic and nuclear medical imaging techniques. Technical aids, such as a scattering grid consisting of lead lamellae in radiological diagnostics or the exclusion of low-energy scattered photons by placing an appropriate energy window in nuclear medicine, can minimize the impact of scattering effects. **Pair formation**: At high photon energies above 1022 keV, the so-called pair formation effect occurs. Here the interaction does not take place in the shell but in the strong electric field of the atomic nucleus. Near the nucleus, the photon can form

an electron-positron pair, consisting of a negatively charged electron and a positively charged positron. The atomic nucleus remains unchanged. Here, in contrast to the pair annihilation, a pair is formed which, however, emits two annihilation quanta of 511 keV each with one electron of the absorber. The energy release via the pair formation effect plays an essential role in radiation therapy when ultra-hard photons are used.

2. **Incident dose:** This describes the dose in Gy that is measured "free air" without stray bodies. By scattering bodies are meant phantoms or also patients, which would lead to a scattering of the radiation. The incident dose depends on the focal distance, energy (in X-rays kV and filter) and the dose rate. The field size has only little influence. **Surface dose: In** addition to the incident dose, the backscatter from the irradiated object, e.g. the patient, is added to the surface dose. On the entrance side, the backscatter can be up to 50%. The backscattering is strongly dependent on the field size. In radiotherapy, the surface dose on the exit side is also important, since this must be taken into account in the case of opposing fields. More about this later. **Depth dose**: The depth dose describes the dose at a certain body depth, measured from the irradiation surface. The relative depth dose indicates the ratio of a depth dose to the dose maximum in percent. The depth dose is particularly important in radiation therapy, since here a specific dose at a specific location in the body, e.g. a lung tumor, is targeted for therapeutic success. At the same time, surrounding healthy tissue should of course not be damaged.

3. **X-ray deceleration radiation is** produced by the deceleration of electrons at the nucleus into which they cannot penetrate. Some electrons release radiation as soon as they hit the anode. Others penetrate deeper into the electron material,

give off part of their energy and produce X-rays only afterwards. As a result, the electrons produce X-rays with different wavelengths. How much X-ray radiation is released depends on how strongly the electron is decelerated. The immediately produced X-ray deceleration radiation has a smaller wavelength than the radiation produced by the initially decelerated electrons. **Characteristic X-ray radiation is** produced in addition to the X-ray deceleration radiation and is a so-called line spectrum, which depends exclusively on the anode material. It is therefore characteristic for this material.

4. Since the **Linear Energy Transfer** (LE) serves rather the physical consideration of the radiation effect, there is also the term **Relative Biological Effectiveness (RBE)**. It is used, among other things, to subdivide the health hazard posed by the various types of radiation. In this context, the effects that can be observed with different types of radiation when the same dose is administered in grays are put in relation to each other.

5. **Stochastic radiation effect**: With regard to the effect of ionizing radiation, each individual X-ray quantum can cause an undesirable, damaging event in the organism. The probability of this event depends on how many radiation quanta strike the organism. Thus, the highest commandment of radiation protection is derived from the stochastic radiation effect: "As Low As Reasonably Achievable" (ALARA principle)—one may only administer as little radiation as absolutely necessary, since there is no threshold dose for a certain radiation damage. **Deterministic Radiation Effect:** This term means something like "delineation" or "determination". In the context of radiation exposure, it is therefore possible to determine the resulting damage to a tissue. It is known, for example, after how much radiation the healthy skin reacts with a skin reaction (burn).

Accordingly, there is a threshold dose. This is defined for each tissue. From the point of view of radiation protection, deterministic damage must not occur. From the point of view of therapy, however, it is precisely this damage that is "desired", since research results can prove when the threshold dose of a tumor is also reached. In radiation therapy, deterministic damage to malignant tumors is specifically set.

- Chapter 2

1. An X-ray **system** always consists of the following components: an X-ray source that generates the radiation, an X-ray generator that supplies the X-ray source with high voltage, an X-ray application device that is used to position the patient, and an X-ray image converter (X-ray film, detector, …).

2. While overexposure, i.e. too much radiation, does not harm the quality of the image, an **underexposed shot** results in an image that shows much less detail. This phenomenon is also called image noise.

3. $V = B/G = b/g$. In X-ray imaging, the distance g is called the **focus-object distance** and the distance b is called the focus-film distance (FFA). The distance $B–G$ is called **object-film distance** (OFA). The variable V indicates the magnification of the image.

4. **Shielding:** When an X-ray is taken, the patient must of course be exposed to the X-rays. However, if possible, all parts of the body that are not being examined should be shielded from the radiation. Most aids for this purpose are made of lead or lead compounds ("lead rubber"). Depending on the organ being examined, the patient can be protected in various ways. In particular, the organs that are sensitive to radiation should be protected. First of all, these are the gonads, i.e. the ovaries in women and the testes in men. However, the small intestine and the hematopoietic tissue are also particularly

sensitive to radiation. Ideally, the patient should always wear a lead apron or a lead coat when the extremities are imaged. Infants can also be completely wrapped in so-called radiation protection wraps. For images of the chest area, a half apron (gonadal protection apron) or a radiation protection skirt must always be worn to protect the lower half of the body from radiation. When taking images of the pelvis or hip, it is not possible to put on a half apron, as this would cover the bone. There are special lead covers for these shots, depending on gender. **Blending in**: One of the most effective methods of minimizing X-ray radiation is to blend in the radiation field. Thus, by blending in, you not only protect the patient, but you also get a better quality x-ray. **Additional filters/compensating filters**: Filters were mentioned at the beginning of this chapter. These also contribute to the radiation protection of the patient. The filters in the depth diaphragm harden the rays so that the radiation that does not contribute to the image formation does not reach the patient in the first place. **Radiation quality**: The dose to the patient can also be minimized by changing the radiation quality. Whereas a few years ago, for example, the fingers were x-rayed with a voltage of 44 kV, the Medical Association now prescribes a voltage of at least 50 kV. This makes it easier for the rays to pass through the bones and the current intensity can be reduced. With the introduction of digital imaging techniques, the lower contrast that results from the higher voltage can be increased again by suitable image processing.

5. A digital image consists of many individual pixels. These are arranged in rows and columns, this arrangement is then called a **pixel matrix** or **matrix** for short. Depending on the system, an X-ray image consists of between 1024 × 1024 and 4096 × 4096 pixels. One speaks of a 1024 matrix or a 4096 matrix.

■ Chapter 3

1. The **Heel effect** refers to the anode-side dose drop.
2. Due to the **compression of the breast,** the tissue is distributed homogeneously both thoracic and mammillary and can thus be assessed more precisely.
3. In **magnification mammography**, the distance between the breast and the image receiver is increased. Due to the imaging laws, this achieves an enlargement of the structures, e.g. in order to better recognize the shape of microcalcifications, even if the geometric blurring becomes somewhat greater. In addition, the grid can be dispensed with for the magnification image, since the scattered radiation is already too far attenuated and no longer reaches the image receiver.

■ Chapter 5

1. Answers:
   (a) Setting fractures,
   (b) Examinations of the gastrointestinal tract and other body cavities (e.g. the gall bladder) using contrast media,
   (c) Examinations of vessels also with contrast media,
   (d) Placement of probes or drains in the body,
   (e) Consideration of real-time processes in the study of the swallowing act and valvular activity.
2. By the function "**Last-Image-Hold (LIH)**" the last image remains on the monitor, can be stored digitally and thus replace an additional X-ray.
3. The **image receiver** and the **X-ray tube** are connected by a **semicircular rail,** which is anchored to the rest of the system by means of a holding module. This holding module can rotate and can also be moved so that the tube can move sideways along the patient (= images in all spatial directions are possible).
4. Digital subtraction angiography **(DSA)** is an application used primarily for the visualisation of vessels using contrast media.

5. These are used in the **seldinger technique**. With them (especially balloons and stents), the wire is only guided through a second lumen of the catheter for the first 20–30 cm, after which it runs freely parallel to the catheter. In addition to the shorter wires, this also allows a faster catheter change, but the guidance of the catheter is somewhat worse, since the wire reinforcement is only given at the catheter tip.

■ Chapter 6

1. Motion artifact, pulsation artifact, metal artifact, partial volume effect, hardening artifact, measurement field overrun, photon starvation artifact, ring artifact, line artifact.

2. In sequential CT examinations, one slice is acquired per rotation, after which the table is advanced before the next examination section is acquired. In **spiral CT**, the table is moved continuously, the raw data is acquired as a helix and an axial image is calculated from this.

3. **Adaptive Array Detector** and **Fixed Array Detector**. In the "Adaptive Array Detector" the detector chambers become wider and wider towards the periphery. This leads to the possibility of interconnecting individual elements and rows with the option of different layer thicknesses. With the "Fixed Array Detector" there are fixed sizes of detector elements per detector row. By selecting certain detector rows, the layer thickness can be determined.

■ Chapter 7

1. With a targeted look at a sure aqueous-filled structure in the image (e.g., CSF or bladder). If the fluid is brightly imaged, the image is **T2-weighted**. If the fluid is dark, the image is **T1-weighted**.

2. A T2 weighting with fat saturation—here fluid—i.e. also an oedema is mapped hyperintensely. The fat saturation helps to distinguish the edema from the fat, which is also hyperintense in T2 weighting.

3. E.g. **intracranial aneurysm clips, pacemakers/ICDs, neurostimulators, insulin pumps, bladder catheters with temperature probes** (there are also MR-compatible materials among the implants mentioned—their suitability must be checked in advance). But also shrapnel or claustrophobia (if there is no alternative examination possibility, sedation of the patient may be necessary).

4. It depends on the region of examination. Smaller arterial vessels (e.g. intracranial) can be imaged with **TOF angiography**. Slow-flow vessels (e.g. sinus veins) can be imaged with **phase-contrast angiography**.

5. In addition to the immediate life-saving measures such as emergency call and CPR, you must now also pay attention to the safety of patients and staff: The patient must be out of the exam room as soon as possible, and if possible, a person should stand guard outside the door for as long as possible. The resuscitation team or paramedics may not appreciate the dangers of the device. If they instinctively run to the patient immediately, emergency cases and oxygen cylinders brought into the examination room become life-threatening projectiles.

■ Chapter 8

1. The **piezo effect** is caused by the contraction and elongation—i.e. compression and expansion—of the crystal during ultrasound. An applied external electrical voltage causes the emission of vibrations, i.e. sound waves (=sound wave emission). If the sound waves encounter an impedance jump (wave resistance) on their way, e.g. at the border between fatty tissue and water, they are reflected and received as an echo or resonance on the quartz crystal. The resulting sound pressure deforms the crystal and the electrical charge is shifted. This piezo effect creates a measurable electrical voltage, which is recorded by the connected electronics and displayed as an image.

2. **A-mode**: The A-mode is the oldest method. "A" stands for amplitude modulation. Today, the method is still used for distance determination in ENT, ophthalmology and neurology. In the early days, before the development of computer tomography, this method was used, for example, to detect a midline shift in a brain tumor. **M-mode**: With the M-mode (from English "motion") the temporal behavior of a tissue can be imaged. It is used in particular in cardiology. A typical example is the imaging of the movement of a heart valve or the myocardium. **B-mode**: The B-mode (English "brightness") is the most frequently used procedure. In the 2D image, the various image points are recorded with different brightness grey dots, depending on the strength of the reflected signal.

3. Blood flow toward the transducer is coded red; blood flowing away from the transducer is coded blue. Faster blood flow is shown lighter than slower flow. In the image on the right, a corresponding coding is shown with an indication of the measured flow velocity.

4. A special form is the so-called **pocket Doppler**, in which the ultrasound probe looks like a thick pen. It is mainly used in vascular diagnostics to measure occlusion pressure.

5. Ultrasound diagnostics is the **primary diagnostic** imaging for abdominal complaints, vascular diseases and for the diagnosis of cardiac function.

- Chapter 9
1. **X-ray contrast agents** are divided into two major groups:
   (a) Substances with lower density than the environment to be imaged = negative contrast media (gases, water, methyl cellulose, sorbitol)
   (b) Substances with a higher density than the environment to be depicted = positive contrast media (differentiation into water-soluble, water-insoluble and oil-containing)

(c) The accumulation of gadolinium in a tissue depends on the general condition of the patient (fever), the waiting time after the injection and the dose ("much helps much"). The contrast medium may "behave differently" in a patient with fever than in patients without fever. This can play a role in the findings.

2. **Double contrast** is the performance of fluoroscopy with a positive CM (usually barium) and a negative CM (e.g. cellulose, water, CO_2).

3. Response:
   (a) Absolute contraindications
       - Severe kidney dysfunction not previously requiring dialysis
       - Manifest hyperthyroidism
       - Sensitivity to iodine-containing KM
       - Certain thyroid carcinomas
   (b) Relative contraindications
       - Heart failure
       - Severe hepatic dysfunction
       - Hematological diseases (Waldenström's disease)

4. 1% CM is found in the **mother's milk**. That this amount has a harmful effect on the infant has not yet been proven. The current recommendation does not call for any special measures. Nevertheless, a 24-hour breastfeeding break can be considered.

- Chapter 10
1. **IMRT:** IMRT (Intensity Modulated Radiotherapy) is a further developed method of conformal irradiation. During irradiation, the multileaf lamellae move across the irradiation field. This is done either in sliding-window technique, the irradiation runs while the MLC move, or in step-and-shoot technique, the irradiation is interrupted during the movement of the MLC. This allows the dose to be varied from point to point. In this way, tumors can be irradiated with a high dose and sensitive

organs that are in close proximity can be spared more effectively because the reduced dose can be shaped more precisely to the organ contour. The disadvantage of this method is the dose load for healthy tissue. **VMAT**: Volumetric Modulated Arc Therapy (VMAT) is a further development of the IMRT technique: The number of small dose-modulated fields increases, which are irradiated in many different gantry positions. For this purpose, the gantry no longer remains stationary at the individual positions, but moves in a circle or semicircle. This significantly shortens the irradiation time.

2. This refers to **radiotherapy** that is **applied in** a **spatially targeted and highly precise manner.** The method was developed for brain tumors, but is now also used in the rest of the body as body stereotaxy, e.g. for primary tumors and metastases in the lungs and liver, as long as the tumor diameter is not larger than 3 cm.

3. **Intracavitary:** The classic indication for intracavitary brachytherapy is vaginal application for irradiation of the vaginal stump in corpus carcinoma. However, it is also possible for small superficial carcinomas in the esophagus or other cavities. **Interstitial:** The radionuclide is introduced into the tissue either temporarily or permanently. The procedure always involves surgery and anesthesia. Under ultrasound control, the radiation sources made of ^{125}iodine (= seeds) are introduced via a hollow needle and remain in the tissue, e.g. in the prostate in the case of carcinoma detection. Depending on the size of the prostate, their number is between 80 and >100, their dose rate is low (Low Dose Rate, LDR, <1 Gy/h), the half-life is 60 days. **Contact therapy:** Contact therapy is rarely performed because the area to be irradiated must be small and superficial. In addition, this very special method is only used to treat tumors that cannot be irradiated in any other way, e.g. with electrons or con-

ventional X-ray therapy, and for which surgery is not an option because the risk of anesthesia is too high or functional impairment, e.g. blindness, is to be expected.

4. The **boost** is applied to a macroscopic tumor or to an area where there is an increased risk of recurrence, e.g. at the site where surgery could only just be resected or not in healthy tissue. Percutaneously, it is applied in several sessions; with interstitial or intracavitary brachytherapy, it is occasionally applied as a single application. It is possible to perform the boost sequentially, i.e. following the radiation series, or during the radiation series either concomitantly or as a simultaneously integrated boost (SIB).

5. **Tumor volume** (GTV = Gross Tumor Volume): GTV includes the macroscopic tumor, be it the primary tumor, be it lymph node metastases or distant metastases. Clinical Tumor **Volume** (CTV): The CTV encompasses the area of macroscopic tumor (GTV) and the region where tumor cells may still be scattered. Planning Target **Volume** (PTV): The planning target volume (PTV) includes the CTV and is expanded with respect to changes that may occur during radiation. These include: Positioning inaccuracies by the MTRA, patient restlessness, organ movements due to breathing, peristalsis (wave movement of the intestine), different filling states of the bladder and rectum, but also weight gain or loss.

■ Chapter 11

1. Distance, stay, activity, shielding, avoid recording.

2. Keep **radiation effect** on persons as low as possible by decontamination, avoid further spreading.

3. Collimator, NaJ crystal, photomultiplier, electronic data processing.

4. Radioiodine therapy with ^{131}NaI. Benign diseases: Thyroid enlargement, autonomy, Graves' disease. Malignant disease: papillary and follicular thyroid carcinoma.

5. Radiology uses **transmission radiation**, nuclear medicine **emission radiation.**

6. Alpha radiation therapy (e.g. bone metastases), beta-minus radiation therapy, beta-plus radiation diagnostics (PET), gamma radiation diagnostics.

7. **Coincidence** refers to the nearly simultaneous impingement of annihilation beams in the PET ring system.

8. **Single photon emission computed tomography (SPECT):** Creation of a three-dimensional image based on images taken at different angles and suitable back projection.

▪ Chapter 12

1. Intolerance reaction to the KM.

2. To a thyrotoxic crisis.

3. In patients at risk, perchlorate (irenate) is used prophylactically before and 1–2 weeks after the examination with a thyrostatic. Perchlorate decreases iodine uptake into the thyroid gland.

4. Cardiac massage: find a hard surface if not already available → pressure point in the middle of the chest (lower half of the sternum) → compression depth approx. 4–5 cm → 100 compressions; ventilation: after the first 30 compressions (frequency 100–120/min) → first ventilation cycle of approx. 1 s with ventilation twice; continue as above in the ratio 30 (cardiac compressions):2 (ventilations).

5. If a tonic-clonic seizure lasts longer than 5 min or if an entire series of seizures occurs without the patient regaining consciousness in the meantime, this is referred to as status epilepticus. The danger here is an undersupply of oxygen (hypoxia) and dangerous cardiovascular stress.

▪ Chapter 13

1. **The** patient should be **informed** about the planned measures in such a way that he/she can decide for him/herself whether the planned procedure makes sense for him/her (**self-determination information**). To this end, the patient must be informed about the risks of the planned treatment, but also about the risks that may arise if the measure is not carried out. The actual treatment information includes the concrete treatment (e.g. computer tomography) with possible risks (e.g. contrast medium incident with anaphylactic shock). In the end, it is not the frequency of risks that is important, but the consequences. For example, possible lethal complications must be mentioned, even if their probability of occurrence is very rare but possible. Information must also be provided on possible alternatives to the proposed procedure, especially if there are in fact two approximately equivalent procedures.

2. The **X-ray Ordinance** regulates areas with X-ray radiation with a limit energy of more than 5 keV and less than 1 MeV. The handling of radioactive substances and ionizing radiation not covered by the X-ray Ordinance is regulated by the Radiation Protection Ordinance.

3. Examinations may only be performed if a competent physician has provided the **"justifying indication"** according to § 23 RöV or § 80 StrlSchV. It must be assessed whether the benefit of the planned examination outweighs the risk of radiation exposure and whether the question cannot be answered by another examination with lower radiation exposure.

4. No, working in the controlled area is possible under certain conditions.

▪ Chapter 14

1. **An epidural hemorrhage is** located under the dura and is limited biconvex. In addition, the cranial sutures are respected. A **subdural hemorrhage** spreads along the dura, which includes the falx cerebri, and can be delineated concavely. Subdural hemorrhages may cross the cranial sutures.

2. Bleeding in the **basal ganglia** and in the **pons** is considered typical and is usually due to hypertension. In other hemorrhage localizations, one must search for a cause for the hemorrhage.

3. **Tumor edema** spreads finger-like into the gyri, the cortex is usually preserved, whereas ischemic edema involves the cortex in most cases.

4. In the case of a **space-occupying lesion** in the **cerebellopontine angle**, one has to think of a **meningioma,** an acoustic neuroma (=wannoma) and/or an epidermoid tumor.

■ Chapter 15

1. DD **mucocele shadowing vs tumor shadowing of** the NNH: thinning of the wall without destruction in mucocele.

2. An **anechoic lumen, a smooth wall structure** and a distal **sound amplification** are shown.

3. Midface fractures are classified according to **LeFort** into:
   (a) LeFort I = basal detachment of the maxilla
   (b) LeFort II = pyramidal detachment of the maxilla including the bony nose
   (c) LeFort III = high avulsion of the entire midfacial skeleton including the bony nose

4. In the case of an **orbital fracture,** if the force is exerted directly on the eye, a so-called blow-out fracture can occur, in which the orbital floor fractures and orbital content can enter the maxillary sinus, which then becomes visible as a so-called "hanging drop".

   In **sialography**, which can also be used to visualize salivary stones, the orifice of the salivary glands is probed with a fine cannula and filled with CM to enable better visualization in conventional X-rays, CT or MRI. This also allows tumors to be visualized.

■ Chapter 16

1. A **breast carcinoma** can be delineated on sonography as an echo-poor, blurred round focus, possibly with dorsal sound extinction and above all with interruption of the longitudinal connective tissue structures (Cooper's ligaments).

2. To an **inflammatory breast carcinoma**. Clinically and mammographically, mastitis and inflammatory breast carcinoma look very similar: in addition to a thickened cutis, a diffusely condensed breast parenchyma can be seen.

3. One possible form of therapy **is** the **embolisation of fibroids**. This involves probing the feeding artery with a catheter and then closing it off with the help of small particles. The fibroid dies from the lack of oxygen and hopefully no longer stands in the way of the patient.

4. You think of an **inflammatory process with accompanying** edema. Your suspicion is adnexitis.

5. The **indications** are: positive lymph node involvement, tumor size: over 4 cm, from FIGO III primary radiochemotherapy is usually performed as combined tele- and brachytherapy, adenocarcinoma, R1/2 or narrow tumor-free resection margin.

■ Chapter 17

1. <10 U = transudate, >10 U = exudate.

2. The X-ray shows the following characteristics:
   (a) Kerley B/C line = interstitial edema in the interlobular septa in the form of a reticular pattern.
   (b) "Frosted glass phenomenon" due to intralobular edema.
   (c) Peribronchial cuffing = oedema formation in the peribronchial interstitium.
   (d) "Washed out" Hilus.
   (e) Subpleural edema.

3. p = pinhead, q = micronodular, r = nodular.

4. **Initial phase = Up to** 1 h; interstitial pulmonary edema with patchy indistinct condensations develops; **early phase = 1–24** h; alveolar pulmonary edema with microthrombi and rapid fusion to homogeneous condensations; **intermediate phase = 1–7** days; microatelectasis, fibroblast proliferation and regression to patchy shadows; **late**

phase => 7 days; pulmonary fibrosis with regression of patchy shadows, reticular pattern (= irreversible fibrosis).
5. In pulmonary embolism. Conventional X-rays show a regional reduction in blood flow, which reduces the diameter of the vessel and results in a secondary increase in transparency (so-called **Westermark sign**). Furthermore, there is a so-called **knuckle sign**, an enlargement with a jump in calibre, which results from the ballooning of the central artery and a resulting clear difference in size to the continuing vessels.

■ Chapter 18
1. **Primary sclerosing cholangitis** is a sclerosing chronic inflammation and destruction of the intra- and extrahepatic bile ducts and is manifested on ERCP (gold standard) or MRCP by a pearl cord-like duct irregularity.
2. Response:
   (a) **Zenker diverticulum**: 70% of all diverticula, cervical pulsatile diverticulum. Preferred in men of older age. Large pseudodiverticulum localized dorsally at the upper esophageal jugular predominantly on the left side.
   (b) **Bifurcation diverticulum**: True diverticulum due to scarring, e.g. after TBC.
   (c) **Epiphrenic pulsatile diverticulum**: Pseudodiverticulum above the hiatus, often combined with hiatal hernia or achalasia.
3. **Krukenberg tumor** is a drip metastasis of gastric carcinoma in the ovaries or in the Douglas space.
4. **Appendicitis** presents as a cocard >7 mm. The wall is thickened to >3 mm. Often an appendicolith is detectable.
5. During the **sigmavolvulus**, i.e. the rotation of the sigmoid colon around its mesenteric axis, the coffee bean sign appears.

■ Chapter 19
1. First, order a urinalysis, especially with the question of hematuria, and a sonography of the abdomen. If the diagnosis of **urolithiasis** remains suspected, perform a low-dose CT of the urinary tract.
2. **Bland renal cysts** are hydrous in all imaging techniques, i.e. anechoic with dorsal acoustic enhancement, in CT with density values around 0 HU and in MRI fluid isointense in all sequences. Complicated renal cysts may be hemorrhaged or septated with corresponding changes such as anechoic contents of the cyst or hyperdense appearance on CT. Contrast enhancement cannot be detected in cysts; should you detect this, it can no longer be assumed to be a cyst.
3. The **benign prostatic hypertrophy** affects the central zone around the urethra and has an inhomogeneous structure, the prostatic carcinoma is located in the peripheral zone and there mainly dorsal. In MRI the carcinoma is T2w hypointense with signal enhancement in diffusion due to cytotoxic edema.
4. Depending on the tumor stage, primary surgery, radiotherapy alone or hormone ablative therapy or a combination of hormone ablative therapy and radiotherapy.
5. Calcifications of the vasa deferens of the seminal vesicles or the interdigital arteries are almost pathognomonic for the presence of **diabetes mellitus**.

■ Chapter 20
1. **Definite fracture signs**: Axial malalignment, open fractures with bone fragments protruding from the wound, steps or gaps in the course of the bone, crepitation. Uncertain fracture signs: pain, swelling, redness, hyperthermia, restricted mobility (functio lesa). X-rays should always be taken in two planes.

2. Type of lesion, bordering of the lesion, cortical changes, periosteal reaction, assessment of the matrix, growth rate as an expression of aggressiveness, localization.

3. **Protrusion**: Bulging disc in which the diameter of the protrusion is greatest at the base. Extrusion: Bulging disc in which the diameter of the protrusion is greater peripherally than at the base (hourglass shape). **Bulging**: broad-based disc protrusion beyond the vertebral body, where the protrusion occupies more than 180 ° of the disc circumference. **Sequester**: extrusion in which at least part of the herniated disc tissue no longer has a connection to the residual disc).

4. **Tumor embolisation**: angiographic embolisation of osseous metastases, e.g. renal cell carcinoma. Pain therapy: PRT for the treatment of herniated discs. CT-guided treatment of bone tumors: thermoablation for osteoid osteoma.

■ Chapter 21

1. **DeBakey**: Type I (ascending aorta affected downstream of the supraaortic vessels), Type II (ascending aorta affected upstream of the supraaortic vessels), Type III (aorta affected distal to the supraaortic vessels). **Stanford**: Type A: Ascending aorta is involved. Type B: Aorta distal to the supra-aortic vascular branches is affected).

2. First determine pretest probability (according to Wells), not high: D-dimer determination, if negative no treatment, high probability: direct compression ultrasound, if negative no treatment, if positive treatment, in case of inconclusive findings supplementary phlebography or control ultrasound in four to seven days.

3. CT and MRI are equivalent in principle, but since there is often an emergency situation, CT is given priority for rapid clarification.

4. **Acute occlusion**: lysis, thrombectomy. **Chronic occlusion**: PTA, stent implantation.

■ Chapter 22

1. Autonomous adenomas.

2. On CT, **adenomas** show hypodense and take up contrast.

3. The **MRI**.

4. An examination with **iodine-containing contrast media** (6–8 weeks before diagnostics) as well as contamination with **iodine-containing food** represent a contraindication of thyroid scintigraphy, because otherwise the applied ^{99m}Tc cannot be transported into the thyroid tissue due to saturation. An undesired medicinal TSH suppression of the patient should be avoided.

5. To detect catecholamine-producing pheochromocytomas, ^{123}J- or ^{131}J-labeled **MIBG** is administered.

6. The most important benign indications for radioiodine therapy are **functional autonomies, Graves' disease and euthyroid strumen**. A corresponding indication for the therapy of malignant tumors is the still existing functional similarity to the thyroid tissue. This is the case with papillary (approx. 70% of malignant thyroid tumors) as well as follicular (approx. 20% of malignant thyroid tumors), the so-called differentiated thyroid carcinomas.

■ Chapter 23

1. As with sonography, computed tomography can detect the fatty hilus as a fatty isodense central zone in the lymph node even in relatively large lymph **nodes** in the groin. This is indicative of benignity of the lymph node. An absent fatty hilus is a sign of pathologic change, such as malignancy or inflammation. The shape also plays an important role in the evaluation of the lymph node as in sonography. A further indication of malignancy or benignity results from the localization of the lymph node.

2. For an **echinococcus cyst**.
3. **Thymomas** and **thymic carcinomas** usually present as a well circumscribed soft tissue mass in the upper anterior mediastinum. Vascular infiltration or sheathing as well as pleural metastases are indicative of malignancy. Magnetic resonance imaging (MRI) of the thorax may be helpful in rare cases to assess vascular infiltration.

■ Chapter 24

1. The **single-flush catheter** is placed over a suitable vein under sterile conditions and should be positioned in front of the right atrium. The beginning of the catheter should always be imaged as well, since the catheter may have already coiled up at the beginning. The **umbilical vein catheter** is placed via the umbilical vein through the ductus venosus Arantii into the inferior vena cava and is used, among other things, for the possibility of an exchange transfusion or for measuring the central venous pressure. The catheter should end 1 cm above the diaphragm. The **umbilical artery catheter** is used to measure pO_2 in ventilated premature infants. The appropriate position should be above the diaphragm, at a safe distance from the outlet of the renal arteries.

2. **Respiratory distress syndrome (ANS)** can occur in premature infants <28th week of gestation due to lung immaturity, in shock situations and, for example, in infants of diabetic mothers. Stage IV corresponds to white lung on X-ray.

3. Your tentative diagnosis is **intussusception**. This is an invagination of a part of the intestine into the following caudal part of the intestine. This leads to strangulation of the mesenteric vessels with edema, stasis hemorrhage, intestinal necrosis due to ischemia.

4. For imaging, an **MRI of the entire craniospinal axis** must be performed. In the T2 image, the solid part of the tumor is predominantly hyper- to isointense to the cerebellar cortex and shows a heterogeneous appearance. The T1-weighted image shows a predominantly hypo- to isointense, heterogeneous tumor.